MALNUTRITION

and RETARDED

HUMAN DEVELOPMENT

MALNUTRITION
and RETARDED
HUMAN DEVELOPMENT

By

SOHAN L. MANOCHA
Yerkes Primate Research Center
Emory University
Atlanta, Georgia

With a Foreword by

G. H. Bourne
Director
Yerkes Primate Research Center

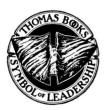

CHARLES C THOMAS • **PUBLISHER**
Springfield • Illinois • U.S.A.

Published and Distributed Throughout the World by
CHARLES C THOMAS • PUBLISHER
BANNERSTONE HOUSE
301-327 East Lawrence Avenue, Springfield, Illinois, U.S.A.

Library of Congress Catalog Card Number: 72–79193

With **THOMAS BOOKS** *careful attention is given to all details of manufacturing and design. It is the Publisher's desire to present books that are satisfactory as to their physical qualities and artistic possibilities and appropriate for their particular use.* **THOMAS BOOKS** *will be true to those laws of quality that assure a good name and good will.*

Printed in the United States of America
EE–11

To all those children who,
through ignorance, prejudice,
or man's inhumanity to man
have suffered the pangs of hunger
and the blight of malnutrition.

FOREWORD

"**S**END WHEAT OR COFFINS!" This was the text of a dramatic telegram sent to Athens by the inhabitants of the Greek island of Syra during the Nazi occupation of Greece during World War II.

The effects of the Nazi occupation on the people of Europe was described in detail in my book *Starvation in Europe,* published by George Allen and Unwin of London in 1943 This book brought attention to the tragic results of starvation and near starvation on a national scale on whole populations, especially on children.

In 1945, after the Japanese surrender, I went to Malaya as nutritional advisor to the Military Administration and was able to see firsthand the drastic effects of severe food deprivation on an infant and child population. When the child welfare clinics were opened, mothers brought children of two, three or four who could not sit up; some could not even cry—they were just skin and bone. Even those who were not in that severe state of malnutrition were stunted, slow in speech, slow in reaction, and slow to learn. One of the most severe deficiencies was that of protein.

But protein deficiency in many parts of the world and even starvation have not necessarily required a war to produce them, and when a war is superimposed again, it makes things even worse. Few of us can think of the children of Biafra without a shudder. The majority of children in developing countries, and even in great countries like India and China, are undernourished; again, protein is the most important nutrient that is lacking. Even in wealthy countries like America, protein deficiency occurs in many areas. In the last decade or so, there is a realization that protein deficiency does more than stunt growth. It also stunts the brain and the mental processes, and the stunting begins in the fetus when the pregnant mother is deprived of protein. Protein-deficient diets are deficient not only in proteins—there are minerals, vitamins, and trace elements to be considered, and these deficiencies all play a part in the malnutritional picture that is presented.

In this fine book, Dr. Sohan Manocha has brought together a mass of scientific data on the effects of malnutrition in retarding human development. He has devoted many years of his scientific life to the study of the morphology and chemistry of the brain, and currently, his energies are devoted to understanding the effects of protein deficiency on the concentration and distribution of enzymes and nucleic acids in the brains of pregnant monkeys and their babies.

This book has involved a tremendous amount of work, and the author is to be congratulated not only on the quantity of material that he has collected together but also upon its quality.

It is an outstanding contribution to our knowledge of the effects of malnutrition on the human brain and its function.

GEOFFREY H. BOURNE

PREFACE

THIS BOOK IS A general discussion on how malnutrition affects the human organism. The problem of malnutrition has become all the more important because of an ever-increasing human population, in the absence of a comparable increase in the food resources required for the well-being of that population. The problem is manifested wherever poverty exists. In the rich industrialized countries of the world, the poor people are increasingly unable to share the benefit of the vast food resources of their regions, and their numbers are growing every year. Furthermore, the impoverished countries are growing poorer because their rate of population growth is greater than the rate of their resource development. More than two thirds of the human population are crowded into these poorly developed areas that cannot provide adequate nutrition to all their members. The resulting widespread malnutrition interacts with similarly poor environmental factors and interferes with optimum development in terms of growth and activity of the population. An example of one such overcrowded country is India. Not long ago, her Family Planning Minister remarked that India produces two babies every three seconds, 55,000 each day, and 1,650,000 every month. At this rate, within the next 28 years India will double her population. Comparable patterns of growth among the poor of the world in general would create additional malnutrition which would adversely affect the physical and mental development of individuals and thereby the group as a coherent society. As a result, the ability of the species to survive without indulging in some form of mass scale self-destruction is lessened. We must not forget the powerful Roman Empire as well as old Greece, before it was the victim of wild, hungry tribes bent on destruction.

At this time the critical concern, in addition to inadequacies of vitamins and minerals, is the inadequate and imbalanced availability of proteins and/or calories. This book stresses the effects of protein or protein-calorie malnutrition on the human body. Episodes of malnutrition leave permanent deficits in the physical and mental development of the individual, which may not be corrected by later nutritional rehabilitation. The growth retardation caused by maternal malnutrition during pregnancy could have more severe consequences than the malnutrition of the infant in his postnatal period. The results are not hard to imagine when it is established that episodes of severe malnutrition during the first years of life leave significant deficits in physical growth as well as behavioral and intellectual capacity. Winick, from his experimental studies, postulated that a prenatally and postnatally deprived animal starts his life with as few as 40 percent of the normal number of brain cells. Other studies show that the children who are rehabilitated in a hospital during the first year of their life and examined several years after recovery show lower heights and weights compared to their controls who were matched for sex, race, and socioeconomic status. These data indicate that, as far as physical dimensions are concerned, an incomplete nutritional recovery occurred.

That malnutrition singularly retards intellectual function has not been firmly established. In human society, malnutrition does not exist without the interaction of other impoverishing factors which contribute to the state of malnutrition. A number of important studies clearly reveal that children raised in poor environments and with insufficient, unbalanced diets score poorly on the intelligence test scores. Poor environments contribute heavily to behavioral deficits, which seem to persist even if the child is nutritionally rehabilitated. On the other hand, there are critical periods of brain development when an irreversible damage to the nervous system would be inevitable even in the presence of stimulating environments. Barnes, Dobbing, Platt, Stewart, Winick and a host of other prominent workers have shown that direct damage to the brain either during intrauterine life or the neonatal period results from malnutrition. Such damage manifests itself in functional impairment that is independent of the environmental condition under which the child is reared in the postnatal period.

The big question that has not been answered satisfactorily is the degree to which recovery occurs after a period of rehabilitation. Is the damage caused by malnutrition permanent? What kinds of behavioral deficits persist after rehabilitation from severe malnutrition in early life? Still another question that is equally hard to answer is the relative importance of malnutrition and of the surrounding environment during the period of rehabilitation, in view of the fact that stimulating environments greatly speed up the nutritional recovery. Some prominent workers have provided evidence that hospitalized children who are given constant attention recover much faster than those who are given the same nutritional rehabilitation but are less stimulated.

The main objective of this monograph is to create an awareness of the problem of overpopulation on this planet and the resultant malnutrition that exists in a large segment of the population. These undernourished and malnourished masses of people not only fail to achieve their growth potential but suffer functionally as well. As a consequence, they are not able to compete successfully in this aggressively competitive world and very soon may create a problem of eugenics for the human species. My appeal for recognition of these problems is directed to the medical and paramedical professions, especially pediatricians, pediatric nurses, psychologists, nutritionists, and all those interested in child development as well as human health and welfare. I hope that this presentation will serve to increase the awareness of such people and thereby contribute to the effort of solving this problem that is so crucial to human survival.

It is indeed a very pleasant opportunity to thank a few individuals whose valuable help went a long way in producing this manuscript. My grateful thanks are due to Dr. G. H. Bourne for his critical evaluation of the whole project and his constant encouragement. To Dr. Z. Olkowski, I am very thankful for his constant reading of rough pages of the manuscript and his valuable suggestions at every step. Thanks are also due to Drs. Josephine Brown, Irwin Bernstein, Totada Shantha, Adrian Perachio, Ronald Nadler, Miss M. Pandit, and Miss R. Rajan for their reading of different parts of the manuscript and for making very helpful corrections. Special thanks go to Mrs. Nancy Hiller for her technical assistance and to Mr. Ngwa Suh, Mrs. Betsy Bradford, Miss Linda Powers and Mrs. Nellie Johns, who rendered valuable technical, typing and library help throughout the preparation of the manuscript. I am also thankful to Mr. Frank Kiernan and Mrs. Helen C. Wells for their photographic and artwork respectively. Lastly, I must express my deep appreciation to my wife, Swaran, for boosting my morale all along, and for giving me sufficient time at home to write this book.

It is a great pleasure to acknowledge the generous help of the following authors and publishers for their kind permission to reproduce their illustrations: Dr. D. B. Jelliffe and the World Health Organization for Figures 3, 4, and 16 and Tables I and VII; Dr. M. Swaninathan and S. Karger Basel for Figure 1 and Table VI; Dr. Ernst Jokl and Charles C Thomas for Figures 2 and 8; Dr. C. D. William and Lancet Limited for Figure 5; Dr. M. Behar and the New York Academy of Sciences for Figure 6; Dr. O. Pineda and Little, Brown and Company for Figure 7; Dr. M. S. Guzman and MIT Press for Table III; Dr. R. E. Brown and *East African Medical Journal* for Figure 9 and Table VIII; Dr. John Dobbing and MIT Press for Figures 10 and 11; Dr. Myron Winick and W. B. Saunders Company for Figures 12 and 13 and Table IV; Dr. F. Mönckeberg and MIT Press for Figures 14 and 15; Dr. J. M. Bengoa and *Journal of Tropical Pediatrics* for Figure 17; Dr. H. A. Prasana and the American Society of Clinical Nutrition, Inc. for Figure 18; and Mr. J. C. Abbott and the American Chemical Society for Table II. The inclusion of these figures has added to the value of this book, and the author is grateful for the help of the above mentioned scientists and publishers.

Finally, the author acknowledges with deep appreciation the help of Grant No. RR-00165 from the Animal Resources Branch of the National Institutes of Health to Yerkes Primate Research Center, and of National Science Foundation Grant No. GB-30358 to the author.

S. L. MANOCHA

CONTENTS

MALNUTRITION

and RETARDED

HUMAN DEVELOPMENT

Chapter 1

NUTRITIONAL DEPRIVATION AND HUMAN DISTRESS

UNDERNUTRITION AND MALNUTRITION among children and adults in a number of countries on all continents of the world has been so acute during the last few decades that the effects of this socioeconomic problem on human eugenics cannot be ignored. Approximately half of the existing population has survived a period of serious nutritional deprivation during childhood,[118] and more than half of all the children in the world are "at risk" from the serious effects of malnutrition. Children in their period of maximum growth suffer most because of their greater nutritional requirements in relation to body weight. In the earlier part of the twentieth century, most concern was concentrated on vitamins and mineral deficiencies and resulting diseases like beriberi, pellagra, rickets, scurvy, iron deficiency anemia, and goiter, which took a heavy toll of human lives. During the recent years, however, we have also been concerned about the total food intake, i.e. the availability, especially to the vulnerable groups, of sufficient quantities of high-quality proteins and calories. In a number of over-populated developing countries where cereals or carbohydrate-rich foods are the staple diets, children as well as adults suffer from varying degrees of protein deficiency. Since low protein foods produce loss of appetite, the total food intake generally decreases, resulting in a deficiency of proteins as well as calories. Protein and protein-calorie malnutrition has become over the years the most widespread nutritional disease of the world and has caused an alarming number of deaths in the developing countries. Kwashiorkor and marasmus, the clinical conditions resulting from protein and protein-calorie deficiencies, will be discussed briefly in a later section. These conditions are most prevalent in children whose postweaning

3

diets consist predominantly of carbohydrate-rich gruels made from rice, sago, yams, bananas, and so on. In certain circumstances, children also suffer in the preweaning stages due to lactation failure or inadequate quantities of breast milk or because they are given a highly diluted formula with up to 75% water content. The latter, even in adequate quantities, fails to provide sufficient calories for the maintenance of basal metabolism. Besides the deficiency of protein and calories, these children suffer from vitamin and mineral deficiencies. Such children succumb to minor infections, which would ordinarily be overcome by healthy children.

The discussion in this volume on malnutrition and retarded human development is centered mainly on the effect of nutritional deprivation of protein or calories or both on children in the period of their maximum growth. The protein requirement of the adult, who has ceased to grow, is probably not more than 30 gm a day (0.4 gm/kg/day), and this quantity can be easily provided by most basic adult diets available throughout the world.[27] However, these amounts may not permit the laying down of labile protein deposits or provide the capacity to resist infections or even allow prolonged physical or mental work. Among children, malnutrition results in growth stunting, behavioral and psychological disturbances and impaired learning ability, which are not observed in the adult population in general, although extreme degrees of undernutrition and starvation resulting from a famine or war may lead to symptoms such as mental confusion, apathy and inability to concentrate. Malnutrition among children cannot, however, be divorced from the nutritional status of the adults as well as the biosocial factors under which the adult population lives. The technological backwardness, the low purchasing power, level of food budget or conditions of employment of adults directly influence the physical, emotional, and mental development of children. For example, the inability of an adult to earn sufficient money in order to buy food for the family may prompt a young member of the family to leave school in order to help increase the purchasing power of the family. The consequences of such early school drop-out are reflected in illiteracy and inadequate training which result in technological backwardness and persistence of primitive concepts of health and disease. The relatively early enrollment of these children in the labor force may lead to an adult life and adult responsibilities of marriage and a family at an early age. This could lead to a vicious cycle of illiteracy, faulty training in social responsibilities and in turn to inadequate child care, and illness and malnutrition in the next generation.[19] According to Cravioto

> Such factors as illiteracy, traditional modes of child care, rearing, attitudes and values toward formal learning, absence of facilitating experiences for the child are severely or in multiple combinations present in the macro- and micro-environments in which significant malnutrition is found.

The general growth and development of a child depends on the parental knowledge of health and use of medical facilities by the parents as well as social status of the family and the current socioeconomic situation of the country. The socioeconomic underdevelopment of groups of people leads to "Low income per capita, illiteracy, low cultural level, bad sanitary conditions, low intellectual performance of the less privileged groups, and finally racial or religious prejudices." [69] Even a casual study makes it evident that most of the retardation, physical as well as mental, occurs among the members of the lower socioeconomic groups. Unfortunately, most of the world population belongs in this category, and it is estimated that more than 350 million children, or seven out of ten children under the age of six in the entire world, are affected by some degree of malnutrition which leads to impaired learning potential and hence deterioration of the genetic quality of the human species. Jelliffe[56] summarizes in a beautiful manner the social, economic, agronomic, and cultural factors which contribute to the etiology of malnutrition (Table I).

Fortunately we have sufficient knowledge of nutrition with respect to the requirements of nutrients and the biochemical processes concerned with utilization of food constituents. The existing malnutrition is mostly a result of inequitable distribution of populations and food sources and our inability to apply existing knowledge of nutrition most effectively. The application of our knowledge is hindered by economic, social, and political

TABLE I

MISCELLANEOUS FACTORS IN THE ETIOLOGY OF PCM [56]

Geographico-climatic	Unproductive soil Climate (high temperatures, extremes of rainfall)
Educational	Too few schools (illiteracy)
Social	Illegitimacy; family instability Absence of family planning (children too closely spaced; population pressure) Poor communications (food distribution) Alcoholism
Economic	National poverty (low gross national products) Family poverty (low per capita income) Low level of industrialization
Agronomic	Old-fashioned methods of agriculture Inadequate protein production (animal and vegetable) Concentration on inedible cash crops Poor food storage, preservation and marketing
Medical	High prevalence of conditioning infections (measles, diarrhea, tuberculosis, whooping cough, malaria, intestinal parasites) Inadequate health facilities (too few; incorrect orientation) Inadequate staff (too few; ill trained in nutrition and child health)
Sanitational	Unclean, inadequate water supply Defective disposal of excreta and rubbish
Cultural	Faulty feeding habits of young children Recent urbanization (changing habits) Limited culinary facilities Inequable intrafamilial food distribution Overwork by women (limited time for food preparation for children) Sudden weaning (psychological trauma)

obstacles. Economically, resources have to be found which will make an increased food production possible. This involves huge capital investments in order to create irrigation facilities and establish agricultural industries, e.g. the manufacture of farm equipment, fertilizers, and pesticides in overcrowded developing countries. Even if the advanced richer countries are ready to help the developing nations in economic terms, can the countries concerned surmount the social and political obstacles? The social awareness that children and pregnant and lactating mothers need more nutritious foods, particularly proteins, than adults, is essential. Such an awareness would modify the distribution of available food in the family in a manner such that milder forms of malnutrition caused by maldistribution of food would disappear. For example, it is all right for adults to consume cassava, yams, and plantains in certain quantities, but children must be given a fair share of meat, fish, or beans.[27] Also, a country has to be convinced at both the social and individual level about the need for curtailing the population. The big question is always sociopolitical: Can a political leader in India institute rigorous measures like compulsory sterilization of males or females after two children? The need of solving the problem of malnutrition is closely integrated with problems of family planning, improvement of medical facilities, and bringing the nutrition knowledge to the general public in a meaningful way. A well-planned educational program will bring about an awareness that life on this planet is worthwhile only when every human being gets the benefit of adequate nutrition, adequate shelter, adequate clothing, and adequate opportunities of developing his or her personality, which are not possible in an overcrowded world.

WORLD FOOD RESOURCES—PROSPECTS AND THE PROBLEM

The problem of undernutrition and malnutrition is directly related to the food supply of this planet versus the number of people to be fed. Great inequities in food availability exist at the present population level. With the projected doubling of the world population by the turn of the century, the problem of malnutrition is likely to get worse unless food is produced at a much faster rate than the rate of increase in the population.

The world population is growing at a rate of 190,000 persons every 24 hours, or the equivalent of 350 moderate-sized cities annually. The tragedy is that more than half of the 70 million or more babies born this year are doomed to suffer from malnutrition within the next 2 years. Annual birth rates in the non-industrialized countries least able to feed their people adequately are about 40 for each 1,000 persons, compared with 20 in the industrialized countries. Death rates in the high-birth-rate countries constantly decrease. As a consequence, populations are growing at rates greater than in any other epoch.[75]

Increased food production and reduced rate of population growth are among the foremost problems of the present world. Knowing that malnutrition affects mental development, we must give even higher priority to reversing the trend towards less food per person.

> Food shortage and rapid population growth are separate but interrelated problems. The solution, likewise, is separate but related. The choice is not to solve one or the other; to solve both is an absolute necessity. The current tendency on the part of the public to think of food production and fertility control as alternate solutions to a common problem is dangerously misleading.[7]

The existing malnutrition is not so much a problem of total food supply of the world versus total population but is a problem of food supply of an area versus the population in which this food has to be distributed. A country like India has two fifths of the land area of the United States but has to support about three times the population of the United States. Southeast Asia is also similarly crowded, resulting in too much pressure on the land. Since the area of land available for agriculture is bound to be limited, a time may come when it is not possible to maintain an increase in agricultural production to match an expanding population. Rao and Swaminathan [80] charted the regional shares of world production and agricultural production (Fig. 1). Whereas North America produces a sizeable surplus of agricultural commodities compared to its population, the picture is the reverse in the Far East, where more people are produced relative to the output of food. Although the picture is not as bad as in the Far East, it is not very promising in Latin America, Africa, and the Middle East. With the growing human population, it is these areas which will feel the pinch of food shortages the most with the prospects of a higher rate of undernutrition and malnutrition. It has been established that malnutrition leads to impaired mental development. By that score, the future of three fourths of the human species is not very rosy, "And since every child born has to be fed more than half a century, we will do well to plan now to stabilize our populations if our children and grandchildren are to enjoy an adequate share of the fruits of the earth." [48]

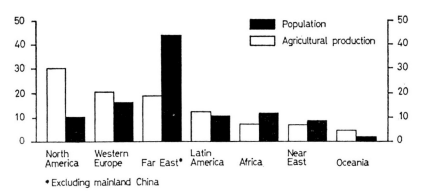

Figure 1. A representation of regional share of agricultural production relative to density of population.[80]

The amount of available food versus population reflects the dietary standards of the population. Whereas an adult living in the United States gets an average of 3,000 calories a day, two thirds of the world population gets a subsistence diet consisting of no more than 1,900 calories per capita a day (Fig. 2). In a country like India, if the population keeps on increasing at the levels of the 50s and 60s, there is no hope that the nutritional standard of the people, which is presently approximately 2,000 calories per day, can ever be substantially improved. Furthermore, the nutritional standard of a population can be more accurately determined by the quality of the diet than by the number of calories per day. Again, there are significant differences in the diets of the inhabitants of different parts of the globe. In North America, an average diet provides 46 percent of the total calories from carbohydrates, 14 percent from protein and 40 percent from fats (23% from unsaturated vegetable fats and 17% from saturated animal fats). This is in contrast to 80 percent of the calories derived from carbohydrates, 10 percent from protein and 10 percent from fats (9% from unsaturated fats and 1% from animal fats) in a typical Far Eastern diet.[59]

The people of North America, Europe, Oceania, and the River Plate countries consume a daily average of 573 g. of milk, 152 g. meat, 30 g. eggs, and 34 g. fish. The people of the poorer countries, mostly in Asia, Africa and Latin America, get an average of only 79 g. milk, 30 g. meat, 4 g. eggs, and 24 g. fish daily. Total intakes of protein are

90 g. per head per day (44 g. of animal proteins) for the wealthy and 58 g. (only 9 g. from animal sources) for the poorer group.[59]

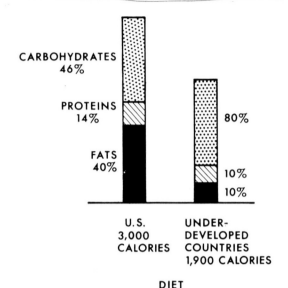

CARBOHYDRATES
46%

PROTEINS
14%

FATS
40%

80%

10%

10%

U.S.
3,000
CALORIES

UNDER-
DEVELOPED
COUNTRIES
1,900 CALORIES

DIET

Figure 2. Dietary analysis showing the total number of calories as well as percent of carbohydrates, proteins, and fat consumed by the American population compared to subsistence diets available in the underdeveloped countries of the world.[59]

Table II explains the per capita protein supply from different sources in different parts of the world.[1] This inequity in the quality of diet in various parts of the world is likely to worsen if the balance in the population versus food supply is not tilted significantly in favor of the latter. In order to provide adequate food to the existing population, the overpopulated countries have no other choice than stabilizing their numbers or even reducing them in view of the urgency to increase per capita food production.

In the developing countries, more and more reliance is being placed on cereals and cereal proteins, whose supply may be adequate, but which are qualitatively deficient in one or two essential amino acids. Fortunately, pulses, oil seeds, and nuts are rich not only in protein (20% to 40% protein on a dry basis), but they also have the substantial quantities of amino acids that are deficient in cereals. The solution to adequate nutrition of populations in the developing countries lies in much higher production of these protein-rich foods along with cereals. This combination of legumes and cereals can play a vital role in relieving malnutrition in those areas of the world, where animal products are scarce and cannot be afforded. Sir Hutchinson [48] believes that the reason for not growing these crops in adequate quantities is due to a lack of appreciation of their dietary importance, and because quantitatively their yields per acre are less as compared to grain and starchy vegetables. Fish, as a conventional source of protein, has not been tapped adequately and contributes only 3 percent as a source of protein all over the world. In the developing countries the problem of malnutrition can be greatly overcome by bringing the consumption of fish to the level of Portugal (23% of the total protein) and Japan (18% of the total protein). Dried fish, as a major source of protein, and fish-protein concentrate, to be mixed with other traditional foods, have a great potential which has not been exploited.

Dr. Bennett,[7] the chairman of a panel of the President's Science Advisory Committee to study the world food problem, believed that hunger, malnutrition, and the population explosion in the developing countries are not the real maladies, but are only the symptoms of poor and "lagging economic development." According to him, "Until the rich nations and the poor nations make a commitment to long-range, coordinated action dedicated to the systematic solution of a series of interrelated problems, none of which can be solved in isolation from its fellows, the situation will continue to worsen steadily." The findings of this committee which surveyed food resources in relation to the projected population were generally pessimistic, and it believed that poor nations have to bear the main brunt of the gigantic efforts needed to change the food shortages to avert famine conditions. The overpopulated countries must not only pay adequate attention to population control as a long-range plan, but they must spend every ounce of their energy to increase the food production from farming and nonagricultural sources of food. Increased food production in the immediate future is essential because the results of family planning become obvious only in the size of the next

TABLE II

PER CAPITA PROTEIN SUPPLIES IN SELECTED COUNTRIES[1]

	Total Protein	Animal Protein	Grain	Starchy Roots	Pulses Oil seeds, and Nuts	Vegetables	Fruit	Meat and Poultry	Eggs	Fish	Milk and Products
Argentina											
grams/day	98	57	34	3	1	2	1	43	2	1	11
% of total protein		58	35		3	1	2	44	2	1	11
Australia											
grams/day	92	61	23	3	2	2	1	37	3	3	18
% of total protein		67	25	3	2	2	1	40	3	3	20
Brazil											
grams/day	61	19	24	2	14	0	2	11	1	2	5
% of total protein		31	39	3	23	0	3	18	2	3	8
Canada											
grams/day	95	63	23	3	3	2	1	29	5	4	25
% of total protein		66	24	3	3	2	1	31	5	4	26
Ceylon											
grams/day	45	9	27	1	7	2	0	1	0	6	2
% of total protein		20	60	2	16	4	0	2	0	13	4
China (Taiwan)											
grams/day	57	14	31	3	12	4	0	11	0	12	2
% of total protein		25	54	5	12	4	0	11	0	12	2
Colombia											
grams/day	48	23	15	2	5	1	2	15	1	0	7
% of total protein		48	31	4	10	2	4	31	2	0	15
Finland											
grams/day	94	53	34	5	1	1	0	12	2	6	33
% of total protein		56	36	5	1	1	0	13	2	6	35
India											
grams/day	51	6	30	0	14	1	0	1	0	0	5
% of total protein		12	59	0	27	2	0	2	0	0	10
Ireland											
grams/day	96	57	29	7	1	2	0	20	5	2	30
% of total protein		59	30	7	1	2	0	21	5	2	31
Israel											
grams/day	84	33	39	2	4	3	2	10	6	3	14
% of total protein		40	47	2	5	4	2	12	7	4	17

Japan	grams/day	67	17	31	1	19	6	0	5	1	18	1
	% of total protein		26	46	3	19	6	0	5	1	18	1
Libya	grams/day	53	10	34	1	4	2	2	4	0	1	5
	% of total protein		20	64	2	7	4	4	8	0	2	9
Mauritius	grams/day	46	11	27	1	6	1	0	2	1	4	4
	% of total protein		23	59	2	13	2	0	4	2	9	9
Mexico	grams/day	68	20	33	0	13	1	1	9	2	2	8
	% of total protein		30	49	0	19	1	1	13	3	1	12
New Zealand	grams/day	105	72	25	3	2	2	1	36	5	3	28
	% of total protein		68	24	3	2	2	1	34	5	3	27
Pakistan	grams/day	46	7	33	0	9	2	0	2	0	2	11
	% of total protein		16	72	0	9	2	0	2	0	2	11
Peru	grams/day	49	12	22	6	5	3	1	6	0	3	3
	% of total protein		24	45	12	10	6	2	12	0	6	6
Philippines	grams/day	47	13	26	2	4	6	2	9	2	15	2
	% of total protein		28	55	4	4	6	2	9	2	15	2
Portugal	grams/day	72	26	29	6	4	5	1	6	1	16	3
	% of total protein		37	41	8	6	7	1	8	1	23	4
Sweden	grams/day	61	52	22	4	1	1	1	17	4	7	24
	% of total protein		64	27	5	1	1	1	21	5	9	30
Turkey	grams/day	91	15	61	2	7	3	2	5	0	1	9
	% of total protein		17	68	1	8	3	2	6	0	1	10
United Arab Republic	grams/day	76	13	51	0	7	3	2	5	1	3	5
	% of total protein		17	67	0	9	3	3	7	1	4	5
U. S. A.	grams/day	92	65	15	2	5	4	1	32	6	3	24
	% of total protein		70	16	2	5	4	1	35	7	3	26

generation. Whereas the successful population control programs may cut down the food needs by about 20 percent in the long run, the task of feeding the existing population is truly immense. This is particularly significant in view of the fact that half of the population in the developing countries is under 15 years of age and is not only economically nonproductive, but because of its growth needs, it requires larger and larger quantities of food to avert undernutrition and malnutrition.

The situation in the developing countries, which are running a desperate race between numbers and food supply, can change for the better only by the mass scale use of modern technology, and it is here that the developed countries have a humanitarian obligation to lend technical assistance without looking for trade benefits and economic rewards. The developing countries are short of capital to invest in agricultural industries and to advance as credit to the farmers to make use of their output. They are also short of trained technical personnel to design and establish such industries and to conduct systematic research to broaden their industrial base. Only massive technical and financial assistance can help the developing countries to achieve self-sustaining economic growth in which they can balance their numbers and food supply in a somewhat comfortable manner. External financial assistance is also needed to add to the circulating money and to create a better purchasing power on the part of consumers to buy the additional commodities. "The problem would be so much easier if the people had the money in their pockets to create a demand for the things which we know they should eat, and we might persuade them to eat and give to their children." [48] In the writer's opinion, although it may already be somewhat late, a comprehensive and coordinated program of action should be undertaken right now before the situation in terms of human numbers and food resources is worsened in the overpopulated developing countries. If the present trend is permitted to continue, even the huge resources of developed countries may not be able to avert the worst disaster the human species has known. The genetic quality of this species may then deteriorate to such an extent that the dead may be considered more fortunate than the half-living malnourished. Even a fractional increase of the world population means an immense demand for protein. If a modest annual growth is envisaged, the demand for protein [1] will be two-and-a-half times that of 1959, calculating a marginal improvement in the existing diets. More than twice as much protein will still be needed if there is no improvement in diets.[33]

MALNUTRITION AND DEFICIENCY DISEASES
Protein and Protein—Calorie Deficiencies

The term protein-calorie deficiency was adopted by the FAO/ WHO expert committee on nutrition in 1962 which suggested the following three categories: (1) kwashiorkor, including marasmic kwashiorkor; (2) marasmus, including athrepsia, cachexia, and extreme wasting; and (3) unspecified, including starvation in adults, famine, and edema.[71] The various categories of protein and protein-calorie malnutrition are widely spread in the Far East, Africa, and Latin America as shown in the map (Fig. 3). The word "kwashiorkor" was introduced by Williams [114,115] as a disease of the weaning child, but since then a variety of names have been used in the literature, which essentially designate the same syndrome, e.g. enfants rouges, culebrilla or "snake skin," referring to the "flaky paint rash," bouffissure d'Annam, syndrome depigmentation oedème, fatty liver disease, dystrofia pluricavencial, syndrome pluricavencial, multiple deficiency disease, Mehlanährschaden, flour malnutrition, nutritional oedema syndrome, malignant malnutrition, and so on. Kwashiorkor is predominantly observed in children one to three years old. Trowell *et al.*[105] analyzed 1,141 cases and found that 45 percent of the children were in the age group of one and two years and 69 percent between one and three years of age. The severity of kwashiorkor in different individuals depends on the extent of protein deficiency, and therefore the resulting clinical symptoms vary from individual to individual. Gopalan [37] showed that the clinical symptoms among kwashiorkor children vary from place to place. For example, in India the kwashiorkor children are lighter in weight in Hyderabad than those in Conoor. However, such children are in general obese.[58] Jelliffe [56] explained that the clinical picture of kwashiorkor varies with factors, such as degree

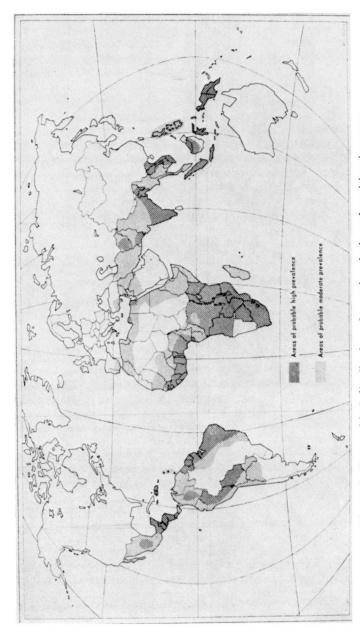

Figure 3. Geographical distribution of protein-calorie malnutrition in young children.[56]

of protein deficiency, velocity of onset, age of occurrence, duration, infections, trauma and genetic characteristics such as skin color and type of hair (Fig. 4). Latham *et al.*[62] summarized some of the important factors in the etiology of kwashiorkor:

1. The rapid growth and relatively high protein requirements of the rapidly growing child;

2. A protein poor, staple food for the child, e.g., manioc, bananas, sugar;

3. Poor infant feeding practices;

4. A lack of protein-rich foods, both animal products (meat, milk, fish, eggs) and vegetables (beans, peanuts);

5. A poor distribution of available foods in the family (e.g. the adults and older children often get the major share of protein-rich foods, such as meat);

6. Seasonal food shortages;

7. Poverty and its attendant ills;

8. Cultural dietary practices, including food taboos which may preclude the child from consuming certain available and desirable foods;

9. Infections, such as diarrhea, measles, whooping cough;

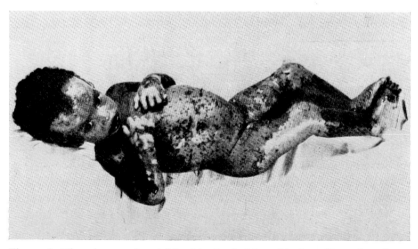

Figure 4. The picture of a child with classical kwashiorkor. Note the misery, edema, and marked "flaky-paint" rash characteristic of this condition.[56]

10. Ignorance or lack of knowledge on the part of parents or guardians of what foods are needed in the child's diet; and

11. Psychological factors which may affect the appetite of the child.

The complex and multiple etiology of malnutrition has been graphically tabulated by Williams [116] and Williams [117] as shown in Figure 5.

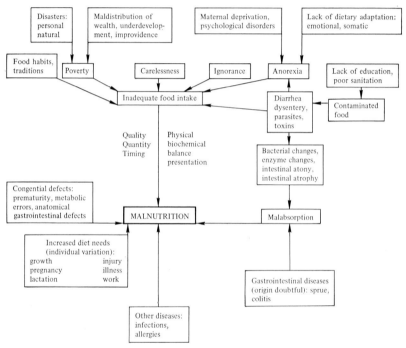

Figure 5. The multiple etiology of malnutrition.[116]

Nutritional Marasmus

Nutritional marasmus refers to a condition accompanied by severe wasting due to grossly inadequate diet. The word "marasmus" is derived from a Greek word *marasmos* which means wasting. "It is applied to the state of chronic total undernutrition in children which represents a deficiency of both proteins and calories in various degrees of severity and produces a gradual wasting away of body tissue with general emaciation." [117] Behar *et al.*[6] gave an excellent schematic interrelationship between the different malnutritional states, as represented by Figure 6. Whereas the kwashiorkor cases manage to get most of the needed calories from their heavy starchy diet and starve because their protein requirements are not met, the marasmic children experience a lack of proteins as well as calories and may have to cannibalize on their own tissues in order to provide the needed energy requirements, leading to a severe form of growth retardation and wasting of muscle and subcutaneous fat. Bottle feeding in preference to breast feeding has especially contributed to an increase in the incidence of nutritional marasmus in a number of developing countries because of recurrent infective diarrheas caused by infected milk.[54,67] Whereas nutritional marasmus occurs in all ages, even amongst adults, its incidence is highest among the preschool children. The parents of these children are often poor and ignor-

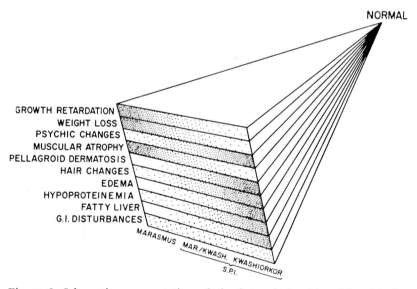

Figure 6. Schematic representation of the interrelationship of kwashiorkor and marasmus. At the left of the pyramidal base, the intensity of the stippling suggests the frequency with which the signs and symptoms listed appear in marasmus. At the right, the occurrence of the same signs and symptoms in "classic" kwashiorkor are portrayed. In between are all combinations between these two extremes. The severity of the signs and symptoms is indicated by the distance from the apex.[6]

ant of food values or may have severe mental and emotional problems, so that they fail to provide the care that the child needs. Most often nutritional marasmus is chronic in poor socio-economic settings, and the child becomes the victim of these circumstances. For a clearer understanding of kwashiorkor and maramus, it may be worthwhile to compare the general symptoms of both conditions (Fig. 7).

KWASHIORKOR	MARASMUS
The onset of Kwashiorkor is fairly rapid. The symptoms may become evident within two to four weeks after an attack of diarrhea or fever in a child with such clinical deficiency state.[14]	The onset of Marasmus is insidious, and the duration of illness is much longer as compared to kwashiorkor.
"Wasting" is not as evident as in marasmus. In chronic cases, wasting accompanied by edema of feet is observed. In general, wasting is marked by edema; otherwise, the muscles of arms and legs are always affected. Edema, a characteristic symptom of kwashiorkor, starts with swelling of the feet, spreading to legs, hands, face.	Marasmus is characterized by extreme degree of wasting, and the patient is grossly underweight with less than 60 percent of standard weight. There is little subcutaneous fat present because of the absence of edema and the whole body appears shrunken to the extent that the skin lays in wrinkles as in old people, especially around the buttocks and thighs.
The patients show a 'moon face' appearance (full, well-rounded, somewhat pendulous and blubbery cheeks), due to increased edema or even increased fat.	The face is generally pinched, accompanied by prominent bony points to the extent that it may look like a 'monkey face'[14] or "wizened little old man."[56]
Growth failure may not be reflected by weight because of edema, but the patient is generally short for his age. In Uganda, certain anthropometric measurements showed that kwashiorkor patients showed 68 percent weight, 91 percent length, 92 percent sitting height, 78 percent calf circumference, and 77 percent arm circumference of the local standard.[56] The appetite is poor.	Growth failure is prominent, and the patient's height is extremely subnormal. The limbs are thin, and the patient is a very poor specimen of a human child. The appetite is better than the kwashiorkor patient.

KWASHIORKOR

The skin changes or dermatosis may or may not be present. Whenever present, they are of classical type: darkly pigmented patches, desquamated like old blistered paint (flaky paint dermatosis). Initially starting as hyperpigmented brownish skin, these areas later desquamate as large tissue paper-thin flakes, leaving damaged atrophic hypopigmented skin beneath. In some cases dermatosis develops in the groins, behind the knees, and other areas of friction.

Prominent in kwashiorkor are hair changes in texture, color, strength, and pluckability. Black hair may turn brown or even be discolored. Dyspigmentation of the hair may result from nonnutritional, environmental, and genetic causes and may be found in children without kwashiorkor.

The kwashiorkor patient is usually apathetic, miserable, inert, anorexic, disinterested in his surrounding environments, and gets irritated at the slightest disturbance. His behavioral development is retarded. Autret and Behar [4] gave an excellent description of typical kwashiorkor patients as, "They are indifferent to their surroundings and remain immobile for hours with open eyes and expressionless features, suggesting a mask rather than a human face. This immobility is often accompanied by a monotonous wailing without tears, and children refuse all food and whimper at the least touch." [56]

A marked disturbance in water and electrolyte metabolism is evident.

MARASMUS

Skin changes are not observed in marasmic condition.

Hair changes are less common in marasmus. Thinning of hair may be observed, but hair changes are never marked.

The marasmic patient is alert and does not show as dull an appearance as a kwashiorkor case. Also, they are not disinterested or irritable.

Sodium depletion may be observed particularly when diarrhea is a com-

KWASHIORKOR	MARASMUS
"Total body water increases and there is a marked reduction of total body potassium and retention of sodium. The sodium partially replaces the last of the intracelluar potassium, a dearrangement that critically affects important cell enzyme systems which are normally dependent upon potassium. Factors probably responsible for these fluid and electrolyte disturbances are hypoalbuminemia, endocrine dysfunction, and circulatory failure. A magnesium deficit, similar to that of potassium, has been described and may also affect cell enzyme function." [117]	plication. No water retention in marasmic cases.
Diarrhea is present in the majority of cases, and the stools are loose, containing undigested food particles and extreme degree of foul smell. Jelliffe [56] explained that the loose stools of kwashiorkor patient seem to have (a) diminished exocrine pancreatic secretion, due to acinar changes in pancreas, (b) intestinal malabsorption due to decreased secretion of enzymes, especially lactase,[9,25] (c) associated enteral infection or changes in bacterial flora of intestines,[89,110] and (d) continued ingestion of unsuitable indigestible food, associated with intolerance of fat, including milk fat, and of sugars including lactose.	Diarrhea not uncommon, but not as much as in kwashiorkor cases.
Anemia is generally present due to the shortage of protein needed to synthesize blood cells. Iron deficiency anemia is also common. The nutritional anemia is masked initially by hemoconcentration, becoming more apparent when hemodilution occurs.[2]	Anemia is present due both to protein and iron deficiency.

KWASHIORKOR

There is a general reduction in total serum proteins. Serum albumin content is much more reduced compared to globulin.

Liver in the kwashiorkor cases is often very much enlarged and is grossly fatty.

The blood lipid transport is abnormal, and there is alterations in fat synthesis and catabolism probably due to deficiency of essential fatty acids. This abnormality in lipid transport may cause the level of fat soluble vitamins to remain low.

Nearly all abnormalities of kwashiorkor are related to insufficient synthesis of proteins, and the tissues with faster protein turnover are most affected. Plasma-free amino acid levels are greatly decreased. A detailed study of Holt *et al.*[46] in nine different countries revealed that the limiting factors in diets that produce kwashiorkor is not an essential amino acid, but the nitrogen per se.

The blood levels of vitamins, especially fat soluble, iron, and copper are low.

Glucocorticoid is low in kwashiorkor, and its secretion generally fails when the diet consists predominantly of calories and is deficient in proteins. The mechanism of this failure is not known.

MARASMUS

Serum proteins may be reduced but not as much as in kwashiorkor cases. The hydroxyproline-creatinine index is low.[111]

No enlargement in size or fatty change is observed in the liver.

Fat absorption, although not normal is not so much damaged as in kwashiorkor. "The enzyme system for digestion, mechanism for transport of fat through intestinal wall, and sufficiency of lipid transport protein are conserved for longer periods in this disease." [117]

Serum protein levels are higher as compared to kwashiorkor cases. Due to general wasting, the liver suffers great protein depletion and loss of its amino acid pool.

Body stores of vitamins and minerals decline gradually. Vitamin A absorption is better than in kwashiorkor.

Glucocorticoid secretion remains high in marasmus.

In both kwashiorkor and marasmus, the following symptoms are considered extremely unfavorable and may have a grave prognosis resulting in death: (1) marked asthenia, persistent

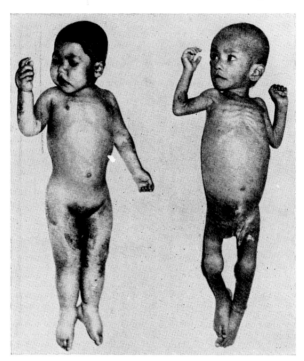

Figure 7. A typical child of the group considered as kwashiorkor (left) and a representative child of the marasmic condition (right).[75a]

subnormal temperature, extensive and refractor edema; (2) progressive wasting and persistent abdominal distension in marasmus; (3) uncontrolled vomiting, obstinate diarrhea and dehydration; (4) pulmonary and skin infections not responding to antibiotics; and (5) uncontrolled fever of unknown nature.[14]

Malnutrition and infections of all kinds go together, mainly because a malnourished child cannot immunologically fight the common infections as effectively as a healthy child can. Control of common infections by early treatment or their prevention by immunizations whenever possible could significantly reduce the mortality rate among malnourished children. Infected as well as malnourished children grow at a very low rate, and in many places such children show two, three or even four years of growth retardation in relation to their chronological age. Edozien,[27] while studying the malnutrition patterns in Africa, observed that children whose infections had been prevented showed much less incidence of protein-calorie malnutrition than a group of control children who had the same diet but whose infections had not been treated. There is an established synergism between infection and malnutrition and most often either malnutrition increases the chances of infection, or infections deplete the organism of moderately nourished child, so that it becomes malnourished.

It may be worthwhile to mention some of the common infections that are usually present and flourish in individuals who suffer from protein or protein-calorie malnutrition. The illnesses associated with malnutrition may be classified as bacterial (e.g. tuberculosis, whooping cough, infective diarrhea), viral (e.g. measles), and parasitic (e.g. malaria and certain helminth infestations). The bacterial infections are mainly a result of unsanitary conditions which prevail in the dwelling places of lower socioeconomic classes of people living in the developing countries where the problems of malnutrition are most acute. Jelliffe [56] stressed that, "Probably three-fourths of the world population drink unsafe water, dispose of human excretion recklessly, prepare milk and food dangerously, are constantly exposed to insect and rodent enemies and live in unfit dwellings." Living under these conditions, these people are highly susceptible to all kinds of infections, and because their protein reserves are low, they succumb to them more readily compared to the well-nourished population. Children in particular show respiratory infections, skin sepsis from scabies, and enteral infections from contaminated water or other unclean sources. Diarrhea and gastroenteritis are the most common complications among malnourished children. Gordon et al.[38] introduced the term "weanling diarrhea" because of its most frequent occurrence among children who are weaned from their mother's breast to starchy foods prepared under very unhygenic conditions. The weanling diarrhea is generally a result of malnutrition and enteral infections.

Measles is a common viral complication which frequently occurs among malnourished individuals, and although there is no direct relationship between measles and malnutrition, it may prove to be a precipitory factor in the etiology of kwashiorkor. The same is true of other infections, such as malaria, ascariasis, and hookworm. For details, the reader is referred to the excellent description by Jelliffe.[56] In malaria, the plasmodia, being the agent responsible for the onset of this disease, may have a direct effect on the host's body and may cause a direct drain on the host's protein and vitamin stores. In malnourished individuals, it may mean further deterioration of the condition and an extensive accumulation of the malaria pigment in the reticuloendothelial system which could direct some of the body's iron into inaccessible deposits and thereby contribute to hemolytic anemia. The manner in which the plasmodia effects the protein metabolism of the host has been explained by Jelliffe.[56]

> The parasite splits the hemoglobin of its host cells into hematin and globin. The globin is hydrolysed or phosphorolysed, and about half of the amino acids so produced are used to make the proteins present in the parasite. Globin, however, contains 1 percent methionine (most proteins contains 3–4 percent), and the parasite supplements its requirements from the host plasma methionine. In such infection the dietary requirements of host and parasite are considerable; for 2 percent of red cells may be destroyed, and about 1 g. of parasite nucleoprotein synthesised every three days.

The nutritional status of the host, who in most instances happens to be already malnourished, is adversely affected by the ascariasis infection. The parasite depletes the host in a variety of ways, such as ingestion of the available food, absorption of carbohydrates, fats and proteins, and by damaging the intestinal walls by physical injury, as well as by the toxic action of its excretions on the smooth muscle of the intestine.[52] The hookworm infection leads to a constant loss of blood, since a single hookworm ingests an estimated 0.38 ml to 0.84 ml of blood daily.[56,82] Depending on the number of hookworms, the consequences of this blood drain could be disasterous to a malnourished child within a short period of time.

Mention may also be made of the "vomiting sickness of Jamaica" and "infective gangrene of the mouth," which may not be directly attributed to malnutrition, but nevertheless is prevalent amongst malnourished children. The former is generally caused by ingestion of some toxic substance in the food which may not adversely affect a healthy well-nourished child, but may induce clinical symptoms such as mental depression, drowsiness, twitching of muscles, and convulsions in malnourished children.[58,96] The illness is generally initiated with vomiting, due to gastric irritation caused by any toxin followed by a "toxic blockage of the hepatic enzymes responsible for gluconeogenesis."[56] The infective gangrene of the mouth is observed in preschool children who are extremely malnourished, since they live mainly on a carbohydrate diet which is generally deficient in protein. Gingivitis leads to the spread of infection along the roots of the teeth. It produces osteomyelitis of the maxilla and mandible and in some cases infects the soft tissue of the cheeks. Penicillin and well-balanced diets improve the condition, but may still leave permanent deformities.[56]

Vitamin Deficiencies

Vitamin A

Varying degrees of vitamin deficiency are observed in groups of people who subsist on unbalanced diets consisting predominantly of cereals with very little animal protein. Vitamin A deficiency is especially common in these groups because of non-availability of preformed vitamin A or retinol (1 mg retinol = 330,000 IU of vitamin A), which is generally present in animal liver, kidneys, meat fat, egg yolk and liver oils from cods, sharks, and so on. A number of vegetables and fruits contain provitamin A or carotenoids, e.g. yellow- and orange-colored fruits and vegetables, carrots, squashes, mangoes, oranges, tomatoes. However, the absorption of provitamin A is less efficient in comparison to the preformed vitamin A which is obtained from animal sources of meat and milk. Night blindness, xerophthalmia and keratomalacia are the main vitamin A deficiency symptoms besides minor complications, such as foamy Bitot's spots in the eye, skin changes, and diarrhea. Abnormal electroretinograms are also observed under the effect of vitamin A deficiency. Night blindness, marked by an inability to see in dim light, is an early sign of deficiency but often goes undetected in young children. When the serum levels of vitamin A are low, the availability of a small amount of vitamin A in the retinal epithelium, required for the deposition of rhodopsin in the rods of the retina, is significantly delayed, and the results are poor night vision. Rhodopsin is decomposed by bright light, but it is quickly regenerated if vitamin A is readily available. Xerophthalmia begins as a result of the drying of conjunctiva and cornea which lose their shining luster, giving a very dull appearance to the eye. If xerophthalmia is not treated in time by regular doses of vitamin A, it could degenerate into a severe form of keratomalacia (dryness with ulceration and perforation of the cornea), a major cause of blindness in many developing countries. This condition leads to metaplasia and degeneration of the corneal epithelium-producing opacities. The cornea becomes vascularized, edematous and infiltrated with leucocytes.[56] Early cases of xerophthalamia can be helped by bathing the eye in water for a minute or two. Moderate forms of xerophthalmia can be easily treated by a regular intake of vitamin A. Care should be taken, however, not to give massive doses of vitamin A because this can lead to conditions like anorexia, growth failure, irritability, skeletal lesions with pain in extremities, periosteal bone thickening, tissues at the corners of the mouth and nose, hair coarsening. These conditions disappear when an excess amount of vitamin A is discontinued.[117] Vitamin A deficiency also leads to pronounced disturbances in the nervous system. It is essential in the formation as well as maturation of the neural tube,[81] and a vitamin A deficiency has been observed to cause degenerative changes in the optic, femoral, and sciatic nerves and the spinal cords in experimental animals.[22]

Severe cases of vitamin A deficiency should be treated as an emergency because of the imminent damage to the eyesight. Latham *et al.*[62] recommended the following treatment: an initial injection of 7,500 IU of vitamin A followed by oral administration of the same amount of vitamin A daily in the form of cod liver oil and 5 mg of riboflavin, three times a day. Both the eyes should be instilled with tetracycline or another antibiotic eye ointment, every four hours the first two days and less frequently during the next five to eight days. To avoid any secondary infection, 600,000 units of penicillin should be injected intramuscularly for seven to ten days. Above all, the patient must be treated for the correction of protein or protein-calorie malnutrition, if present. Skin changes (dry or rough skin with small papillar eruptions at the sites of hair follicles), generally referred to as phrynoderma or "toad skin" caused by vitamin A deficiency, disappear after the administration of the appropriate doses of vitamin A. Vitamin A deficiency is fairly widespread over the globe. In overpopulated regions, such as India, China and Indochina, numerous children suffer from vitamin A deficiency. More than 1 percent of the population of India is blind or nearly blind, and this is attributed to the widespread deficiency of vitamin A.[78]

Vitamin B Complex

A sufficient amount of thiamine, a water-soluble vitamin, is essential for complete metabolism of carbohydrates as a coenzyme in glucose metabolism. Thiamine deficiency causes beriberi and Wernicke and Korsakoff syndromes involving different body tissues, particularly in the neuromuscular system.

The nervous system changes include a reduction in the thiamine content of different areas of the brain. This results in specific histological abnormalities (e.g. leukocyte infiltration, cytoplasmic eosinophilia of neurons and glia, condensation of chromatin material, vacuolization of the neuropil) which can be observed in the thalamus, the hippocampus, and the basal ganglia.[16] Since thiamine has a direct inhibitory action on cholinesterase, its deficiency reduces the amount of acetylcholine.[64] In the thiamine deficiency state, the activity of some important enzymes in the brain, e.g. 6-phosphogluconate and pyruvate, is elevated,[16] whereas the activity of pyruvate dehydrogenase and transketolase is greatly reduced.[45]

Beriberi is generally observed among those people who prefer to eat polished rice, as thiamine is lost during the process of refining. Clinical beriberi may be differentiated into wet and dry kinds of infantile beriberi. The infantile beriberi is found in infants whose symptoms are due to a thiamine deficiency in the milk of the mother, who in turn may be living on a diet deficient in this vitamin. The incidence of infantile beriberi is most common during the first year of a child's life, particularly between two and six months of age. In the chronic form of beriberi, the infant shows signs of aphoria (low fever, cough, choking, as observed in the infection of respiratory tract), wasting of muscles, diarrhea, vomiting, acute edema, and cries continuously without much sound. In the acute form, the infant may develop dyspnea, cyanosis, and may experience cardiac failure. The cardiac condition develops rapidly in acute cases and may prove fatal. The symptoms of thiamine deficiency start with restlessness, sleepiness, and bouts of screaming which develop into anorexia, vomiting and breathlessness. "Most of the physical signs are related to acute cardiac dilation and failure and consists of tachycardia, enlargement of the heart to the right, a systolic murmur, pulmonary edema with rales, tender enlargement of the liver, edema and oliguria." [56] In young adults, wet and dry beriberi starts with a generally tired condition, mild swelling around the ankles, "pins and needles" in legs, and occasional palpitation of the heart. The dry form does not show edema, which is characteristic of the wet form, and the edema generally accumulates in the legs, face, and scrotum. In somewhat acute form, the pulse is rapid, irregular, and the heart is enlarged. The urine output is very low, and in the wet form may contain no albumin despite the edema. In the adult beriberi, the symptoms become evident because of the involvement of the peripheral nerves and the related muscle function, so much so that the patient may not be able to get up easily from a squatting position. Loss of tendon reflexes and paralysis is evident, and death may occur due to cardiac failure or some chronic infection. The treatment recommended by Latham et al.[62] may be pointed out here. In the infantile beriberi, a 5 mg injection of thiamine for four days to the child should be accompanied by 10 mg of thiamine orally twice a day for the mother, if the child is breast fed. In the adult dry and wet beriberi, 10 to 20 mg of thiamine injections in the initial stage and oral administration in the later stage accompanied by a nutritious diet rich in B Vitamins and low in carbohydrates is highly desirable. The dry beriberi may, however, need further physiotherapy.

Beriberi in the endemic forms is likely to be present in areas where the consumption of refined forms of cereals are becoming popular. Numerous cases of beriberi have been reported in Japan, Indonesia, China, Malaya, India, Burma, Philippines, and Brazil.[117] Among Western countries, beriberi is observed more among alcoholics and very poor people who are malnourished in other nutrients besides thiamine. Alcoholics are particularly susceptible to Wernicke's disease (Wernicke-Korsakoff syndrome) which

> Is characterized by eye signs (nystagmus, diplopia, paralysis of the externi recti muscles and sometimes ophthalmoplegia) ataxia and mental changes. Korsakoff's psychosis leads to a loss of memory of the immediate past, and often an elaborate confabulation which tends to conceal this amnesia.[62]

Alcoholic polyneuropathy, a condition similar to neuritic beriberi is also caused by thiamine deficiency. The condition responds favorably to the administration of thiamine, even if the consumption of alcohol is continued. However, besides the provision of thiamine in food and the administration of thiamine orally and in the injection form, it may be worthwhile to fortify alcoholic beverages and snacks generally eaten with alcohols with thiamine.[60]

Ariboflavinosis, caused by deficiency of riboflavin, results in seborrheic dermatitis in skin folds, e.g. nose edges and behind the ears, cheilosis (swelling or reddening of the lips) and eye lesions, frequently with irritation and itching. Although no evidence of nervous system disturbances because of riboflavin deficiency exists for humans, experimental evidence obtained from dogs and rodents indicates a myelin degeneration of the peripheral and posterior columns of the spinal cord.[122]

Riboflavin is commonly found in milk, meat, fish, leafy vegetables and legumes, and poorer socioeconomic sections who cannot afford to eat substantial quantities of these items suffer from it. Indonesia, parts of Africa, and India report a large number of cases. It is virtually absent in the United States, although a few decades ago it was not uncommon in the Southern states.

Niacin deficiency leads to pellagric conditions and, like ariboflavinosis, was common in the Southern states of the United States, but it has been eliminated in recent times. Diets consisting predominantly of corn were responsible because they raised the normal requirements of the body in some unknown manner.[56] The amino acid tryptophan is easily converted into niacin in the body, and corn is deficient in this amino acid. The major complication in pellagra is skin lesions (dermatitis) ; however, in the severe form, pellagra patients have acute diarrhea and dementia, and this may prove fatal. Dermatitis is most common in exposed parts of the body and becomes very painful on exposure to the sun. In addition, the mouth and tongue are sore, and the latter is red and raw looking. The nervous system is affected in the more severe forms, and the symptoms include irritability, loss of memory, lassitude, apprehension, delusion, insomnia and anxiety leading to dementia.[29] Mild sensory and motor changes may occur, but complete paralysis is rarely seen.[62] Brain abnormalities under the effect of niacin deficiency include tigrolysis of brain stem, especially atrophy of nerve cells, vasodilation, and chromatolysis.[26] An intramuscular injection of 50 to 100 mg of niacin for one to four days followed by oral administration is recommended. A deficiency of B_6 leads to reduced levels of gamma aminobutyric acid (GABA) as pyridoxine is essential for the decarboxylation of glutamic acid and 5-hydroxytryptophan to GABA and 5-hydroxytryptamine in the brain.[104] The abnormal metabolism of 5-hydroxytryptamine is generally related to certain mental disorders.[29] A single massive dose of niacin may lead to a dramatic improvement in the psychological performance of the patient.[28] Tranquilizers in the initial stages of treatment may be prescribed for those who experience mental disturbances.

All the vitamins of the B complex are essential for normal functioning of the nervous system, but vitamin B_6 is especially important. Convulsions of epilepsy [103] may result due to deficiency of vitamin B_6. Babies fed formulas deficient in B_6 are irritable, sensitive to noises, and show abnormal electroencephalograms. Certain genetic defects may be responsible for poor utilization of B_6 and, therefore, increase its dietary requirement.[18] It is, however, not wise to give large doses of vitamin B_6 alone; the other B vitamins should also be supplied because of their increased need. Conditions like chorea and Parkinson's disease have greatly improved after giving 10 to 100 mg of vitamin B_6 daily, and the patients showed increased mental alertness and decreased muscular cramps.[24] Pyridoxine is present in a wide variety of foods, and since only 2 mg a day is enough for body needs, a deficiency of this vitamin is unlikely if a balanced diet is eaten. A deficiency of folic acid leads to macrocytic megaloblastic anemia, whereas a deficiency of B_{12} will lead to pernicious anemia. Folic acid deficiency may be due to low dietary intake, poor absorption or increased metabolic demands, for example, in late pregnancy and early infancy. The symptoms of folic acid deficiency include general weakness and/or degeneration of surface mucosal tissue, resulting in ulceration and secondary infections, a sore tongue, and gastrointestinal problems, e.g. diarrhea.[117] Folic acid deficiency leads to delayed maturation of EEG, and persons with inborn errors of folic acid metabolism show signs of mental retardation.[3,78] Pernicious anemia is characterized by general weakness, dyspnea, and palpitation accompanied by an enlargement of the liver and spleen; macrocytic anemia may be corrected by 5 to 20 mg daily of folic acid, whereas complete prevention of pernicious anemia may not be possible. Injections of B_{12} will, however, help greatly. It is interesting as well as fortunate that the breast milk of the poorly nourished mothers contains adequate quantities of folic acids, even if the concentration of other vitamins is decreased.

Vitamin C

Vitamin C deficiency over prolonged periods of time leads to scurvy. Dietary intake of subnormal amounts for months may not become apparent in any physical condition, since scurvy develops only after the tissue stores of this vitamin are exhausted. The symptoms of scurvy include tenderness of the extremities, swollen and easily bleeding gums, loose teeth, hemorrhages of the skin, nose, under the nails and subperiosteal areas, delayed healing of wounds, anemia, and shortness of breath. Follicular hemorrhages of the skin and deep hemorrhages of the muscle tissue are very common. The joints are particularly susceptible, and hemorrhages in the cavities of the joints lead to painful swelling and immobility. In infants this condition leads to a characteristic posture "supine with knees partially flexed and thighs extremely rotated," often referred to as scorbutic pose.[117] The patient, although not appearing very seriously ill, may suddenly die of a cardiac failure. Infantile scurvy is observed in infants two to 12 months of age. Scurvy is also not uncommon among adults.

Among adults, general "weakness, lassitude, irritability and vague dull aching pains in the muscle and joints of the lower extremities" [117] are characteristic; whereas infants suffer acute pains of the limbs and joints due to swellings and hemorrhages in the legs and bruising of the body. The growing end of the bones are particularly susceptible, and the infant is in a perpetual state of agony, crying at the slightest touch or movement. Normally, infants are born with adequate amounts of vitamin C, which could easily last for a few months under normal circumstances. Infants of six months or more do consume supplementary foods which provide their vitamin C needs. Citrus fruits and a large number of fruits and vegetables are rich in vitamin C. The treatment of scurvy consists of administration of large doses of ascorbic acid (1,000 mg followed by 250 mg, 4 times daily for 6 to 7 days). Latham *et al.*[62] recommended a vigorous treatment in view of the danger of sudden death, even in a patient who apparently looks all right. However, the disease dramatically responds to ascorbic acid treatment, and it has been observed that gum and nose bleeding stops within 24 hours, and that a patient may be completely recovered within two to three weeks.

Vitamin D

Vitamin D deficiency leads to rickets and osteomalacia. Both of these conditions are caused by impaired metabolism of calcium and phosphorus, and since vitamin D is directly responsible for their retention and absorption, they are considered disorders of vitamin D deficiency. Vitamin D may be obtained from a dietary source, but this vitamin can also be manufactured by the body from exposure of the skin to sunlight (vitamin D_3 produced by irradiation with ultraviolet light of the provitamin, 7-dehydrocholesterol). Naturally occurring foods are not rich in this vitamin, but at the present a number of foods, especially milk, are supplemented with vitamin D. The main symptom in the development of rickets is the rarefaction of bone tissue and the deformity of bones under the weight of the body or even the pull of the attached muscles. Besides showing changes in the skeleton which need x-ray examination, children suffering from vitamin D deficiency are slow in learning to sit, to walk, or to get their teeth, and show a flabby toneless state of their muscles. External signs include swelling of the epiphysis of the large bones, resulting in the formation of bowed thighs and knocked knees, swelling of the costochondral junctions and their bead-like appearance. Even the spine may get curved, and the child tends to slump when in a sitting posture. The toneless muscles of the abdomen also bring about a protuberance of the abdomen. The head appears bigger due to softening of the occipital and parietal bones of the skull and delayed closing of the anterior fontanel. Whereas rickets are observed in young children, osteomalacia is observed in adults, especially among women in whom calcium stores have been depleted due to repeated pregnancies, and who also show a deficiency in vitamin D. Osteomalacia is characterized by the softening and bending of the bones with more or less severe pain. The bones are soft because they contain osteoid tissue which has failed to calcify. A constant pain in the pelvis, lower back, and legs is felt by the patient. The severe form of osteomalacia may lead to spontaneous bone fractures and other skeletal complications. The treatment of rickets as well as osteomalacia consists of making heavy doses of vitamin D available to the patients. To children 3,000 IU of vitamin D may be enough, but to adults 50,000 IU daily should be given. The diet also should have a good calcium source, such as adequate quantities of milk intake, and above all, parents should be instructed to the benefits of skin exposure to the freely available sunshine. Latham *et al.*[62] also stressed good obstetrical care of women who had pelvic abnormalities due to osteomalacia. Rickets and osteomalacia are common in only those areas where as a result of certain cultural or social reasons, the children as well as adults are not exposed to sunlight. For example, in the old Muslim culture, women are not allowed to move around without a black cover "burka" over their entire body. The houses are dark, without many windows and sunlight, which increases the chances of the development of osteomalacia. Women in such a culture can produce children with deficient vitamin D and calcium stores.[56] Bicknell and Prescott [8] have described the situation very graphically as follows:

> With each child the condition takes a step forward as the body is
> further drained of its minerals and vitamins. And with each child the

condition becomes more piteous; the mother is more imprisoned in the house by pain and deformities; her chances of earning more money, of gaining more food, more sunlight, are curtailed; her pelvis collapses further and further, making her next confinement even worse than the last. Sometimes her downward progress halts between her pregnancies; sometimes she may even improve if fortunately she does not suckle her infant in the vain hope of thus warding off her tragic fertility.

Vitamin E

Vitamin E is required for the normal maintenance of reproductive processes, musculature, central nervous function, and the prevention of liver necrosis. Vitamin E deficiency is associated with biliary atresia, cystic fibrosis of the pancreas and neuronal dystrophy characterized by loss of nerve cells in certain nuclei of the medulla oblongata.[39,78] Vitamin E is believed to function as an antioxident in the prevention of lipid peroxidation. Gallagher [35] described how generous amounts of vitamin E make animals resistant to cancers. A cancer tissue placed in blood stream rich in vitamin E does not grow, but this tissue placed in serum without vitamin E grows readily. Besides maintaining normal reproduction and musculature (people with vitamin E deficiency complain of stiff legs), this vitamin is also related to hematopoietic factors and has a certain relationship to folic acid and vitamin B_{12}. The erthrocyte survival time is greatly decreased because of vitamin E deficiency, thereby helping to create anemic conditions.[65]

Vitamin K

Vitamin K deficiency is uncommon among adults, first, because it is abundant in green leaves and vegetables, and second, it can be synthesized by the body. The only susceptible population is the neonate, who not only lacks stores of this vitamin but also cannot synthesize it due to his sterile gastrointestinal tract devoid of bacteria. According to an estimate, one in every 1,000 newborn infants dies from hemorrhage,[117] which is the principal complication of vitamin K deficiency. In the newborn, vitamin K is essentially needed for the formation of prothrombin—a substance necessary for blood clotting. Prothrombin is produced in the liver in the presence of vitamin K. At the site of injury, the pro-thrombin reacts with the blood and changes into thrombin which further changes fibrinogen to fibrin. The latter produces a clot by its sticky cobweb-like structure.[35] In the newborn, hemorrhage can be easily prevented by giving small doses of vitamin K. Excess doses may be toxic and even fatal. The American Medical Association Council on Drugs recommends 1 mg of synthetic vitamin K for prophylaxis and treatment.

Deficiency of Minerals

About 15 minerals make up 4 percent of the body weight, out of which calcium alone accounts for one half of the mineral matter. Even though some minerals are present only in trace amounts, their absence can cause serious problems and their excess may prove toxic.

Calcium and Phosphorus

The metabolism of calcium is intimately linked with phosphorus and vitamin D. Since phosphorus is present in almost all the foods consumed by human beings, its deficiency is very unlikely. However, groups of people who consume cereals without many green vegetables and do not eat animal products can develop calcium deficiency. The main sources of calcium are animal foods, dairy and meat products, and leafy vegetables. Inorganic calcium salts are also ingested along with drinking water. In infants, the calcium obtained from breast milk, particularly of undernourished mothers, may be somewhat insufficient to maintain the growing skeleton, and if the vitamin D intake is low, the situation could be further complicated because vitamin D is mainly responsible for the retention and absorption of calcium. A high calcium intake by a mother during pregnancy as well as lactation is, therefore, essential. Osteomalacia, the adult version of rickets and osteoporosis (skeletal atrophy) among persons of older age, especially women, is mainly a result of calcium and vitamin D deficiency, although other factors, such as protein malnutrition, can also contribute. In osteoporosis, the decline in secretion of hormones by sex glands and the pituitary gland is also responsible. This condition can best be combated by the administration of combined male and female hormones along with increased dietary intake of calcium and vitamin D.[117] Calcium requirements for growing children are estimated to be around 0.7 gm, but as stressed by Jelliffe and other workers in the tropical and subtropical countries, children on poor calcium diets are adapted to its lower availability and appear as healthy as children with sufficient calcium in their diets. Veen [108] remarked:

> The calcium problem in some tropical countries is of interest. If calcium requirements were always as high as accepted in the U.S.A. and Western Europe, and if they were absolutely rigid and not influenced by such factors as adaptation, race, environment, etc., it would be rather difficult to explain why, for example, nearly all the Javanese, Sudanese and Madurese, or about fifty million people do not exhibit calcium deficiency problems.

Tetany is an important disorder caused by deficiency of calcium salts and is marked by intermittent tonic muscular contractions, accompanied by fibrillary tremors, paresthesias and muscular pains. There is increased irritability of the motor and sensory nerve to electrical and mechanical stimuli. Tetany in neonates may be the result of a high phosphate content obtained from whole cow's milk. An increased level of serum phosphate leads to a decreased level of serum calcium.[117] Gastric tetany may develop as a result of a loss of chloride ions which reduces the serum chloride level and increased bicarbonates, which elevate the blood pH. Similarly, bicarbonate tetany may be produced by excessive intake of sodium bicarbonate which elevates the blood pH as well as the blood carbon dioxide content.[117]

Iron

Iron deficiency leads to anemia, which is characterized by general weakness, pallor, fatigability, headaches, and palpitation. The main criteria for the establishment of iron deficiency anemia is the reduced hemoglobin content compared to the red blood cell count. In extreme anemic conditions, the hemoglobin value may be as low as 5 gm/1,000 ml compared to normal values of 14 $\pm$ 1 gm and 16 $\pm$ 2 gm for women and men respectively. Iron deficiency is one of the most common nutritional disorders over the world. Iron from cereals is poorly absorbed, whereas it is well absorbed by the body from meats. In the developed countries of the West, its prevalence is mainly due to ignorance, food fads, and very low intake of total food for fear of obesity, particularly among women with blood losses during menstruation when their needs are twice as high as those of adult males. During the period of pregnancy, the demands for iron are increased tremendously due to stress of the growth of the fetus and the increased volume of blood. Among infants, especially those born to anemic mothers, anemia is common because milk is a poor source of iron, and unless supplementary foods containing iron are given, anemia may develop in the latter part of infancy.

Besides general tiredness and shortness of breath, the common symptoms of iron deficiency anemia are flat brittle fingernails with pale nail beds, a sore mouth, difficulty in swallowing, papillary atrophy of the tongue, gastritis and enlargement of the liver and spleen. Anemia among adults may result from blood losses due to hookworm or other infectious or chronic illnesses. For example, chronic blood losses due to gastrointestinal bleeding may drain the body reserves. Under normal circumstances, infants and young females, especially during menstruation and pregnancy, should be careful about their iron needs and increase its intake either through diets or iron supplements.

Iodine

The main complication of iodine deficiency is the swelling of the thyroid gland. The enlarged gland presses on the trachea, thereby creating respiratory complications, such as hoarseness of voice and cough. The patients feel great discomfort in swallowing. The enlargement of the thyroid in the absence of available iodine is a result of a compensating mechanism intended to produce the maximum possible thyroxine (a hormone containing 65% iodine) for normal functioning. Iodine deficiency may result from a lack of mineral iodine in the water supply of an area due to certain goitrogenic factors which hinder the absorption of dietary iodine. Such goitrogenic substances are found in cabbage, brussel sprouts, soybeans, peanuts, turnips,[34] and so on.[117] Approximately 10 percent of the world population seems to exhibit iodine deficiency, and widespread deficiency of this mineral has been reported in Indonesia, Thailand, Indochina, Ceylon, Northern India, Western China, South America and Central and West Africa.[56] Cretinism, which is characterized by a stunted growth, dwarfism, and various degrees of mental retardation, abnormalities in hearing and speech, neuromuscular disorders, impairment of somatic development, is a result of severe iodine deficiency over several generations of mothers and infants.[91]

> The infant might appear normal at birth, but is slow to develop, small in size, mentally dull, has a thick skin and characteristic face with depressed nose and often a protruding, enlarged tongue. Deaf mutism and mental retardation are found more frequently in the children of mothers with enlarged thyroid glands.[62]

Cretinism is more common in areas of endemic goiter, where the iodine content of the thyroid of an average person, particularly females, is reduced to a mere 1 to 2 mg as compared to a normal level of 8 to 10 mg. The iodine intake of a normal person is proportional to the blood concentration of the thyroid hormone. The protein bond is reduced in hypothyroidism and increased in hyperthyroidism.

The most important preventive measure of goiter is the use of iodized salts, which theoretically appears simple but may be difficult in actual practice.[56] The affected population could also be encouraged to use larger quantities of seafoods which are rich in iodine. In New Guinea and Andean Ecuador, iodized oil has been tried with beneficial results.[12] In severe cases and for immediate improvement, Latham *et al.*[62] suggested the administration of small doses of thyroid extracts in thyroxine, starting from 1/2 grain daily, increasing to 2 grains daily.

Sodium, Potassium, Magnesium and Trace Elements

For proper functioning of the nervous tissue, particularly nerve irritability and muscle contraction, depends on exact amounts of sodium, potassium, magnesium, and calcium since they control the passage of substances into and out of the cells and regulate the transmission of nerve impulses. Sodium ions, present extracellularly and potassium within the cell, maintain the fluid balances, and a disturbance leads to either edema or dehydration. Sodium and phosphate compounds also maintain the acid-base balance and blood pH and sodium salts are important buffers of plasma, extracellular fluid and urine. The deficiency of sodium results in the slowing of growth and lack of appetite. In tropical countries, manual laborers working outdoors under the hot sun lose large quantities of sodium through sweat, and the electrolytic imbalance results in muscular cramps and mental apathy. Excess carbohydrates cannot be changed into fat without sodium, nor can the synthesis of protein take place. Potassium is essential for the synthesis of protein and for enzyme functions within the cell. Potassium is widely present in food, and a deficiency is unlikely to occur. However, potassium depletion is a major biochemical byproduct in kwashiorkor and is a direct result of protein deficiency. In a malnourished edematous child, potassium deficiency may be more prominent than protein deficiency. Potassium deficiency results in constipation, slow growth, nervous ailment, sleeplessness, slow heart beats, enlarged kidneys and fragility of bones. In the Philippines, Stransky *et al.*[94,95] found that out of 88 children in the first years of life, 74 showed low sodium levels and several indicated hypopotassemia. Great care is needed in early childhood to see that the sodium and potassium balance of the body is not upset.

Next to potassium, magnesium is the predominant metallic cation in living cells, regulating nervous irritability, muscle contraction and activating many of the enzymes involved in energy metabolism. A deprivation of Mg^{++} may contribute to the growth retardation found in kwashiorkor; the intracellular magnesium level is greatly reduced; [63] and a large quantity of magnesium is lost in the loose stools of diarrhea.[70] A good supply of magnesium, potassium, and protein is essential for adequate growth.[63] In general, magnesium deficiency causes depression, muscular weakness, vertigo and liability to convulsions.[44] People whose hands twitched and trembled so severely that their handwriting was illegible showed immediate improvement after getting magnesium, and their handwriting became steady. Davis [24] described that a tiny bit of magnesium changed "a trembling, irrational, noisy, combative and wildly restless individual into a charming delightful gentleman free from symptoms in 18 hours."

Chromium is a trace element, and its importance in human nutrition has been well recognized. It has been shown that in the presence of insulin, chromium enhances the transport of glucose across the cell and the mitochondrial membranes.[68] The impaired glucose utilization observed in kwashiorkor is greatly corrected by oral administration of 250 mg of trivalent chromium.[85]

Zinc is another trace element which is a constituent of a number of metallo-enzymes and is believed to be essential for the growth and gonadal function in man.[76,77] Zinc deficiency has been observed to delay normal healing.[93] Diseases generally associated with alterations in zinc metabolism include postalcoholic cirrhosis, pernicious anemia, and a chronic myeloid leukemia.[76,77] Milk is a good source of zinc. Copper deficiency in experimental animals leads to demyelination of the brain.[31,49]

There is no indication that fluoride, although present in many tissues in small quantities, is essential for normal health. It is believed that fluoride deficiency causes dental caries, but it is also well known that dental caries are due to many other causes. Numerous studies have been conducted on the effect of fluoride on dental caries only to add more confusion to the already confused state of affairs. In an examination of caries in children born prior and during the first nine months following fluoridation of a water supply, no significant reduction in caries was observed. Too much fluoride during the formation of the teeth causes the enamel to become mottled, corroded, structuarlly weak and finally to deteriorate. Other studies strongly support the reduction of caries after prolonged drinking of fluoridated water. At present in the United States there are more than 60 million people who drink water with a 1 ppm fluoride content.

Obesity

Obesity is a form of malnutrition which for a long time has been mistaken for good health by physicians and laymen alike in many countries of the world. During recent years, there has been a growing appreciation of the fact that obesity, which is a result of a very high level of caloric intake, combined with low levels of energy expenditure, predisposes a person to cardiovascular and pulmonary diseases, hypertension, diabetes, peripheral vascular and orthopedic disorders and shortens the life span.[62] Obese persons are a surgical risk and are more prone to respiratory problems, such as emphysema, chronic bronchitis, asthma, than normal healthy individuals.

The problems of obesity look simple, and it appears that obesity can be solved by restricting the intake of carbohydrates, fats, and calories and increasing the energy expenditure levels. This caloric restriction or fasting takes into account only the physical factors. Physiological, social, psychological, and genetic factors may be equally important in dealing with the problem of obesity. Physiologically, there are critical periods when obesity is developed. In the science section of *Newsweek* of October 19, 1970, Drs. Jerome Knittle and Jules Hirsch of Rockefeller University discussed that the seeds of obesity are sown in early childhood, when the mother forces a large quantity of food on the child, and the child responds to the large food intake by making an excessive number of fat containing cells in the body. These cells never disappear even under a strict dietary regimen. During starvation and food restriction periods the fat cells shrink in size and the obese person loses weight, but these fat cells always return to their full size as soon as the period of self-deprivation ends. Most obese persons have always been fond of food, such persons are perpetually at the mercy of fat cells, and according to Dr. Knittle, "Must face a choice between constant vigilance and undisguised fatness."

Goldblatt and co-workers [36] studied the social factors in obesity and found that a larger number of obese persons were found in the lower socioeconomic groups than in the higher ones. They found that with increasing upward mobility, the incidence of obesity declined, especially among women. "With increasing social status, the women moved from the 'obese' to the 'thin' category; the men moved from the 'obese' to the 'normal' category." [117] This study indicates that material affluence does not contribute to obesity, and that genetic or psychologic factors may be more important than socioeconomic factors. Surveys have shown that if one of the parents is obese, 40 percent of the children are obese, but if both parents are obese the number of obese off-springs goes as high as 80 percent.[117] It is probable that besides genetic factors, the food habits which in the first place contributed to the obesity of the parents are to a great extent responsible for the obesity of the children. Emotional factors, such as disappointments, fears, and anxieties, also lead to overeating and reduced activity level with the resulting upset in the balance of caloric intake and energy expenditure. In certain instances, food deprivation may increase the emotional instability because of the association of food with the sense of security and well-being. A change of attitude towards life and motivation is extremely important in any successful treatment of obesity. A study of emotional and psychological factors among adolescents and adults reveals that the success or failure of the treatment of obesity is directly related to the emotional stability of the subjects.[121]

It should be stressed in any weight-reduction program that a rapid weight loss may greatly weaken the motivation of the patient because it might be accompanied by general weakness and dizziness. The slower the weight loss, the easier it may be to maintain the regimen for prolonged periods of time.[119] As a matter of fact, the dietary regimen intended to reduce the caloric intake must provide all the essential nutrients in sufficient amounts. Since one pound of body fat represents about 3,500 calories, a daily deficiency of 500 calories could lead to one pound loss every week. A cycle including the sudden loss of weight at one time and regaining it and going back to lose it may prove more harmful than maintaining a steady weight even at levels of moderate obesity.[62] Salt restriction may also be recommended to those obese subjects who show a tendency to retain excessive amounts of fluids.

Cardiovascular Disease Related to Nutrition

Cardiovascular diseases, including arteriosclerosis which involves the coronary and cerebral circulation, rank first in causing deaths to millions of people, particularly in the technologically developed countries of Europe and North America. Heart disease has been referred to as the disease of the affluent countries. It is interesting, therefore, to examine briefly what contributes to this ever-increasing number of people exhibiting coronary heart disease, particularly men in their forties and fifties. Over the years, a number of exhaustive studies have established the fact that cardiovascular diseases are not a consequence of either age or hereditary tendencies, but that diet, through its lipid metabolism and circulating lipids, is an important environmental element in its causation. Other factors may be hypertension, smoking, obesity, and probably alcoholism. In a typical United States diet 40 percent of the calories are derived from fats compared to 10 percent fat calories in the underdeveloped world. Out of 40 percent, 17 percent of the calories come from saturated fats derived from animals meat, eggs, and dairy products as compared to 1 percent in the developing countries (Fig. 2) . Such differences are reflected in the incidence of heart diseases. Figure 8 depicts the mortality rate from coronary heart diseases in the year 1948–49 and shows a direct correlation between death rate from degenerative heart disease and fat calories consumed in the diet. The picture in recent years is no different. An analysis of 1968 figures of death by cardiovascular diseases reveals that in the United States 927,660 people died of arteriosclerosis; 26,580 deaths were attributed to hypertension; and the cause of 67,140 deaths was diagnosed as chronic rheumatic heart disease and other diseases of arteries, arterioles, and capillaries. The total deaths directly related to cardiovascular diseases were estimated as 1,021,380 which is 49.6 percent of all deaths that took place in the United States in 1968. With these grim figures, any way in which the situation can be remedied or improved is worth the effort. Of all the factors, an overall awareness and change in dietary habits so as to reduce the amount of circulating blood lipids is the most practical approach. There is solid evidence that a cholesterol reduction in the diet significantly reduces the incidence of coronary heart disease. The level of beta lipoproteins, which are complexes of triglycerides, cholesterols, and phospholipids, are closely associated with the

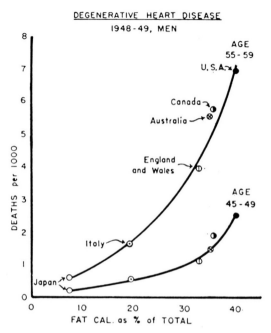

Figure 8. Mortality rate from coronary heart disease in different countries as related to percentage of fat calories consumed in the diet.[59]

onset of degenerative cardiovascular diseases. Some investigations have shown that a 12 percent reduction of serum cholesterol through dietary regimen among 1,000 "high risk individuals" greatly decreased the incidence of heart disease. It has also been shown among a group of men who survived from a myocardial infarction that by reducing the serum cholesterol level up to 17 percent through a strict dietary control, they showed significantly reduced incidence of cardiovascular problems over a five-year follow-up period, as compared to a counterpart control group. Latham *et al.*[62] described a dietary management which, by reducing the serum cholesterol level, reduces the chances of a cardiovascular disorder. The first main requirement is a reduction in the intake of saturated fats. Animal foods (meat, dairy) are the main sources and should to a great extent be replaced by fish and poultry, which are comparatively low in saturated fats. The fats from the dairy products are easily extractable, and the use of skim milk, nonfat powdered milk, for example, should be encouraged for all members of the family. In contrast, the intake of polyunsaturated fats, the main source of which is vegetable oils, may be increased. To lessen the serum cholesterol content, certain foods rich in cholesterol should be either avoided or reduced to a minimum level, e.g. the use of egg yolk should be limited to two or three a week. In addition to their rich cholesterol content, egg yolks are also implicated in the impairment of iron absorption.[62] An excessive use of eggs may not only raise the blood cholesterol level but also contribute its share in the development of iron deficiency anemia. The whole strategy should be to increase the ratio of polyunsaturated fats to saturated fats and at the same time to cut down the total fat intake to a level of 35 percent fat calories or even less. Lessening the fat calories should also be accompanied by an increase in the level of physical activity.

Latham *et al.*[62] also suggested that in cases of hypertension and congested heart condition, it is important to reduce the dietary sodium intake. The

> net body loss of sodium in the individual with a failing heart reduces extracellular fluid volume, correcting edema and its complications and by reducing circulating fluid volume. All these tend to lessen the work of the heart. The resulting improvement of organ perfusion, especially of the kidneys, results in the ability of intrinsic homeostatic mechanisms to regain control of sodium balance and improves exercise tolerance.[62]

The aim of this sodium reduction intake should be to induce a negative sodium balance in the body which can be best achieved by reducing the intake of common salt (sodium chloride) from the average level of 3 to 7 gm to about 1 gm or even less per day. However, it must be emphasized that common salt is not the only source of sodium chloride. Animal food sources, such as meat and dairy products, are also rich in sodium. Most preserved frozen foods have salt added to them. A number of other foods used daily in the menu also contain sodium. Therefore, it is recommended that if a reduction in sodium intake is necessitated because of hypertension or failing heart condition, foods should be prepared on a "no added salt" basis. The sodium content of the foods should be enough to maintain a good sodium level of the body.

MALNUTRITION AND GROWTH RETARDATION

Normal growth among humans is directed by genotype and nutrition. The latter includes favorable and unfavorable environment and nutritional state with respect to the quality of proteins as well as the quantity of available nutrients (carbohydrates, fats, vitamins, and minerals). Environment and nutrition play an important role among children whose growth under adverse conditions could be temporarily or permanently hindered. Growth as defined by Cheek and Cooke[15] relates to

> the physiological accretion of new tissue, which is reflected in the acquisition of protein and water. This leads to increases of length, weight and volume, which progress actively from the fertilization of the ovum to the period of sexual maturity when millions of cells are present in a state of advanced organization.

Good nutrition promotes the production and activities of the growth hormone, which influences the metabolism of proteins, carbohydrates, fats, and minerals and promotes nitrogen retention.[84,87] A lack of adequate nutrition will hinder such a natural growth pattern, and a stunted physical growth may be accompanied by physiological abnormalities or even retarded mental development. Many babies, particularly in developing countries, suffer from severe retardation of growth between six months and two years of age. Even after this period, they are generally fed less than the optimum requirements and face recurrent deprivation. Such malnutrition in a growing child leads to a condition which is a result of multiple disturbances in metabolic pathways and enzymatic activity affecting almost every organ and system. The resulting small size may lead to functional impairment. Tanner[98] observed that short people have on the average a lower intelligence than taller ones, which may be the result of impaired neurological development in early life. Thomson[99] concluded that growth stunting between the critical six months and two years of age caused by malnutrition tends to become a permanent retardation even if the child is fed adequately afterwards .

The neonate who has been well nourished *in utero* has 5.7 percent of his adult weight, 30 percent of his adult height and 63 percent of his adult head circumference. At one year, the child has 16.3 percent, 44.1 percent, and 83.6 percent of his adult weight, height, and head circumference respectively, and at three years, 24 percent, 57 percent and 90 percent of them.[40] Infants who have been malnourished *in utero* as a result of a lack of adequate nutrition or other intrauterine disorders suffer a significant deficit in height and weight. Graham [41] closely watched 60 infants and children suffering from severe malnutrition for a period of 24 months and concluded that a severe degree of malnutrition or caloric deprivation during the first year of life would lead to permanent reduction in height as well as head size. When the child in its first year of life is malnourished or starved, the growth failure in terms of weight, height, or head circumference is so significant that it may be impossible for the child to catch up from this deficit under the best of circumstances.[40] Stoch and Smythe [92] reported significant and long-lasting reductions in the height, head circumference, and mental achievements of a number of malnourished infants, and Cabak and Najdanvic [13] observed in similar cases a striking degree of retardation in mental development. "Looked at from either end of the growth span, there is thus a good deal of evidence which seems to support the hypothesis that impairment of early growth in man, from any cause, may result in permanent anatomical stunting and reduction of physiological efficiency." [99] Srikantia [90] emphasized that the supplementary feeding of preschool children does not greatly help to correct the growth retardation experienced at an earlier age. He believed that the lesser growth rates are a legacy from the early life of the child. The generally small size of the adult population may be the result of a combination of primary early malnutrition and continuing secondary malnutrition. An interesting parallel to nutritional deprivation has been observed in a study of monozygotic and dizygotic twins. In such cases, the smaller partner suffers to some extent intrauterine malnutrition because it is believed to be maintained by a small fraction of the placenta. Professor Falkner in Louisville, Kentucky, studied 160 pairs of such twins and found that between them the smaller of each pair behaved like a "small for date" baby and after six years was smaller in size and trailed behind the bigger one in psychological development.[41]

Growth retardation is a result of the inability to gain weight and leads to skeletal immaturity as well as physical, mental, and emotional inactivity. With respect to skeletal immaturity, Guzman,[49] Rohmann [83] and collaborators observed significant degrees of bone retardation in the Guatemalan children of low socio-economic groups. Specific changes related to a lesser number of ossification centers in different parts of the skeleton. Growth retardation due to malnutrition may begin in the intrauterine life, if the mother's diet during the latter part of pregnancy is not adequate in high-quality protein and other nutrients. Commenting on the relationship of maternal diet and the growth of the baby in terms of its birth length, De Silva and Baptist [87] believed that

> the length of the baby at birth is influenced more by the amount of protein in the maternal diet than by the mother's height. A diet well supplied with protein-rich foods tends to produce a long baby, while a low-protein diet would in all probability result in a relatively short baby irrespective of the mother's height. It would appear correct to assume that the amount of total protein in the prenatal diet is a more influential factor in determining the birth length of the infant than either calcium or riboflavin.

In general, growth retardation among children of postweaning age is caused by dietary deficiencies of specific nutrients, such as vitamins or minerals, or a general lack of body-building proteins and/or calories for maintaining basal metabolism as well as allowing for further weight gain. In most developing countries, it is the inadequate availability of high-quality proteins as well as fats and carbohydrates which precipitate malnutrition. During infancy, when the mother's milk provides a balanced ratio of amino acids as well as other nutrients, most children in the developing countries show growth rates comparable to those of advanced nations of the West. Such a growth pattern is, however, not continued in the postweaning period because most children, particularly those belonging to lower socioeconomic groups, get an unbalanced and insufficient diet with respect to one or more essential amino acids and/or other nutrients. The parents of the unfortunate children do not have a full appreciation of the growth needs of these preschool children. They do not understand that when adequate quantities of protein and calories are not made available in the diet, the child is likely to be affected in growth. Sufficient amount of calories in the diet are as essential as good quality proteins. Proteins badly needed for tissue building may be used up as a source of energy. Conditions of malnutrition and kwashior-kor are particularly the result of an imbalance of carbohydrate to protein.

Udani [107] conducted a survey on the physical growth of children in different socioeconomic groups in Bombay, India, and con-cluded that there are significant differences in the weight and height of neonates, as well as children of one to 11 years of age, belonging to upper, middle, and poor socioeconomic groups. Udani calculated from his statistical data that in terms of weight and height a one-year-old child of the upper socioeconomic groups is equivalent to a one-and-a-half-year-old child in the middle class and a two-year-old child in the lower socioeconomic groups. Simi-larly, a six to seven-year-old upperclass child is equal to a nine-year-old middle class and an 11-year-old lower class child with respect to weight and height. The differences are the result of a diet deficient in calories and proteins as well as chronic or re-current acute or parasitic infections which result in socioeconomic malnutrition for generations. This may lead to "genetic malnutri-tion" or poor constitution. Similar conditions exist in some other developing countries. A survey showed that two thirds of the population of Haiti suffer from varying degrees of protein calorie malnutrition as judged by growth retardation. Surveys on nutri-tion in Central America lead to similar conclusions.[5] A dietary survey of the Mayan Indian community of the Guatemalan high-lands over a period of three years revealed that at two years of age, the diet given to children provided one half of the number of needed calories and 55 percent of the needed protein.[5] Obvi-ously, this amount of total food intake will also be inadequate in quantities of vitamins and minerals. These insufficient diets, generation after generation, lead to a progressively smaller-sized adult population than that of the industrialized countries of the West. Table III illustrates the height and weight of children from high and low socioeconomic groups in some selected countries at different ages.

TABLE III
HEIGHT AND WEIGHT OF CHILDREN OF DIFFERENT SOCIOECONOMIC
BACKGROUNDS AT DIFFERENT AGE GROUPS [42]

Population	Height (cm)						Weight (kg.)					
	1 mo	6 mo	12 mo	6 yr	10 yr	14 yr	1 mo	6 mo	12 mo	6 yr	10 yr	14 yr
High Socioeconomic Group												
U. S. White [51]	54	68	76	116	139	159	4.2	8.1	10.5	21.0	31.0	48.0
U. S. Negro [86]	54	67	76	0	0	0	4.1	8.0	10.2	0	0	0
Guatemala [47]	54	68	76	0	0	0	4.1	7.6	10.1	0	0	0
Guatemala, private schools	0	0	0	114	135	154	0	0	0	21.0	30.0	45.0
Panama, private schools	0	0	0	117	135	157	0	0	0	22.2	32.6	48.9
Japan [72]	53	66	76	0	0	0	4.2	7.7	9.0	0	0	0
India [21]	55	66	77	0	0	0	4.0	7.4	10.0	0	0	0
Low Socioeconomic Group												
U. S. Negro [120]	0	61	69	0	0	0	0	6.3	7.9	0	0	0
Guatemala (urban)	54	65	72	0	0	0	4.0	6.8	8.3	17.6	22.8	35.6
Guatemala (rural)	53	63	68	108	121	140	4.0	7.2	8.2	17.6	22.8	35.6
Guatemala, public schools	0	0	0	108	123	145	0	0	0	17.3	24.0	36.1
Thailand [88]	55	65	71	104	124	144	4.1	6.17	9.0	15.9	22.8	33.7
Malaya [109]	0	0	0	0	122	142	0	0	0	0	24.2	35.3
India [21,79]	52	64	73	106	126	146	3.6	6.4	7.3	16.0	22.0	31.0

0 = Data not available.

The association between adult stature and the socioeconomic status has been established by observation of a number of workers.[100,101] The small stature of the women, which is probably a result of undernutrition or malnutrition during infancy, is of great obstetrical importance. The onset of menses is delayed by two or more years in undernourished girls. Burrell [11] and Oettle [73] estimated that the median age of menses in the South African Bantu girls of low socioeconomic groups occurred at about 14.5 years compared to less than 13 years in the well-nourished girls. "In the former group a slow growth during puberty indicates an altered function associated with growth retardation." A number of observations also suggest that shortness of the mother is "Associated with a greatly increased liability to delivery by cesarean section because of cephalopelivc disproportion and of perinatal deaths due to birth trauma." [99] Thomson *et al.*[100] observed a high incidence of delivery by cesarean section and of perinatal deaths among the small-sized Chinese women of Hong Kong. In certain countries the small size of the women and their inability to provide an adequate nutrition to the fetus and an adequate milk supply to the neonate is the result of certain religious beliefs, traditional social observances, superstitions, taboos, and fears. Collis and Janes [17] made a detailed study of the Algerian conditions and documented that

> In certain areas of Algeria, pregnant women are not allowed to eat vegetables or fruits. Even after delivery, they are not allowed soup containing meat or fish. Children also suffer an imposing variety of prohibitions. They must not drink coconut milk, or they will become morons. They must not eat eggs because they will become liars or thieves.

All these restrictions lead to growth retardation of the members belonging to the vulnerable groups. Lower socioeconomic classes in the developing countries are the special targets of malnutrition because of their ignorance, illiteracy, and the relative ease with which the social and religious leaders of the area exploit them to their advantage and impose upon them some irrelevant social and religious customs.

Social conditions under which groups of men live determine primarily the food habits and their nutritional state irrespective of race, e.g. in Costa Rica, the lower-income classes are generally of European origin, and they also show the same growth retardation as the low-income members of Mayan Indian origin in Guatemala. Social conditions, although not a primary factor, are to a significant degree responsible for growth retardation or even retarded mental development under the impact of malnutrition. Cravioto *et al.*[20] made an experimental and ecological study of the relationship between nutrition, growth, and neurointegrative development and concluded that "(1) social conditions are the primary factors influencing both malnutrition and mental development, and (2) that malnutrition is the central factor, influenced by social conditions, but itself the primary factor influencing both physical and mental development." [17] Malnutrition, although the causative factor in the physical growth retardation is a result of social conditions. The possibility cannot be excluded that nutritional and social conditions influence physical growth as well as mental development independently, although they interact with each other significantly. Guzman [42] hypothesized that the general growth retardation observed among the malnourished people would be self-corrective if social and economic conditions are improved. Collis and Janes [17] after a detailed investigation of the causative factors in malnutrition and retarded growth in Nigeria concluded that

> insufficient money to buy the necessary food was the biggest single factor in causing malnutrition in children of the urban populations studied, whereas ignorance was the biggest factor in certain of the rural areas. For example, the western region villagers had more land than the eastern villagers, but their children were on the whole more poorly nourished than those of the other regions. They did not know the cassava, yam, and maize were bad staples, and they did not use green vegetables as the eastern villagers did. The northern villagers, although much poorer with regard to money, had a far better knowledge of good foods, such as guinea, corn, millet and rice.

It is evident, therefore, that retarded physical growth caused by mental and psychological development is not solely a lack of adequate nutrition, but also the result of a widespread ignorance about food selection. Think about the Chinese millionaire, whose child is dying of beriberi, or an Indian maharaja, whose wife is wearing diamond necklaces worth millions of rupees and is suffering from nutritional anemia or marasmus, or the rich members of the Masai tribe in Africa, who own hundreds of cattle but whose children suffer from severe forms of malnutrition.[48] As Collis and Janes [17] put it, "This is a curious reflection on *homo sapiens,* who in losing the innocence of the animal world seems also to have lost the inherent instinct for correct food."

REFERENCES

1. Abbot, J. C.: In Robert F. Gould (Ed.) : *World Protein Resources.* Washington, American Chemical Society (1966).
2. Allen, D. M. and Dean, R. F. A. *Trans. R. Soc Trop. Med. Hyg., 59:*326 (1965).
3. Arakawa, T., Fujii, M., and Hayashi, T.: *Tohoku J. Exp. Med., 91:*143 (1967).
4. Autret, M. and Behar, M.: *Bull. W.H.O., 11:*891 (1954).
5. Behar, M.: In N. S. Scrimshaw and J. E. Gordon (Eds.) : *Malnutrition, Learning and Behavior.* Cambridge MIT Press (1968).
6. Behar, M., Viteri, F., Bressani, R., *et al.: Ann. N.Y. Acad. Sci., 69:*956 (1957).
7. Bennett, I. L.: *World Review of Nutrition and Dietetics.* Basel, S. Karger (1969), vol. 2, p. 1.
8. Bicknell, F., and Prescott, F.: *The Vitamins in Medicine,* 3rd ed. London, Grune, Heinemann (1953).
9. Bowie, M. D., Brinkman, G. L., and Hansen, J. D. L.: *J. Pediatr., 66:*1083 (1965).
10. Brock, J. F. (Ed.) : *Recent Advances in Human Nutrition.* Boston, Little, Brown (1961).
11. Burrell, R. J. W., Healy, M. J. R., and Tanner, J. M.: *Hum. Biol., 33:*250 (1961).
12. Buttfield, I. H. and Hetzel, B. S.: *Bull. W.H.O., 36:*243 (1967).
13. Cabak, V. and Najdanvic, R.: *Arch. Dis Child., 40:*532 (1965).
14. Chaudhuri, R. N.: *Trans. R. Soc. Trop. Med. Hyg. 57:*448–457 (1963).
15. Cheek, D. B. and Cooke, R. E.: *Annu. Rev. Med., 15:*357 (1964).
16. Collins, R. C., Kirkpatrick, J. B., and McDougal, D. B.: *J. Neuropathol. Exp. Neurol., 29:*57 (1970).
17. Collis, W. R. P. and Janes, M.: In N. S. Scrimshaw and J. E. Gordon (Eds.) : *Malnutrition, Learning and Behavior.* Cambridge, MIT Press (1968).
18. Coursin, D. B.: In N. S. Scrimshaw and J. E. Gordon (Eds.) : *Malnutrition, Learning and Behavior.* Cambridge MIT Press (1968).
19. Cravioto, J.: In P. Gyorgy and O. L. Kline (Eds.) : *Malnutrition is a Problem of Ecology.* Basel, S. Karger (1970).
20. Cravioto, J., Delicardie, E. R., and Birch, H. G.: *Pediatrics,* 38 (Suppl. 2, pt. 2) : 319 (1966).

21. Currimbhoy, Z.: *Indian J. Child Health, 12:*62 (1963).
22. Dam, H. and Sondergaard, E.: In G. H. Beaton and E. W. McHenry (Eds.) : *Nutrition.* New York, Academic Press (1964), vol. 2.
23. Darling, C. G. and Summerskill, J.: *J. Am. Diet Assoc., 29:*1204 (1953).
24. Davis, A.: *Let Us Get Well.* New York, Harcourt, Brace & World (1965).
25. Dean, R. F. A.: In D. Gairdner (Ed.) : *Recent Advances in Pediatric.* London, Churchill (1965).
26. Denton, J.: *Am. J. Pathol., 4:*341 (1928).
27. Edozien, J. C.: In P. Gyorgy and O. L. Kline (Eds.) : *Malnutrition is a Problem of Ecology.* Basel, S. Karger (1970).
28. Efremov, V. V.: In *Nutrition and Health.* Proceedings VII International Congress Nutrition, Hamburg. New York, Pergamon Press (1967), vol. 1.
29. Eiduson, S., Geller, E., Yuwiler, A., and Eiduson, B. T.: *Biochemistry and Behavior.* Princeton Van Nostrand (1964).
30. *Endemic Goitre,* W.H.O. Monograph, Series No. 4, Geneva, W.H.O. (1960).
31. Everson, G. J., Shrader, R. E., and Wang, T.: *J. Nutr. 96:*115 (1968).
32. *FAO Tech. Rep. W.H.O. 295:* (1962).
33. *FAO Third World Food Survey.* Rome (1963).
34. Follis, R. H.: *Preschool Child Malnutrition.* Publ. 1282, Washington, Academy of Sciences (1966), p. 87.
35. Gallagher, G. H.: *Nutritional Factors and Enzymological Disturbances in Animals.* Crosby, Lockwood & Son (1964).
36. Goldblatt, P. B., Moore, M. E., and Stunkard, A. J.: Social factors in obesity. *J.A.M.A. 192:*1039 (1965).
37. Gopalan, C.: *J. Trop. Pediatr., 9:*67 (1963).
38. Gordon, J. F., Chitkam, I. D., and Wyan, J. B.: *Am. J. Med. Sci., 245:* 345 (1963).
39. Gordon, H. H. and Nitowsky, H. M.: In M. G. Wohl and R. S. Goodhart (Eds.) : *Modern Malnutrition in Health and Disease.* Philadelphia, Lee & Febiger (1968.)
40. Graham, G. G.: *Fed. Proc., 26:*139 (1967).
41. Graham, G. G.: R. A. McCance and E. M. Widdowson (Eds.) : *Calorie Deficiencies and Protein Deficiencies.* Boston, Little, Brown (1968).
42. Guzman, M. A.: In N. S. Scrimshaw and J. E. Gordon (Eds.) : *Malnutrition, Learning and Behavior.* Boston, MIT Press, (1968).
43. Guzman, M. A., Rohmann, C. G., Flores, M., Gravu, S. M., and Scrimshaw, N. S.: *Fed. Proc., 23:*338 (1964).
44. Hanna, S., MacIntyre, I., Harrison, M., and Frazier, R.: *Lancet, 2:*172 (1960).
45. Holowach, J., Kauffman, F., Ikossi, M. G., Thomas G., and McDougal, D. B.: *J. Neurochem., 15:*621 (1968).

46. Holt, L. E., Snyderman, S. E., Norton, P. M., Roitman, E., and Finch, J.: *Lancet, 2*:1343 (1963).
47. Hurtado, V. J. J.: *Guatemala Pediatrica, 2* (7) :78 (1962).
48. Hutchinson, J.: In R. A. McCance and E. M. Widdowson (Eds.) : *Caloric Deficiencies and Protein Deficiencies.* Boston, Little Brown (1968).
49. Inns, J. R. M. and Shearer, G. D.: *J. Comp. Pathol., 53*:2 (1940).
50. Interdepartmental Committee on Nutrition for National Defense. *The Kingdom of Thailand, Nutrition Survey, October–December 1960.* A Report by the Interdepartmental Committee on Nutrition for National Defense. February 1962. Washington, U. S. Government Printing Office, 1962.
51. Jackson, R. L. and Kelly, H. G.: *Pediatr., 27*:215 (1945).
52. Jelliffe, D. B.: *Docum. Med. Geogr. Trop. (Anst.), 5*:314 (1953).
53. Jelliffe, D. B.: In *Malnutrition in African Mothers, Infants, and Young Children.* Report on 2nd Inter-African (CCTA) Conference on Nutrition, Gambia (1954), p. 230.
54. Jelliffe, D. B.: *Am. J. Clin. Nutr., 10*:19 (1962).
55. Jelliffe, D. B.: *Am. J. Public Health, 53*:905 (1963).
56. Jelliffe, D. B.: *Infant Nutrition in the Tropics and Subtropics,* 2nd ed. Geneva, W.H.O. (1968).
57. Jelliffe, D. B.: In P. Gyorgy and O. L. Kline (Eds.) : *Malnutrition is a Problem of Ecology.* Basel, S. Karger (1970).
58. Jelliffe, D. B. and Stuart, K. L.: *Br. Med. J., 1*:75 (1954).
59. Jokl, E.: *Nutrition, Exercise, and Body Composition.* Springfield, Thomas (1964).
60. Latham, M. C.: *Present Knowledge in Nutrition.* New York Nutrition Foundation (1967).
61. Latham, M. C.: In R. A. McCance and E. M. Widdowson (Eds.) : *Caloric Deficiencies and Protein Deficiencies.* London, Churchill (1968).
62. Latham, M. C., McGandy, R. P., McCann, M. D., and Stare, F. J.: *Nutrition Scope Manual.* Kalamazoo, Upjohn (1970).
63. Linden, G. C., Hansen, J. D. L., and Karabus, C. D.: *Pediatrics, 31*:552 (1963).
64. Mann, P. J. G. and Quastel, J. H.: *Nature, 145*:856 (1940).
65. Marvin, H. N.: *Am. J. Clin. Nutr., 12*:88 (1963).
66. McLaren, D. S.: *Malnutrition and the Eye.* New York, Academic Press (1966).
67. McLaren, D. S.: *Lancet, 2*:485 (1966).
68. Mertz, W. and Roginski, E. E.: *J. Biol. Chem., 238*:868 (1963).
69. Monckeberg, F.: In P. Gyorgy and O. L. Kline (Eds.) : *Malnutrition is a Problem of Ecology.* Basel, S. Karger (1970).
70. Montgomery, R. D.: *J. Pediatr., 59*:119 (1961).

71. Morley, D.: *Trans. R. Soc. Trop. Med. Hyg., 62* (2):200 (1968).
72. Nakayama, K. and Arima, M. (Eds.) : Child Health in Japan: An exhibition at the XI International Congress of Pediatrics. Nov. 7–13, 1965. Tokyo, Japan.
73. Oettle, A. G. and Higginson, J.: *Hum. Biol., 33:*181 (1961).
74. Oomen, H. A., McLaren, D. S., and Escapini, V.: *Trop. Geogr. Med., 16:*271 (1964).
75. Pearson, A.: *Proc. R. Soc. Med., 59:*55 (1966).
75a. Pineda, O.: In R. A. McCance and E. M. Widdowson (Eds.) : *Calorie Deficiencies and Protein Deficiencies.* Boston, Little, Brown and Co. (1968).
76. Prasad, A. S.: *Am. J. Clin. Nutr., 20:*648–652 (1967a).
77. Prasad, A. S.: Nutritional metabolic role of zinc. *Fed. Proc., 26:*172–185 (1967b).
78. Rajalakshmi, R. and Ramakrishnan, C. V.: Nutrition and brain function. *World Rev. Nutr. Dietet.* Basel, S. Karger, (In Press) vol. 14 (1971).
79. Rao, K. S.: In *Review of Nutrition Surveys Carried out in India.* Indian Council of Medical Research. Special Report Series No. 36. New Delhi, Indian Council of Medical Research (1961), p. 26.
80. Rao, Narayana, M. and Swaminathan, M.: In *World Rev. Nutr. Diet., 11:*106 (1969).
81. Richter, D.: *Br. Med. Bull., 21:*76 (1965).
82. Roche, M. and Leyrisse, M.: *Am. J. Trop. Med. Hyg., 15:*1032 (1966).
83. Rohmann, C. G., Garn, S. M., Guzman, M. A., *et al.: Fed. Proc., 23:* 378 (1964).
84. Root, A.: *Pediatrics, 36:*940 (1965).
85. Sandstead, H. H.: *Present Knowledge in Nutrition.* New York, Nutrition Foundation (1967).
86. Scott, R. B., Cardozo, W. W., Smith, A., and Delitty, M. R.: *J. Pediatr., 37:*885 (1950).
87. DeSilva, C. C. and Baptist, N. G.: *Tropical Nutritional Disorders of Infants and Children.* Springfield, C. Thomas (1969).
88. Smith, B. J. and Hauck, H. M.: *J. Trop. Pediatr., 1:*55 (1961).
89. Smythe, P. M.: *Lancet, 2:*724 (1958).
90. Srikantia, S. A.: In N. S. Scrimshaw and J. E. Gordon (Eds.) : *Malnutrition, Learning and Behavior.* Cambridge, MIT Press (1968).
91. Stanbury, J. B. and Ramalinyaswami, V.: In G. H. Beaton and E. W. McHenry (Eds.) : *Nutrition.* New York, Academic Press (1964), vol. 1.
92. Stoch, M. B. and Smythe, P. M.: *Arch. Dis. Child., 38:*546 (1963).
93. Strain, W. H., Pories, W. J., and Hinshaw, J. R.: *Surg. Forum, 11:*291 (1960).

94. Stransky, E., Davis-lawas, D. F., and Vicente, C.: *Acta Med. Philipp.,* 6:351 (1950a).

95. Stransky, E., Davis-lawas, D. F., and Vicente, C.: *J. Trop. Med. Hyg.,* 53:170 (1950b).

96. Stuart, K. L., Jelliffe, D. B., and Hill, J. R.: *J. Trop. Pediatr., 1:69* (1956).

97. Symposium: Iron deficiency and absorption. *Am. J. Clin. Nutr., 21:* 1138 (1968).

98. Tanner, J. M.: *Eugen. Rev., 58:*122 (1969).

99. Thomson, A. M.: In R. A. McCance and E. M. Widdowson (Eds.): *Calorie Deficiencies and Protein Deficiencies.* Boston, Little, Brown (1968).

100. Thomson, A. M. and Billewicz, W. Z.: *Proc. Nutr. Soc., 22:*55 (1963).

101. Thomson, A. M., Billewicz, W. Z., and Holliday, R. M.: *Br. J. Prev. Soc. Med., 21:*137 (1967).

102. Thomson, A. M., Chun, D., and Baird, O.: *J. Obstet. Gynaecol. Br. Commonw., 70:*871 (1963).

103. Tower, D. B.: *Nutr. Rev., 16:*161 (1958).

104. Tower, D. B.: *Am. J. Clin. Nutr., 12:*308 (1963).

105. Trowell, H. C., Davies, J. N. P., and Dean, R. F. A.: *Kwashiorkor.* London, Arnold (1954).

106. Udani, P. M.: *Indian J. Child. Health, 11:*498 (1962).

107. Udani, P. M.: *Indian J. Child. Health, 12:*593 (1963).

108. Veen, A. G.: *Am. J. Trop. Med., 31:*158 (1951).

109. Wadsworth, G. R. and Lee, T. S.: *J. Trop. Pediatr., 6:*48 (1960).

110. Weijers, H. A. and Kamer, J. H.: *Nutr. Abstr. Rev., 35:*591 (1965).

111. Whitehead, R. G.: *Lancet, 2:*567 (1965).

112. *W.H.O. Chron., 19:*429 (1965).

113. *W.H.O. Chron., 19:*485 (1965).

114. Williams, C. D.: *Arch. Dis. Child., 8:*423 (1933).

115. Wiliams, C. D.: *Lancet, 2:*1151 (1935).

116. Williams, C. D.: *Lancet, 2:*342 (1962).

117. Williams, S. R.: *Nutrition and Diet Therapy.* St. Louis, Mosby (1969).

118. Winick, M.: *Med. Clin. North Am., 54(6):*1413 (1970).

119. Wohl, M. G.: In Wohl and Goodhart (Eds.): *Modern Nutrition in Health and Disease.* Philadelphia, Lea and Febiger (1968).

120. Woodbury, R. M.: *Children's Bureau Publication,* No. 87. Washington, U. S. Government Printing Office (1921).

121. Young, C. M.: *Am. J. Clin. Nutr., 5:*186 (1957).

122. Zimmerman, H. M.: In Erduson *et al.* (Eds.): *Biochemistry and Behavior.* Princeton, Van Nostrand (1964).

Chapter II

MALNUTRITION AND REACTION OF
THE BRAIN

IT IS EXTREMELY difficult to conduct experimental studies
in humans to investigate the morphological and biochemical
changes in the brain that have been reported in the experimental
animals. At the same time, it is important to know the effect of
malnutrition (deficiency of protein, protein-calorie as well as other
nutrients, such as vitamins and minerals) on the human brain
either by direct studies or by an indirect extrapolation of results
from the experimental studies on animals because of the magnitude of the problem and significance of the brain, being solely
responsible for perception, learning, problem solving and regulating a number of vital physiological and endocrinological functions of the body.[54] Estimates indicate that 60 percent of the
world population of children between birth and five years suffer
from varying degrees of malnutrition. Millions of children are
born to mothers who are weak and depleted; the fetuses in their
body do not get adequate nutrition, and after giving birth, the
mothers are unable to nurse their infants at all or at best can do
so in a totally unsatisfactory manner for a few weeks. Supplementary foods and sterile milk are virtually impossible to get for
lack of availability or the money to purchase. The infants in these
circumstances go through a period of severe degree of malnutrition, which most often is accompanied by infection. A large number of such infants die, but a large number of them also survive,
and it is with these survivors that we are most concerned here.
We are particularly concerned on how satisfactory their brain
growth is in spite of the lack of adequate nutrients. Howard,[46]
however, commented that because of the high tissue metabolic
rate of the nervous tissue, the latter will get a priority on the avail-

able metabolites and may thus be spared from the drastic effects of malnutrition.

This is an oversimplification of the problem, as far as infants in their early period of brain growth are concerned. In the adults, during a period of malnutrition or starvation the loss of body weight is generally dramatic, whereas the effect on the brain weight is negligible. It has been observed that severe malnutrition among adults may lead to as much as 40% to 50% loss in body weight, but the brain weight may remain unaffected or at best affected by 5 to 10 percent. In older children, although the severity of brain reaction may be more severe than in adults, the brain may be spared to a great extent and continue to grow or maintain its weight or lose by only a small margin.[31] However, when we discuss the infants in their early part of life, the story is quite different. First of all, an infant may be at a nutritional disadvantage right from the start because of bad pregravidic health of the mother and an unbalanced or inadequate diet during pregnancy. In that case, the fetal neuronal development may be interfered with, and even though the brain may not be as badly affected as the other organs, the severity of changes in the nervous system may be enough to set a certain rate of brain growth which is far below the normal. Such a fetus may at birth be equipped with much less number of nerve cells and have a significantly reduced brain weight. It may be a good strategy to protect the children in early postnatal life in order to overcome the deficits of early malnutrition, but in our enthusiasm we must not forget the mother, whose nutritional deficiencies may preset the infant on a path of permanent re-tardation.

If the mother's pregravadic health is reasonably good, the infant is born with a mature brain as compared to experimental animals on which we depend for the collection of our data. In humans the peak period of brain growth is in the prenatal life, whereas most experimental animals (e.g., rodents) have their maximum brain growth in the postnatal life. In the experimental animals, malnu-trition after birth will, therefore, have more dramatic conse-quences[29] in terms of brain weight increases[75] or cellular proliferation.[1,93] For the same reasons, in an infant born in a healthy state and malnourished in postnatal life, the anthropometric measurements generally used to assess its effect on brain growth are only of marginal advantage. Robinow [77] believed that the technical limitation of using measurements of head circumference as an index of satisfactory brain growth could be misleading due to a well-formed human brain at birth and the absence of standard correlation between bone growth, head size, and intelligence.

The author is working on the brain of primates, in which known degrees of malnutrition have been experimentally induced. Since the primates are closer to humans taxonomically, it is hoped that the results obtained from these studies can be extrapolated in a more meaningful manner to human situations.

EXTERNAL MANIFESTATIONS OF INVOLVEMENT OF THE BRAIN

Retardation in body weight and head circumference in the prenatal and postnatal life due to malnutrition are the commonly accepted parameters of external change. It is, however, neither simple nor conclusive to rely on external manifestations of change and believe that the brain has been adversely affected physically and physiologically. The infants who are born with significantly less than average weight and height are generally those who have suffered varying degrees of intrauterine growth retardation due to maternal nutrition or other factors. Malnutrition during this period of active growth would physically hurt the brain and inhibit growth, resulting in a reduced size.[85] These infants, if they are not carefully nursed, are those who will suffer from a permanent stunting experience. Carothers [10] emphasized that the interruptions of brain maturation during its peak period of growth interfere with the neuronal development process and myelination and impair the growth of the nerve, which could significantly reduce the brain weight. This may be externally manifested in the reduction of head circumference.

In the normal infants, the head circumference increases from about 14 inches at birth to around 19 inches at two years of age, indicating a rapid brain growth. The brain during the same period adds to nervous tissue three times its weight at birth. These

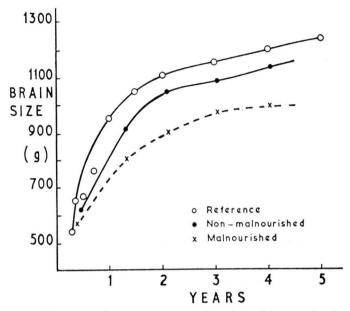

Figure 9. A diagrammatic representation of brain weight as related to age in the malnourished and nonmalnourished children compared to a standard reference.[7]

changes may be considered revolutionary compared to any other years during any subsequent period of human life. Graham's [41,43] detailed investigations on heights, weights, and head circumference of the malnourished children in Lima, Peru, showed that severe degrees of malnutrition during the first year of life cause permanent deficits in height and head size; the latter may reflect the size of the brain or the weight of the brain or even the extent of maturity of the brain (Fig. 9). In a group of 20 marasmic children, Stoch and Smythe [85] observed a smaller mean head circumference and smaller brain size in terms of brain mass. They calculated that these children had an intracranial volume 13.7 percent or 163 cc less than the matched control group drawn from the local population. According to these authors,[83-85] the head circumference of originally malnourished groups constantly remained smaller than the well-nourished children over an eleven-year period of study, and 60 percent of the malnourished children failed to reach the lowest levels of controls. Similar differences in head circumference of persons having good to poor nutritional background, but otherwise comparable genetically, have been reported from Uganda, Peru, Mexico, and Asia by a number of prominent workers. "To the extent that brain growth is impaired concurrently with early retardation in linear growth, the population at risk includes more than half of the world's population." [80]

Accepting head circumference as an indicator of brain size could become a controversial subject. First of all, the head circumference could be reduced during the period of malnutrition due to thinning of the skull bones [43,55,77] and wasting of the temporal muscles. There is no established correlation between head circumference and I.Q. One can come across intelligent people with a small stature and correspondingly small head size and also a big person with large-sized head having an average I.Q. This also does not mean that suboptimal brain growth due to malnutrition is not closely related to a failure to achieve the full potential in I.Q.[83] Rajalakshmi and Ramakrishnan [75] observed a mere 5% reduction in head circumference, when the malnourished child lost as much as 30 percent of his weight. At this stage of knowledge, it is difficult to decide the issue that among the malnourished group, reduced head circumference reflects reduced brain size or reduced intelligence, although a number of autopsies have revealed reduced brain weights in children who died of malnutrition.[7,88] Is it not possible that dehydration of the whole body, evident in severe marasmic cases, played some part?

The most interesting news came from Dr. Mönckeberg,[56] who reported at the Western Hemisphere Nutrition Congress in 1970 the development of a new tool to measure the severity of protein-calorie malnutrition in young children in relation to the nervous system. He used a 500 watt bulb to examine the contents of the cranial cavity. In the case of healthy children, the brain completely fills the cranial cavity, whereas in malnourished children, gross changes in the physical size of the brain become obvious. In patients suffering from severe forms of kwashiorkor, the brain size is decreased and parts of the cranial cavity are filled with the spinal fluid. Such a simple method of examination could not only be a sensitive index of the severity of malnutrition but during rehabilitation could also prove a reliable method of the rate of recovery of the patient.

RATE OF BRAIN GROWTH

The peak period of human growth is a few weeks prenatal and a few weeks postnatal, after which the growth process slows down. In the prenatal period, the growth of the brain reaches a peak about the fifth fetal month, and the tempo is maintained from then onwards till birth. In the postnatal period, a significant growth rate is maintained for a period of six months, after which it falls in parallel to the rate of general body growth (Fig. 10). Coppoletta and Wolbach [15] calculated that the human brain weighs 335 gm at birth, grows to 1064 gm at two years, 1191 gm at four years, and 1351 gm at 12 years of age. Putting it in another manner, the brain at the time of birth weighs about 40 percent of its adult weight. No other organ or tissue in the body is so far advanced in development at the time of birth. Graham [42] showed that "at birth man has reached 5.7% of the adult weight, 30%

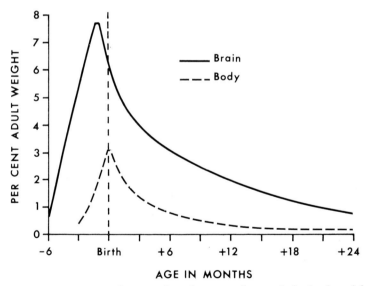

Figure 10. Rate curves of prenatal and postnatal growth in fresh weight of the human brain and body. Increments are expressed as percentages of the adult value (brain, 1.35 kg; body 65 kg.) .[29]

of the adult height and 63% of the adult head circumference. At one year he has 16.3, 44.1, and 83.6% and three years 24, 57, and 90% of these same measurements."

* The growth of human brain involves enormous proliferation in the cell cytoplasm of neurons, the extension of axons and dendrites, and the process of myelination. All these processes involve a large amount of protein synthesis. During its peak growth period, synthesis of proteins and lipoproteins make up to 90 percent of the dry weight of the brain.[17] It has been estimated that protein substances increase more than 2,000 times during the process of maturation of a neuroblast into an interior horn cell, and if this figure is magnified for the entire brain, the latter at the time of birth of the baby is gaining weight at a rate of 1 or 2 mg/min.[18] For all this transformation, an adequate supply of nutrition is essential for the proper development of intelligence, memory, and behavior.[11]

Since most of the histological, cytochemical, and biochemical data on the healthy and malnourished brains is obtained from the experimental animals, it is worthwhile to examine the species difference in the timings of brain growth spurt in relation to birth. Dobbing[29] and Davison and Dobbing[22] have given the rate curve of brain growth in different species (Fig. 11), which indicate that whereas the peak of brain growth in human species is prenatal, the rat (10 days postnatal) and dog (7 to 14 days postnatal) have their maximum brain growth in their postnatal life. The pig has its maximum brain growth period spread over five weeks prenatal and five weeks postnatal life.[70] This would mean that as a result of malnutrition after birth, these animals would suffer much more severe consequences than would a human baby. Understandably, there are also corresponding differences in the timing of behavioral development in relation to birth.[37,39] We must extend the scope of these observations further in order to understand that a direct extrapolation of studies may be dangerous and misleading. Quoting a few important studies on rats and dogs, Culley and Lineberger[19] found in the rats that even by limiting the nursing time from the fifth to seventeenth day of life (in rat the peak growth of brain is in postnatal life), a drastic 27

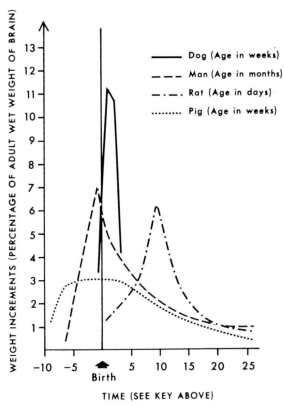

Figure 11. The timing of brain growth in different experimental animals compared to humans in relation to birth.[31]

percent reduction in brain weight can be obtained, and even if these rats are fed ad libitum during the next 93 days, the brain still weighed 18 percent less than the controls. Platt and Stewart [68] mated the congenitally malnourished bitches with obvious lower brain weights with normal healthy dogs. It was found that the brains of the offspring were smaller than the matched controls. Similar results have been obtained in other species as well, from which the conclusion emerges that when malnourished female offspring attain adulthood and become mothers, their offspring show brains of smaller weight, even when mated with healthy males. This could mean a continuation of major impairment in terms of learning capacity. However, when nutritional deprivation is initiated at the time or after weaning, no change in brain size is observed.[32] It may be added here that in certain respects, the brain weight is a poor indication of the extent to which the brain has been affected due to malnutrition. This is especially true during one aspect of brain maturation, i.e. the replacement of water by myelin. A disproportionately higher water content of the brain may give the impression of satisfactory brain weight. As has been discussed in a later section, in such instances the level of cholesterol may be a better indication of the concentration of lipid or myelin as the true weight of the brain.

Compared with the animal studies, it would seem that in humans, the adult neuronal cell number and metabolic stability of myelin sheaths are achieved at a relatively younger age. It may be reiterated that the brain increases in weight in incremental stages, but due to the metabolic stability of many of its constituents, once laid down, it may become inaccessible to the general metabolic pool of the body in the times of shortage. Unlike other organs, the weights of which can increase and decrease, the size of the brain cannot be markedly reduced.[7] The deleterious effects of malnutrition can be manifested only during the period of active brain growth, when its constituents have not acquired the metabolic stability mentioned above. This is precisely the reason why brain size in the experimental animals is not reduced on nutritional deprivation after the weaning period, because the brain is largely protected and its acquired metabolic stability cannot be disturbed easily.

While discussing the effects of malnutrition on the growth of the brain, we have to be concerned with only certain periods of life. In humans, this period includes a few weeks prior to birth and the early part of infancy. It is only during the period of active brain growth that the process can be interrupted or it has to make severe physiological adjustments. After the brain has been nearly complete, and if it is allowed to acquire about 90 percent of its growth by four years, the effect of malnutrition on the brain will be negligible. Statistics of malnutrition collected from all over the world indicate that our concern with malnutrition affecting the brain should be rightfully concentrated on the children in their preschool years.

In view of this growth pattern of the brain, it is not difficult to imagine the consequences of protein-calorie malnutrition in terms of mental development and intellectual functioning, if the deficiency is initiated during the critical periods of brain development. During this period, malnutrition could result in permanent personality retardation from which the baby could not be rehabilitated. Brown [7] found that in Africa the brain weights of children who died of kwashiorkor or marasmus were significantly less compared to their local controls, who, although they did not suffer episodes of severe malnutrition, were nevertheless chronically undernourished (a pattern for the area in question). The brain values of controls were also less than healthy children of other areas. Also the children who die of kwashiorkor show lot of edema and congestion of the brain.[7] If we eliminate the contribution made by extra water to the brain, its actual weight would be much less, and as the various observations show, the brains of malnourished children, despite edema, weigh less than the normal. If these observations are broadly applied, is it not possible that the smaller-sized population of underdeveloped countries with smaller head circumference compared to American standards is a result of smaller-sized brains which are due to generation after generation of chronic undernutrition in these areas?

Some other important studies have shown that the under-nourished children have smaller brains than the well-nourished children of the same age and ethnic group.[9] Those children when given adequate diet at a later stage may reach the weight dimension of the well-nourished children but do not overcome the deficit in brain weight, which probably results in a permanent stigmata if these children suffered malnutrition early enough during their peak period of brain growth. Nelson and Dean [61] observed well-defined focal disturbances in the temporal areas of the brains in about 11 percent of their malnourished patients. Although the selective sensitivity of the temporal lobe cannot be explained satisfactorily, it could mean that the malnutrition during the first year of life could curtail the rate of increase in head circumference.[90] As mentioned earlier, a number of studies have shown that the head circumference of malnourished children is poorer in contrast to matched controls.[80] The important question that has not been answered is whether or not the deficit in brain weight caused by nutritional deprivation at an early period has any direct bearing on the behavioral deficits that are generally found in individuals who so suffered.

Having painted a somewhat gloomy picture, it is also pertinent to point out that prenatal peak of brain growth in human species might be a blessing, and it may be because of this early brain growth that the prevalence of mental retardation and consequent retardation in human personality is not as much evident as is the widespread undernutrition and malnutrition. Also, compared to other experimental animals, the primate fetus appears to have a greater resistance to maternal malnutrition, due to its slower rate of growth and its comprising a smaller proportion of the maternal organism.[31,66] Both these factors play an important role in facilitating the availability of reasonable amounts of nutrients in the forming fetus, even if the mother is undernourished. The peak of brain growth in the prenatal life brings the human baby into the world in a state of advanced development. Even during the postnatal life, in an overwhelming majority of cases, the mother is able to provide at least a bare minimum of all the essential nutrients through her breast milk for a period of six months or more. This gives sufficient period for the brain to develop to a reasonable stage of maturity. Malnutrition after this period would affect the brain and to some extent the mental development, but not to the degree to which it would have been subjected if these protective periods had not been built in the beginning part of human life. It is for this reason that, although malnutrition is a widespread phenomena among the children in most underdeveloped countries (about 60% children between the age of birth and five years) , the mental retardation and abnormally functioning individuals are not as common.

HISTOPATHOLOGICAL OBSERVATIONS ON THE CENTRAL NERVOUS SYSTEM OF MALNOURISHED PERSONS

The central nervous system reacts to episodes of malnutrition in a variety of ways when a person suffers from it. During the adult life, when the brain development has been fully completed, there are pronounced biochemical changes. The histology of the brain makes certain adjustments which probably returns to normal when the episode of malnutrition is over and a balanced diet is made available. The story, however, is different when the body suffers malnutrition at a time when the brain is developing. In that case the central nervous system has to make severe forms of adjustments, and in the process some of the histopathological or biochemical changes may become irreversible, even on later rehabilitation.

The various components of the central nervous system grow at different rates under normal conditions, and it may be quite natural that their response to the state of malnutrition is also variable. The brain increases its weight greater than the spinal cord, and during the peak period of growth (50 days prenatal and 40 days postpartum) the brain tissue grows at the rate of 5 to 6 percent of its adult weight every fortnight.[21] The spinal cord, although a part of the central nervous system, does not follow the growth pattern of the brain but shows growth characteristics resembling the general body and grows in step with the body length. The cerebellum also shows a characteristically different rate of growth compared to the rest of the brain. It shows a much higher rate of growth during the peak period of brain growth and reaches its adult proportions sooner than the rest of the brain.

During the period of malnutrition, the changes are most marked in the anterior horn cells of the spinal cord. The neurons of the lumbar and cervical enlargements show chromatolysis of severe degree even to the stage of ghost cells, which gives the appearance of degenerate looking neurons. The perineuronal oligodendrocytes and astrocytes sharply increase in number, and there is a marked proliferation of astrocytic fibers. The cerebellum, because of its fast growth rate during its development, appears to be the most sensitive to malnutrition, and the nonavailability of nutrients hits the cerebellum the hardest compared to any other nervous tissue. The Purkinje's cells are especially sensitive and show distinct chromatolysis, loss in number, and appear to be sunken in the granular layer. The cells of the granular layer are less densely packed compared to the normal brain. The individual cerebellar folia are reduced in size and the reduction is shared almost equally by granular, molecular, and the fibrous layers.[70] The number of Bergmann's cells is increased and the deep cerebellar nuclei, especially the dentate, show varying degrees of chromatolysis and satellitosis. Before discussing the brain, it may be appropriate to comment on the synaptic areas. The formation of synapses is a critical factor in the process of maturation of the brain. The functional proficiency of the brain depends to a great extent on proper organization of its constituent parts, especially by the pattern of synaptic connections between cells and the efficiency of such synapses in interneuronal communications.[13] So in certain respects the synaptic formations may be more important than the process of myelination or acquisition of DNA. There are indications that in the malnourished animals the interneuronal communication is not as efficient. It is not, however, clear how nutritional deprivation affects, if at all, the formation of synapses and organization patterns of the nervous tissue.

The various parts of the brain react in a different manner to malnutrition. However, the changes in the brain are not as well marked compared to the cerebellum. Experimental work on the animals show that the thalamic, caudate and lenticular nuclei are greatly affected in terms of loss of Nissl's granules and increased satellitosis. The anterior nucleus of the thalamus appears to be more sensitive than the others.[82] The giant cells of the reticular formation show changes similar to anterior horn cells but only in a moderate degree. The cerebral cortex shows greater stress to the dietary abuse. Not only are the gyri less plump than the normal, probably due to reduced amount of white matter, but the neurons of the cortical region show so much reduced cytoplasm and chromatin that they appear to be naked and could be confused for enlarged neuroglial nuclei.[70] A 20 percent reduction in the cortical neurons, which is quite a probability, may appreciably depress the intelligence level. Reduced number of neurons per unit volume of gray matter has been reported by a number of workers. The giant cells of the reticular formation of the brain stem show similar changes (loss of Nissl's granules, increase in perineuronal glial cells, increase in number and caliber of astrocytic fibers) but not as much as in spinal cord, Purkinje's cells or cortical neurons. The neuroglial cells proliferate and appear to be clustered around the severely affected neurons. Most of the additional glial cells are oligodendroglia and astrocytes, the latter show highly enlarged astrocytic fibers. There has been a controversy on the significance of increased number of glial cells. Andrew [2] believed that the additional glial cells have a phagocytic role, whereas Platt *et al.*[67] considered these cells to be auxiliary metabolic units. Some studies indicate that the glial cells proliferate in order to cope with the extraction from blood of additional nutrient supplies and/or their metabolism and can be induced by restricting blood supply, increasing physical work or training or malnutrition.[23,49,87]

> The increased number of glial cells in the central nervous systems of the malnourished animals may, therefore, be no more than an adaptation to an altered environment—an attempt to obtain or metabolize sufficient nutrients from a good supply of poor quality blood instead of, as in Tureen's experiments, a poor supply of good quality blood.[70]

Chromatolysis or glial activation may not leave permanent sequelae of great severity. In most cases, these changes disappear on rehabilitation. According to Meyer *et al.*,[53] the endoplasmic reticulum is the source of the proteins, and the glial cells are concerned with the transfer of substances from blood to the neurons. The effect on them due to malnutrition may be considered as an adjustment or adaptation to a new physiological state. In the congenitally malnourished animals this adaptation may turn into desperation. The nuclei of cells become enlarged, vesicular or horseshoe shaped, accompanied by drastic changes in microglia in severe cases of malnutrition.[69]

Stewart and Platt [82] believed that most of the histological changes would be reversible, but they were not certain about gliosis formed in malnourished pigs in view of their impaired maze-solving performance even after rehabilitation.[4] Although most of these histological and histopathological changes have been documented in the experimental animals, which had been deprived nutritionally under controlled laboratory conditions, a great deal of evidence is available to suggest that the human brain reacts in a manner similar to those of experimental malnourished animals.

The white matter of the spinal cord of malnourished edematous pigs showed lacunae or spaces lined by single layer of flattened cells, which indicate fluid accumulations. Myelin sheaths are swollen, and the amount of myelin per fiber is reduced or less dense, especially in the congenitally malnourished dogs.[70] The myelin sheath in the malnourished animals is often swollen without increase in the number of Schwann's cells in the sheath wall. This might be an indication of less advanced wrapping or the chemical alteration of myelin. Udani [88] found the results obtained from experimental animals and humans quite comparable, and that the children who died of kwashiorkor had the chemical composition of myelin similar to the immature myelin of malnourished animals.[21] Garrow [40] showed potassium deficiency in the brain of such children. Reduced amounts of gangliosides, concentrated in the dendritic formations of nerve cells, have also been observed. Since the number of neurons is reduced in a state of malnutrition, initiated during the period of active brain growth, the loss of gangliosides in the dendritic projections would mean loss of interaction and disturbance in the intersensory and emotional functions.[70]

The brain of the adult, in contrast, does not suffer as much under severe degree of malnutrition. The brain weight is not affected appreciably even if the body weight is reduced as much as 40 to 50 percent. Reports of investigations from situations in which certain men were trapped (German concentration camps, prisoners of war in Japanese camps) or who in addition suffered from tremendous emotional stress as well as malnutrition indicate symptoms such as irritability, emotional instability, headaches, insomnia, defective memory, and depression. These results are as severe as those observed in the young children except that in adults, they seem to disappear completely on rehabilitation.

ELECTRICAL ACTIVITY OF THE BRAIN

The electroencephalograms (EEGs) taken on healthy and malnourished children clearly reflect the degree to which the latter are impaired functionally. In children suffering from kwashiorkor as well as marasmus, a number of prominent workers reported EEG abnormalities in a large number of these cases which did not come to normal even if the children were apparently well rehabilitated.[59-61] Lubchenko *et al.*[51] examined ten-year-old children who weighed around 1500 gm at birth and obviously suffered intrauterine growth retardation or prenatal malnutrition and found abnormal EEGs in 33 out of 55 cases. Engel[34] found grossly abnormal EEGs in seven fatal cases. Some of the patients who showed mild to moderate EEG abnormalities (16 cases) were those who were rehabilitated successfully in the later period, thereby showing some correlation between the EEG pattern and the extent of mental impairment. Engel believed that severe EEG abnormalities in spite of no prognostic value could raise the possibility of permanent brain damage. He was particularly impressed by the dominant rhythm, which always coincided with the stage of mental apathy in severe forms of kwashiorkor. Even after clinical recovery, the dominant frequencies are mostly below the range of healthy American children of the same age.[3] It appears that the EEG abnormalities caused by severe forms of malnutrition become a semipermanent or permanent part of the life, as is evidenced by the reports of some workers [34,38,39,57,78] who reported abnormal EEGs in 18-year-old adults who suffered malnutrition in their early life and considered it as a residual effect. Naeye[58] suggested that the residual abnormalities in the adult brain may be partly due to endemic infantile undernutrition in the area from which the subjects are chosen. Mundy-castle[57] proved the above point and observed abnormalities in EEG patterns in most Ghanian children of lower socioeconomic groups, which may be explained on the basis of poor nutrition and greater frequency of malnutrition in these areas compared to the European populations.

Electroencephalographic changes and changes in behavior go parallel to each other. After complete recovery, the EEGs also show reversion to patterns and amplitudes that are closer to healthy children.[33] It is interesting that Nelson and Dean[61] showed that in 17 of the 47 children with kwashiorkor, abnormal electrical activity originated in the temporal or post-temporal areas.

The electrical activity of the brain in experimental animals show abnormalities comparable to such data obtained on human children. Platt *et al.*[67] reported significant and striking decrease in the faster and increase in the slower components of the electro-encephalograms of the malnourished pigs. Similar and actually more marked EEG abnormalities have been reported in the congenitally malnourished dogs. The EEGs in the malnourished pups showed a number of prominent abnormalities, such as irregular slow activity of large amplitude and multifocal discharges.[65] Meyer *et al.*[53] described that "the deficient animals exhibit a slow, irregular activity, with an amplitude two or three times that of the controls. The congenitally malnourished animals being more severely affected than those deprived only after weaning." Multifocal discharges are seen in the malnourished animals and the fast low-amplitude components are diminished. On rehabilitating these animals, the response of the EEG is greatly improved but does not come to normal. Altered electroencephalograms have not been described in animals who suffered episodes of malnutrition in their adult life.[70]

CYTOCHEMICAL AND BIOCHEMICAL PARAMETERS OF BRAIN REACTION

DNA Content and Cellularity

The brain is not only affected morphologically, but extremely important biochemical changes take place which have a significant bearing on the functioning of the nervous tissue. Experimental animals are ideal for these studies because human material cannot be used for such experimental procedures unless meaningful data can be collected from the autopsied material. Estimation of DNA content of the brain in the healthy and malnourished animals as well as on human cases dying of malnutrition compared to a healthy child dying of an accident have been used to estimate the cell population of the brains under these two conditions. While doing so, it is presumed first that the estimation of tissue DNA is an index of total number of cells. Secondly, we know that the number of cells within the brain increases linearly until birth and then more slowly until about six months of age, after which there is hardly any increase in the number of cells of the brain. Most histological studies indicate that at the time of birth most of the neuronal cell division has stopped. Experimental work has indicated that the smaller weight or brain size caused by malnutrition is generally due to reduced cellularity rather than to smaller cells.[70] Winick and his collaborators [91-96] and Novakava et al.[63] have done extensive studies in this area, and they have concluded that malnutrition in early life retards the rate of cell division and reduces the ultimate number of cells in the cerebrum, cerebellum, and brain stem. The cerebellum in particular is more sensitive than the other areas (Fig. 12). The earlier the period

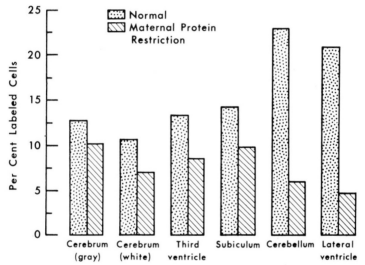

Figure 12. Effect of prolonged maternal protein restriction on various brain regions in 16-day rat embryo.[92]

of malnutrition, the more serious the cell deficit is likely to be. In the case of severe forms of maternal malnutrition, the growing fetus is also affected, and if the prenatal malnutrition of the fetus is continued to the postnatal life, the consequences could be disastrous. It has been calculated that prenatal malnutrition may be responsible for a 15% to 20% deficit in cell number. A postnatally deprived baby also experiences about 15% to 20% deficit. But if a child has been deprived prenatally as well as postnatally, the deficit may be as much as 40 percent in cell number (Fig. 13).

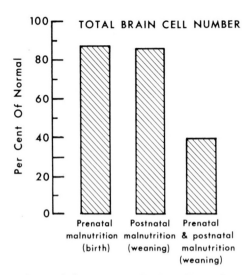

Figure 13. Comparison of the effect on brain cell number of prenatal malnutrition, postnatal malnutrition and a combination of pre and postnatal malnutrition.[92]

Winick [91] reported that malnourished mothers produced offsprings whose brains contain a reduced number of cells, and even if such young ones born with cellular deficits are nursed adequately, they do not recover their loss and are left with a smaller cellular endowment permanently. In certain cases when the prenatally deprived animals are malnourished postnatally, the impact is doubled. Such doubly deprived animals may not have more than 40 percent of the expected number of cells. Winick's remark is quite pertinent: "It is as though prenatal malnutrition has conditioned these animals and made them hypersensitive to postnatal malnutrition." [91] Winick and associates [96] showed that in nine children who died of infantile marasmus during the first year of life their brains contained significantly less number of cells compared to the average of the same area. In three cases, the DNA content was about 40 percent of the normal, indicating a severe reduction of brain cellularity. Concomitantly, the brain weight and head circumference is decreased. They emphasized that a reduced head circumference during the first six months of life reflects a reduced number of cells in their brains.

The cellular changes during the growth of the human brain are qualitatively similar to those observed in the rat brain. In the whole rat brain the DNA synthesis stops at 17 days, whereas the net protein continues to increase up to 99 days. The different regions of the brain also show great variation in their pattern of cell duration or acquisition of DNA. Cerebellum shows the fastest rate of cell division and abruptly stops at 17 days, whereas in the cerebral cortex the rate of mitosis is slower and continues to 21 days. In brain stem and hippocampus there is a cellular increase until 14 to 17 days. Nonavailability of nutrients during this period will result in interference in the proces of cell division and reduced amount of DNA. Overnutrition during the same period results in increase in number of cells, DNA values, as well as brain weight.[90] Winick and Rosso [96] described that in humans,

> DNA reaches a maximum content after birth but prior to the cessation of total brain growth. The increase in total brain DNA content is linear until birth; it then slows down until 6 to 8 months of life, after which there is no further cell division in human brain. The latter part of growth (after 6 to 8 months) is characterized by an increase in total organ weight and protein, as well as RNA content, without concomitant increases in DNA content. During this phase the quantity of protein and RNA per cell is increasing. Regional growth patterns differ qualitatively in human brain from the patterns in the rat brain. In the human, the cell division is equally rapid in the cerebrum and the cerebellum postnatally and stops in both at about 6 to 8 months of age. In the brain stem the rate of cell civision is quite slow but continues until 12 months of age.

The detailed investigations of Winick indicate that the brain growth through the process of cell division is greatly modified among the children who suffer from severe marasmus during their first year. Different regions of the brain show significant reduction in their cell number, which will be found in a child who has been adequately breast fed. Chow [14] explained at the Gordon Research Conference on nutrition that these children develop a permanent impairment in their ability to utilize nitrogen.

The persistent deficits in the amount of DNA-P and cholesterol even after rehabilitation have been observed in a number of experimental animals. If these results are extrapolated to apply to human children, it would mean that the brains of babies who suffered from malnutrition in their early infancy do not completely recover biochemically. This may have been the reason for persistent I.Q. deficiencies in rehabilitated children reported by Stoch and Smythe.[83] In young rats, marked changes in the chemical composition of the brain became evident even by a mild degree of malnutrition during the first week of their life.[29] The cholesterol level and amount of DNA (as an indicator of reduced number of cells and gangliosides) are particularly effected adversely and never come to normal levels even on rehabilitation for prolonged periods of time if the episode of malnutrition in early life had been severe enough.[26,29,44,47] Dobbing did not observe any change either in brain weight or the level of DNA in the brain of adult rats, even when they are subjected to such a severe degree of malnutrition as to lose as much as 46 percent of the body weight. However, the brain cholesterol may be permanently depressed by malnutrition during the critical period of myelination. This conclusion is based on extensive studies in rats and pigs.[19,29,30,47] These results are extremely important in view of their gravity. However, a small word of caution is also important here, and Dobbing[29] has rightly stressed on it. In normal development, the DNA value per gram wet weight of the brain falls due to increase in cell size as well as by the growth of the cellular processes and noncellular myelin accumulation. The concentration of DNA may, therefore, prove to be a poor guide to the total cell number. The DNA content per whole organ may better prove to make a comparative estimation of cellularity.

Myelination of the Brain during the Period of Malnutrition

The rapid growth of the brain consists partly of accumulation of myelin—metabolically a very stable material, which at a later date has a protective influence on the nervous system. Myelin is a complex lipid and in rat brain 70 percent of cholesterol, sulfatides, and sphingomyelin, nearly all cerebrosides, and most of plasminogens are present in this substance that is defined under the name myelin.[21] Myelin is metabolically so stable that once formed, it will not be easily affected. Its metabolic stability makes it possible to use analytic methods to measure brain growth. Histological exam-

ination shows that brain growth takes place in several stages starting from the formation of cells to the growth of cells, its axons and
dendrites and later by myelination. The latter will also include the
proliferation of oligodendroglia, which is known to precede the
synthesis and deposition of myelin.[5] Myelination involves thickening of sheaths by adding laminae and addition of myelin sheaths
to the elongating axons during the development of the neurons,
and as the axons are elongated, they are becoming myelinated in
their extra length. The thickening of the sheaths, on the other
hand, takes place by an increase in concentration of lipids per
gram wet weight of the brain. While assessing the degree of myelination, it may be justified to use "concentrations per gram wet
weight more as an index of myelination maturity than whole brain
amounts, which are more an index related to growth in size."[31]
Most rapid period of myelin synthesis is around birth, but there is
evidence that sufficient synthesis of myelin is taking place even at
two years of age. Myelination proceeds at different times in different areas of the brain and is preceded by a proliferation of
oligodendroglia and the accumulation of hydrophobic lipid drop-
lets in the neuropil, first in the spinal cord and later in the brain.[21]
Such a proliferation of oligodendrocytes occurs most rapidly during a certain period, which varies from one species to the other.
In the case of the human brain, myelin sheaths appear in the
spinal cord tracts during the twenty-second and thirty-sixth week
of fetal life and is followed by the process of myelination in the
other parts of the brain. Much of the increase in wet weight of the
brain is due to myelin deposition, and this process at a slower rate
continues for a long time in the case of human development.
Since the human brain increases in weight well into adolescent
years, it cannot be said with certainty when this process stops.

If the child suffers from malnutrition during the period of
active growth when myelin is being laid down, the result is reduced
myelin content, which starts a chain of metabolic events within
the oligodendrocytes responsible for the synthesis of myelin. In
other words, nutritional deprivation results in faulty myelination.
It also results in significant decrease in the amount of proteolipids,
cerebrosides, plasmalogens and cholesterol, which are closely asso-

ciated with myelin.[27,29] Such effects, especially in its critical periods (prenatal and postnatal periods of active myelination), could produce significant reduction in brain weight. The period of myelination may not only be considered as a vulnerable period in the development, but at the same time the degree of myelination may prove to be a good estimate of the characteristics of myelin lipid in a brain sample and could provide useful information on the effects of malnutrition and the maturation process of the brain.[24,25,29,30] Chase *et al.*[12] believed that even a small degree of nutritional deprivation during the vulnerable period of myelination could have lasting effects on the physical growth of the brain. Davison and Dobbing [22] showed that the myelin of children who die of kwashiorkor show chemical characteristic of the immature myelin.

The effect of nutritional deprivation in the experimental animals on the process of myelination and how its normal schedule is modified under the impact of dietary abuse during the period of maximum brain growth has been studied by a number of workers.[6,21,90] In the congenitally malnourished animals, the amount of white matter is small and the diameter of the myelinated fibers of the cross pyramidal tract is smaller than average, than those of the age controls. The reduction in the diameter of the small fibers is mostly at the expense of myelin walls rather than the axons.[69] No evidence of degeneration of the tracts is seen, but the myelin sheaths of the spinal cord of malnourished animals are often swollen without much thickness, giving the picture of a less dense myelination. Buchanan and Roberts [8] reported a relative myelin deficiency of as much as 20 percent in the optic tracts of malnourished rats, which can be detected without the use of electrophotometer, as compared to their control littermates.

In an effort to understand the sequence of changes in myelination under the impact of nutritional deprivation, especially in its peak period of brain growth, a number of studies have indicated that the rate at which myelin is synthesized and laid down in the brain is greatly reduced, thereby reducing the total myelin content of the brain. Whether it is a change in brain metabolism, as the enzymatic studies of Chase *et al.*[12] would suggest, or simply a reduction in the number of myelin synthesizing cells is not known.[92] The accumulation of cerebrosides and proteolipids takes place simultaneously with the process of myelination,[36] and purified fractions have shown that these are myelin constituents.[62] An interruption in the process of myelination would, therefore, lead to very complex biochemical changes. In undernourished animals, the brain cholesterol and total phospholipids of one-year-old animals corresponded to a normal pig of only 12 weeks of age.[31]

Because of this close association with the myelin, cerebrosides could be a good indication of myelination. Dobbing [29] observed that cerebrosides are depressed up to 36 percent of their normal amount in the brains of pigs which were undernourished from two weeks age to one year. Correspondingly, the cholesterol was depressed 21 percent, total phospholipids, 12.0 percent, and DNA-P, 29 percent. After rehabilitation, the amount of cerebrosides, cholesterol, and DNA-P were still 14 percent, 12.5 percent, and 14 percent less than the normal age controls. It may be interesting that a group of myelin lipids, plasmologens, are not effected as much as other myelin lipids such as cholesterols and cerebrosides.

Pigs were malnourished during the first year of their life to such an extent that they weighed only 3 percent of the weight of their controls. Their brain weight corresponded to nine- to ten-week-old animals. At the same time the brain cholesterol and total phospholipid content corresponded to 12 weeks age. Dobbing [31] showed that a "three year old rehabilitated brain had a cholesterol concentration equivalent to a two year old normal pig but a DNA (cell) content of only a normal one year old." This clearly shows the drastic biochemical reaction of the brain to undernutrition.

Dickerson *et al.*[24,25] showed that during rehabilitation although the level of cholesterol in the brain rose to a great extent, the amount in the forebrain, brain stem, and spinal cord always remained subnormal for the chronological age. An important study of Dobbing [29] on pigs showed that the decreased quantity of cerebrosides and cholesterols never regain their previous levels on rehabilitation. The deficiency of DNA-P was more pronounced than that of cholesterol. In the adult animals, DNA-P cholesterol does not show much variation, even when undernutrition resulted in a loss of 46 percent of the body weight.

It is not the intention here to say that myelin is the basis of mental development. However, it must be said that it is after the successful completion of the process of meylination that the brain is said to be mature and that it is somewhat immune to changes under the impact of undernutrition. The myelin content is not appreciably changed once it is laid down and hence may be a stabilizing factor in protecting the brain. The process of myelination is also an index of the successful period of glial cell proliferation, and even if the myelin is not linked to sensory or motor function, the adequate performance of the later function may very well depend on the extent to which myelination imparts a metabolic stability to the brain. "Whether interference with myelination will result in an impairment of future brain function, or whether there are other systems in the brain (developing coincidently and similarly vulnerable) which are more important, remains to be discovered." [21] It cannot be ignored, however, that the effect of malnutrition during the period of active myelination is to slow down the process of laying down the myelin, which could result in permanent deficits in brain size, brain weight, and probably the intellelctual capacity. At this time it cannot be said with certainty if these restrictions during the process of myelination have any immediate or long-lasting effects on subsequent intellectual capacity and physical growth of both brain and body,[21] and according to Davison and Dobbing,[21] who have to date made the most extensive investigation on the process of myelination of the brain, this aspect needs to be thoroughly and systematically investigated.

Biochemical and Metabolic Disturbances

It has been shown that the various organs respond to protein malnutrition or nitrogen loss by losing proteins. The brain constituents, on the other hand, are quite stable metabolically and do not decrease in size as do the other organs. However, at the present stage of knowledge it is not completely understood how the pattern of biochemical changes that the nervous tissue exhibits along with histopathological alterations discussed earlier relate to mental changes or the level of intellectual functioning. Several studies indicate that these biochemical changes are a form of physiological adaptation and are reversible on dietary rehabilitation.

The rate of protein synthesis is directly dependent on the availability of adequate quantity of amino acids. A limitation in the availability of any essential amino acid is likely to affect the formation of new protein structure. The developing brain during the period of maximum growth (late fetal and early infancy) rapidly synthesizes proteins, which make up to 90 percent of the dry weight of the brain.[76] While the brain proteins are more resistant to depletion compared to other tissues of the body during a period of malnutrition, their depletion from the rest of the body could be as hazardous as the depletion from the brain, in view of the fact that amino acids necessary for growth are also essential for maintenance of nitrogen equilibrium. The exclusion of any essential amino acid would produce changes in appetite, sensations of fatigue, and marked nervous irritability.[17]

As far as the concentration of essential amino acids is concerned, the brain does not differ from the liver or the plasma. The brain, however, appears to have a higher concentration of glutamic acid and gamma aminobutyric acid (GABA).[89] The latter along with glutamic acid affect the electrical ability of the brain in the sense that they have facilitatory and inhibitory action on the dendritic activity.[48] Since the learning process involves repeated firing of neuronal groups,[45] a low electrical activity could have a disorganizing effect on the neurons, since the response of dendrite varies with the strength of the impulse. Rajalakshmi and Ramakrishnan[73] presumed that "an optimum level of dendritic activity is crucial for efficient CNS function. This may involve the maintenance of critical levels of glutamic acid and GABA." The animals deprived of proteins show lower levels of glutamate dehydrogenase and glutamate decarboxylase, and they perform less well on visual discrimination and reversal learning testing procedures.[72] "Decreased enzyme levels were associated with impaired performance in behavioral measures such as performance on the water maze, the Hebb Williams maze, visual discrimination and reversal learning, locomotion scores and tasks involving motor coordination." [75]

The glutamic acid metabolism has been studied in detail by Rajalakshmi and associates, and the reader is referred to their detailed description.[73,75] Mandel and Mark [52] observed no change in glutamate and GABA level after depriving the animals of protein in their diet. However, beneficial effects have been reported if the diet is supplemented with glutamic acid.[98,99] Some important enzymes belonging to certain metabolic pathways by which the nervous tissue feeds and functions are also affected. Rajalakshmi *et al.*[73] showed reduced amounts of glutamate dehydrogenase, glutamate decarboxylase, glutamic pyruvic transaminase and glutaminases.

Glutamate dehydrogenase was affected in cerebellum, midbrain, corpus callosum, olfactory lobes and the thalamic-region, whereas the levels of glutamate decarboxylase were affected in basal ganglia, hypothalamus, medulla, and visual cortex and thalamic region.[75] Sereni *et al.*[81] showed that malnutrition does not affect the activity of succinic dehydrogenase—an enzyme required for cellular oxidation. A satisfactory explanation for those observations with respect to its impact on the learning performance under the impact of protein deprivation is not available at this time. It is possible, however, that the lower levels of glutamic dehydrogenase and glutamate decarboxylase in the brain of malnourished animals may be responsible for lower level of psychological performance.[71]

Some of the vitamins, e.g. group of B_6 vitamins, also play a role in protein or lipid metabolism. Coursin [16] explained the role of pyridoxal phosphate which serves as a coenzyme in a number of enzymatic reactions, such as transamination, decarboxylation, desulfhydration, amine oxidation, involving the amino acids. It is also an integral part of phosphorylase, which is responsible for degradation of glycogen to glucose. In a state of malnutrition, this sequence of metabolic events could be completely disturbed. This could lead to clinical symptoms similar to those of inborn errors of metabolism such as the metabolism of phenylalanine and histidine. "Impairment of metabolic conversion of the amino acids in malnourished infants leads to a rise in their levels and symptomatology—hypotonia, brown sparse hair, depigmented skin, mental regression—identical to phenylketoneuria and histidinimia." [11] In a new born baby, diet deficient in pyridoxal phosphate would result within six weeks in hyperirritability, convulsive seizures, abnormalities in development, and behavioral disorders. A prolonged deficiency of this chemical would result in irreversib!e damage to cerebral function and mental retardation.[33] Cravioto *et al.*[18] pointed out that the high ratio of phenylalanine to tyrosine in the children suffering from severe protein-calorie malnutrition may indicate enzymatic dysfunction and inability to convert phenylalanine to tyrosine. It has been observed that in malnourished infants the metabolism of phenylalanine to tyrosine is depressed, which could be of far reaching biochemical significance,[33] especially when it is evident that the brain is particularly subject to functional dearrangement by alterations in its metabolic environment.

Malnutrition induces gross disturbances in the content of water and several electrolytes in the brain tissue, and Flexner *et al.*[35] believed that these changes are a result of interference with protein synthesis, which further complicates the disturbed biochemistry of the brain.

CONCLUSIONS

The brain responds to dietary deprivation depending on the severity as well as the age of the individuals. If it takes place during the critical stages of its rapid growth and differentiation, the central nervous system is extremely vulnerable and may result in physical, histopathological and biochemical alterations in its composition.[12,20,21,27,28] However, if an adult person suffers from the same degree of malnutrition, the effects on the brain may be minimal.

During the early period of life, the brain reacts to malnutrition, resulting in hampered physical growth and subsequent intellectual capacity. The specific reaction of the brain includes loss of brain weight, interruption in the process of myelination, EEG disturbances and anatomical and biochemical changes in the neurons and neuroglial cells. Prominent histopathological changes in the brains of malnourished individuals, compared to healthy controls, have been observed by a number of workers and include such changes as chromatolysis, foaming of the cytoplasm, swollen appearance of myelin sheath, increase in oligodendroglial cells, neuronal loss, and fibrous gliosis.[70] Protein deficiency also results in demyelination. Electroencephalograms of the malnourished children show striking abnormalities, which do not revert to normal at a later date or after rehabilitation. If the period of malnutrition happens to be a few weeks prior to birth (due to severe maternal nutritional deprivation) and is continued to a few weeks or months of postnatal life (due to lactation failure or nonavailability of good quality uncontaminated milk), the brain is left with a permanent deficit in cell number, incomplete organization, and serious and most probably permanent impairment of its functional ability. Experimental studies on rats show that the prenatally and postnatally deprived animals show as little as 40 percent of the expected number of cells. Besides, a lag of psychomotor development, retarded I.Q. potential, and behavioral abnormalities at a later life could also be traced to a result of malnutrition in early life and adverse reaction of the brain to it.

REFERENCES

1. Adams, D. H.: *Biochem. J.*, *98*:636 (1966).
2. Andrew, W.: *Am. J. Pathol.*, *17*:421–436 (1941).
3. Baraitser, M. and Evans, D. E.: *S. Afr. Med. J.*, *43* p. 56 (1969).
4. Barnes, R. H., Moore, A. U., Reid, F. M., and Pond, W. G.: *J. Am. vol 43 Diet. Assoc.*, *51*:34–39 (1967).
5. Bensted, J. P. M., Dobbing, J., Morgan, R. S., Reid, R. T. W., and Payling, G.: *J. Embryol. Exp. Morphol.*, *5*:428 (1957).
6. Benton, J. W., Moser, H. W., Dodge, P. R., and Carr, S.: *Pediatrics*, *38*:801 (1966).
7. Brown, R. E.: *East Afr. Med. J.*, *42*:584 (1965).
8. Buchanan, A. R. and Roberts, J. E.: *Proc. Soc. Exp. Biol. Med.*, *69*:101 (1948).
9. Cabak, V. and Najdanvic, R.: *Arch. Dis. Child.*, *40*:532 (1965).
10. Carothers, J. C.: *The African Mind in Health and Disease.* W.H.O. Monograph Series (1953).
11. Chandra, R. K.: *Indian J. Pediatr.*, *35*:70 (1968).
12. Chase, P. H., Dorsey, J., and Mckhan, G. M.: *Pediatrics*, *40*:551 (1967).
13. Cheek, D. B. and Cooke, R. E.: *Annu. Rev. Med.*, *15*:357 (1964).

14. Chow, B. F.: In N. S. Scrimshaw and J. E. Gordon (Eds.) : *Malnutrition, Learning and Behavior.* Cambridge, MIT Press (1968) .
15. Coppoletta, J. M. and Walbach, S. B.: *Am. J. Pathol., 9:*55–70 (1933) .
16. Coursin, D. B.: *Fed. Proc., 26:*134 (1967) .
17. Cowley, J. J. and Griesel, R. D.: *J. Genet. Psychol., 103:*233–242 (1963) .
18. Cravioto, J., Delicarte, E. R., and Birch, H. G.: *Pediatrics, 38:*319 (1966) .
19. Culley, W. J. and Lineberger, R. O.: *J. Nutr., 96:*375–381 (1968) .
20. Culley, W. J., Yuan, L., and Mertz, E. T.: *Fed. Proc., 25:*674 (1966) .
21. Davison, A. N. and Dobbing, J.: *Br. Med. Bull., 22:*40 (1966) .
22. Davison, A. N. and Dobbing, J.: In A. N. Davison and J. Dobbing (Eds.) : *Applied Neurochemistry.* Philadelphia, Davis (1968) .
23. Diamond, M. C., Law, F., Rhodes, H., *et al.: J. Comp. Neurol., 128:* 117–125 (1966) .
24. Dickerson, J. W. T. and Dobbing, J.: *Proc. R. Soc., 166B:*384–395 (1967a) .
25. Dickerson, J. W. T. and Dobbing, J.: *Proc. Nutr. Soc., 26:*5 (1967b) .
26. Dickerson, J. W. T. and Jarvis, J.: *Proc. Nutr. Soc., 27:*4A–5A (1970) .
27. Dobbing, J.: *Proc. R. Soc. Med., 159:*503 (1964) .
28. Dobbing, J.: *Biol. Neonate, 9:*132 (1965) .
29. Dobbing, J.: In N. S. Scrimshaw and J. E. Gordon (Eds.) : *Malnutrition, Learning and Behavior.* Cambridge, MIT Press (1968a) .
30. Dobbing, J.: In A. N. Davison and J. Dobbing (Eds.) : *Applied Neurochemistry.* Philadelphia, Davis (1968b) .
31. Dobbing, J.: In W. A. Himwich (Ed.) : *Developmental Neurobiology.* Springfield, Thomas (1970) .
32. Dobbing, J. and Widdowson, E.: *Brain, 88:*357 (1965) .
33. Eichenwald, H. F. and Fry, P. C.: *Science, 163:*644 (1969) .
34. Engel, R.: *Electroencephalogr. Clin. Neurophysiol., 8:*489 (1956) .
35. Flexner, J. B., Flexner, L. B., dela Haba, G., and Roberts, R. B.: *J. Neurochem., 12:*535 (1965) .
36. Folch, J.: In H. Waelsch (Ed.) : *Biochemistry of the Developing Nervous System.* New York, Academic Press (1955) .
37. Fox, M. W.: *Brain Res., 2:*3–20 (1966) .
38. Gallais, P., Bert, J., Corriol, J., and Miletto, G.: *Electroencephalogr. Clin. Neurophysiol., 3:*110 (1951a) .
39. Gallais, P., Miletto, G., Corriol, J., and Bert, J.: *Med. Trop., 11:*128–146 1951b) .
40. Garrow, J. S.: *Lancet, 2:*643–645 (1967) .
41. Graham, G. G.: *Nutritional Symposium.* Annual Meeting of Federation of American Societies for Experimental Biology (1966) .
42. Graham, G. G.: *Fed. Proc., 26:*139–143 (1967) .
43. Graham, G. G.: In R. A. McCance and E. M. Widdowson (Eds.) : *Caloric Deficiencies and Protein Deficiencies.* London, Churchill (1968) .

44. Guthrie, H. A. and Brown, M. L.: *J. Nutr., 94*:419 (1968).
45. Hebb, D. O.: *The Organization of Behavior, A Neuropsychological Theory.* New York, Wiley (1949).
46. Howard, E.: *Neurochem., 12*:181 (1965).
47. Howard, E. and Granoff, D. M.: *J. Nutr., 95*:111–121 (1968).
48. Jasper, H. H., Khan, R. T., and Elliott, K. A. C.: *Science, 147*:1448 (1965).
49. Kulenkampff, H.: *Z. Anat., Entwicklungsgesch., 16*:304 (1952).
50. Lehr, P. and Gayet, J.: *J. Neurochem., 10*:169 (1963).
51. Lubchenco, L. O., Horner, F. A., Reed, L. H., *et al.: Am. J. Dis. Child., 106*:101–115 (1963).
52. Mandel, P. and Mark, J.: *J. Neurochem., 12*:987 (1965).
53. Meyer, A., Pampiglione, G., Platt, B. S., and Stewart, R. J. C.: *Excerpta. Med. Amst., 39*:17 (1961).
54. Miller, N. E.: In N. S. Scrimshaw and J. E. Gordon (Eds.): *Malnutrition, Learning and Behavior.* Cambridge, MIT Press (1968).
55. Mönckeberg, F.: In N. S. Scrimshaw and J. E. Gordon (Eds.): *Malnutrition, Learning and Behavior.* Cambridge, MIT Press (1968).
56. Mönckeberg, F.: *Western Hemisphere Nutrition Conference* (1970).
57. Munday-Castle, A. C., McKiever, B. L., and Prinsloo, T.: *Electroencephalogr. Neurophysiol., 5*:533–543 (1953).
58. Naeye, R. L.: *Arch. Pathol., 79*:284–291 (1965).
59. Nelson, G. K.: *Electroencephalogr. Clin. Neurophysiol., 11*:73 (1959).
60. Nelson, G. K.: *CSIR Res. Rev., S. Africa, 9*:144–146 (1959b).
61. Nelson, G. K. and Dean, R. F. A.: *Bull. W.H.O., 21*:779–782 (1959).
62. Norton, W. T. and Autilio, L. A.: *J. Neurochem., 13*:213 (1966).
63. Novakova, V., Koldovsky, O., Hahn, P., and Krecek, J.: *Nutrition and Health,* Proceedings of VII International Congress Nutrition. London, Pergamon Press (1967), vol. 1, p. 342.
64. Oiso, T.: Ann. Rep. National Institute of Nutrition, Tokyo, Japan (1969).
65. Pampiglione, G.: *Kellaway and Peterson Neurological and Electroencephalographic Correlative Studies in Infancy.* New York, Grune and Stratton (1964).
66. Payne, P. R. and Wheeler, E. F.: *Nature, 215*:1134–1136 (1967).
67. Platt, B. S., Pampiglione, G., and Stewart, R. J. C.: *Dev. Med. Child. Neurol., 7*:9–26 (1965).
68. Platt, B. S. and Stewart, R. J. C.: *Dev. Med. Child. Neurol., 10*:3 (1968).
69. Platt, B. S. and Stewart, R. J. C.: *Dev. Med. Child. Neurol., 11*:174 (1969).
70. Platt, B. S. and Stewart, R. J. C.: In G. H. Bourne (Ed.): *World Review of Nutrition and Dietetics.* vol. 13. Basel, S. Karger (1971).
71. Rajalakshmi, R.: In N. S. Scrimshaw and J. E. Gordon (Eds.): *Malnutrition, Learning and Behavior.* Cambridge, MIT Press (1968).

72. Rajalakshmi, R., Govindarajan, K. R., and Ramakrishnan, C. V.: *J. Neurochem., 12:*261 (1965).
73. Rajalakshmi, R. and Ramakrishnan, C. V.: In *Nutrition, Learning Performance and Brain Biochemistry.* Project Report of PL 480 Project FG–IN–176 of U.S. Dept. of Agriculture (1969).
74. Rajalakshmi, R. and Ramakrishnan, C. V.: Terminal Report of PL 480 Project FG–IN–224, Baroda University, Baroda, India (1969b).
75. Rajalakshmi, R. and Ramakrishnan, C. V.: In G. H. Bourne (Ed.): *World Review of Nutrition and Dietetics* vol. 14 Basel, S. Karger (1971).
76. Richter, D.: *Br. Med. J., 1:*1255 (1959).
77. Robinow, M.: In N. S. Scrimshaw and J. E. Gordon (Eds.): *Malnutrition, Learning and Behavior.* Cambridge, MIT Press (1968).
78. Sarrony, C., Saint-Jean, M., and Clause, J.: *Algerie Med., 57:*584 (1953).
79. Scott, J. P.: *Am. Rev. Psychol., 18:*1–40 (1967).
80. Scrimshaw, N. S.: *Am. J. Clin. Nutr., 20:*493 (1967).
81. Sereni, *et al.: J. Pediatr., 67:*948 (1965).
82. Stewart, R. J. C. and Platt, B. S.: In N. S. Scrimshaw and J. E. Gordon (Eds.): *Malnutrition, Learning and Behavior.* Cambridge, MIT Press (1968).
83. Stoch, M. B. and Smythe, P. M.: *Arch. Dis. Child., 38:*546–552 (1963).
84. Stoch, M. B. and Smythe, P. M.: *S. Afr. Med. J., 41:*1027–1030 (1967).
85. Stoch, M. B. and Smythe, P. M.: In N. S. Scrimshaw and J. E. Gordon (Eds.): *Malnutrition, Learning and Behavior.* Cambridge, MIT Press (1968).
86. Thomson, H. T., Schurr, P. E., Henderson, L. M., and Elrehjem, C. A.: *J. Biol. Chem., 182:*47 (1950).
87. Tureen, L. L.: *Arch. Neurol. Psychiatr., 35:*789–807 (1936).
88. Udani, P. M.: *Indian J. Child Health, 2:*498 (1962).
89. Waelsch, H.: In D. Richter (Ed.): *Metabolism of the Nervous System.* London, Pergamon Press (1957).
90. Winick, M.: Fifty-third Annual Meeting of Federation of American Society for Experimental Biology, Atlantic City, New Jersey (1969).
91. Winick, M.: *Med. Clin. North Am., 54:*1413 (1970).
92. Winick, M.: *Pediatr. Clin. North Am., 17:*69 (1970).
93. Winick, M. and Noble, A.: *Dev. Biol., 12:*451 (1965).
94. Winick, M. and Noble, A.: *J. Nutr., 89:*300 (1966).
95. Winick, M. and Noble, A.: *Nature, 212:*34, 5057 (1966b).
96. Winick, M. and Rosso, P.: *J. Pediatr., 74:*774 (1969).
97. Winick, M. and Rosso, P.: *Pediatr. Res., 3:*181 (1969).
98. Zimmerman, F. T., Burgemeister, B. B., and Putnam, T. J.: *Am. J. Psychiatr., 105:*661 (1949).
99. Zimmerman, F. T. and Ross, S.: *Arch. Neurol. Psychiatr., 57:*441 (1944).

Chapter III

MALNUTRITION AND MENTAL DEVELOPMENT

T HERE IS GROWING concern among nutritionists, psychologists, biochemists, and clinicians over the possible effects of malnutrition on mental development and morphological or biochemical damage to the brain. Of special concern is the most vulnerable period of brain development, which is roughly three months before and six months after birth. It is during this period that maximum brain growth takes place. It includes not only growth of the physical size of the brain, but also of its component parts, especially cell size and numbers. A prenatal curtailment in the cell numbers and differentiation could compound the tragedy if nutritional deprivation is continued into the postnatal period. During this period, nonavailability of all the nutrients, especially protein, would have an adverse effect on the normal course of growth trajectory. For the period three months prior to birth, it is the maternal health and diet that determines the brain growth of the baby, whereas in the postnatal period, the child's growth depends on the maternal lactating ability. This is especially true in most of the developing countries, where well-prepared and well-preserved baby foods are nonexistent. The market milk is adulterated and contaminated and the child depends solely on mother's milk. In this vulnerable period (prenatal and postnatal), the child's growth, well-being and mental development depend greatly on the mother—her pregravidic health, nutritional status during pregnancy, lactating ability, and educational background for child care. In certain places, carbohydrate rich diets with very little protein are culturally accepted baby foods, for example, plantain in Uganda. If the mother's educational background is such that she believes that the plantain would satisfy the child's nutritional requirements, the child is bound to suffer with respect to his physical and mental well being. In addition to choice of foods, the maternal handling and culturally based child-rearing practices will also affect the ultimate personality development of the child and mold his subsequent behavior and learning capacity.[71] Like other organs, the central nervous system requires adequate nutrition for optimal growth and development. A number of workers have pointed out the "brain sparing" effect of undernutrition. While there may be some preferential protection of the brain, this cannot be absolute because an episode of malnutrition during the critical period of brain growth could cause maximal damage to its physical and biochemical structure as well as functional capacity.[18] In that case, malnutrition would adversely influence the mental development of the child.

A significant number of the children who are severely malnourished in their early infancy die due to a variety of reasons, which may include simple exhaustion or inability to combat a minor infection. The dead may be more fortunate in a certain sense compared to the survivors, who experience physical and mental retardation and loss of learning ability during the most critical years of mental development. It has been estimated that 75 to 85 percent of all mentally defective children are born in an environment of poverty.[79] Lowe stated, "It is our conviction that nutrition is the key to normal development of infants and children. In effect, the quality and quantity of nutrition given during the first 2 to 4 years of life may have the effect of programming the individual for the rest of his life." [68] Malnutrition in this early period of life will cause an all-round retardation in physical, motor, and intellectual development [128] and a number of field studies extending to a period of many years from Mexico, Guatemala, Chile, Colombia, South Africa, and other parts of Africa and Asia tend to confirm these observations on specific learning disabilities.[78]

It has been pointed out that structurally the development of the brain is completed by four to five years of age, but the process of mental development continues for a long time.[101] Undernutrition beyond five years of age, unless of a very severe degree, probably would not affect the brain or its function. But if malnutrition is accompanied by extremely depressing environmental conditions, the behavioral and mental development as well as intellectual functioning of the organism could be adversely affected.[50a] Rajalakshmi and Ramakrishnan [100] measured the mental performance of a number of people whose ages ranged from five to 70 years. They pointed out that psychological functions in humans reach a peak in the twenties. Persons between 20 to 25 score the highest, when measured by several Wechsler adult intelligence tests. Such performance measures included measurements of paired associate learning, re-paired learning, coding, recoding, tachistoscopic form discrimination and Wechsler block design tests. Under ideal circumstances when the diet and environmental conditions are in the normal range, the mental performance of individuals kept on increasing from the lowest age till the peak was reached between 20 to 25 years. From this it may be presumed that a nutritional and/or environmental deprivation during this long period of up to 25 years of life may have an adverse effect on the mental development as well as on the intellectual functioning of the individual. "It is not inconceivable that a lack of receptivity and maturation during this period caused by hunger and malnutrition would reflect indirectly on the development." [100]

The International Conference on Malnutrition, Learning and Behavior sponsored by the Nutrition Foundation laid stress on the results obtained from the human as well as animal studies which strongly suggest a relationship between malnutrition in the early life and derangement of mental functions, which may take the form of neurological, developmental, or behavioral disorders.[81]

The studies of Cravioto and Robles [37,38] clearly suggested that an interruption in the maturation of nervous system during its peak period of growth may leave defects in psychomotor development, which may not be corrected even with an adequate diet later on. Generally, the motor development is not retarded as much, and the greatest difference is observed in the ability to learn language. Cravioto *et al.*[34] believed that protein deficiency could result in structural lesions of the nervous system, which would lead to mental damage. Barnes *et al.*[5] posed some very important questions which have not been satisfactorily answered and cannot be done unless a multidisciplinary approach is adopted and vigorous steps are taken to study the problem seriously while attempting at the same time to alleviate the conditions of the victims. These questions are

> Does severe malnutrition in early life cause a measureable retardation in learning behavior following complete dietary rehabilitation? Does malnutrition result in a retardation in the individual's capacity to learn? In his motivation to learn? Are behavioral abnormalities long lasting, or are they only transient during the acute nutritional crisis? What are the relative contributions of the early malnutrition, and what are the effects of continuing social, cultural, educational, and economic deprivations that extend from the child to the adult? What effects, if any, result from the milder forms of malnutrition that undoubtedly affect a large proportion of the children in developing countries and, in fact, may involve many of the underprivileged classes in our economically highly developed countries? If milder forms of malnutrition, such as marasmus, exist during very early life, are there temporary or perhaps even long lasting effects on behavioral development? If there are such effects, are they traceable to a direct influence of malnutrition or, as many child psychologists believe, to social and family deprivations, such as result from early weaning from the breast? Does malnutrition of the mother during gestation affect behavioral development of the offsprings?

The answers to these questions are extremely difficult to find. However, the experimental evidence on a variety of animals clearly suggests that malnutrition causes retardation in learning pattern, motivation and behavioral development. To some extent, these results are applicable to humans as well. The behavioral changes and consequent retarded intellectual development are long lasting and may become permanent if the episodes of malnutrition are experienced during the period of active brain growth. In such individuals, the behavioral changes would be most prominent and would reflect changes in emotionality and elevated response levels to adverse stimuli.[2,5]

MENTAL RETARDATION AS RELATED TO PHYSICAL GROWTH STUNTING OF THE BODY

The visible manifestation of severe protein or protein-calorie malnutrition includes the stunted height of a child, and it is commonly used as an indicator of nutritional status. Malnourished children are shorter in stature in preschool years as well as in adolescence compared to those who are brought up under better dietary care. Chronic undernourishment leads to growth retardation, which may be reduced as much as 30 to 35 percent in weight and 10 to 15 percent in height. This pattern of height and weight may continue into the second, third, and succeeding generations due to a persistent pattern of undernutrition throughout this period. It is because of this that millions of adults belonging to the lower socioeconomic classes show smaller heights and lower weights compared to people in the same area but belonging to the upper socioeconomic classes. Richardson,[102] however, rightly pointed out that great caution is needed in using height as a sole indicator of nutritional status, because this will give the impression that among the people of smaller stature, the level of mental development is lower than in those of the taller people. Such a conclusion may be completely false. The height of a person or that of a child is determined by a number of factors, especially hereditary ones. The pertinent question that remains unanswered unequivocally is whether or not there is any association between height, weight, and intelligence.

In order to study the effects of malnutrition on mental development one has to study its prevalence in a particular area. The simplest and most sensitive method may be to undertake a study of the patterns of physical growth and development of the preschool children, particularly those under five years of age. Guzman [65] believed that if nutrition requirements of children are fully met, the growth performance of children under five years of age is not affected by racial, climatic, or other environmental differences. The influence of these factors become evident after the age of five years. The growth pattern of young children is generally determined by the quality and quantity of available nutrition. If this criteria of physical growth is accepted, it is estimated that 50 to 80 percent of all the preschool children in the developing countries experience protein-calorie malnutrition to the extent that their physical growth patterns are less than normal and, by inference, may have suffered some disturbance in learning capacity and behavior.[49]

Quite a few prominent workers have reported a direct association between physical growth stunting and lower levels of mental
performance from a number of technologically less developed
countries among malnourished children. Gesell tests were per-
formed on African malnourished and healthy children in Uganda,
and similar studies have been used by Robles, Cravioto, and
collaborators in Mexico.[104] All these investigations found a striking contrast in the learning skills, psychomotor development, and
motivation of the malnourished children compared to their local
controls. In extreme cases of malnourishment, the height may
therefore be used as one of the indicators of retarded growth and
may be helpful to point out the suspected cases in which to look
for certain degree of lag in mental development. It is often observed that most of the very small children are born to small and
unhealthy mothers. Because of the poor health of these mothers,
especially during pregnancy, there is always a possibility that
along with deficits in physical growth the development of the
brain may have deflected from its normal course of growth and
thereby might have resulted in some brain damage and lower
levels of intelligence. Such extreme cases, however, do not warrant a general conclusion that there is a positive correlation between the height of a person and his level of intelligence. Because
of better nutrition all through the growing years, the children of
the upper classes are able to achieve their maximum hereditarily
controlled growth potential and are taller than the members of
the lower economic classes. However, this may not mean that
the members of the upper classes are more intelligent than those
of the lower ones. The extra stature in the members of the upper
classes may also be due to the fact that they have better educated
mothers, who not only feed their children more wisely but also
stimulate them in some other ways which help to unfold their
personalities.

Since it is of utmost importance to have a reasonably precise
estimate of the prevalence of malnutrition in young children,
interest in anthropometry is also increasing. These techniques are
also based on the same assumption that under optimum conditions
of nutrition, children of all races and genetic background grow

within certain norms, and any growth failure or bodily disproportion resulting from nutritional deficiency could be easily picked
up by a series of anthropometric body measurements. These techniques are simple, cheap, and quite satisfactorily objective.[70]
These measurements may be age dependent or age independent.
The former may include weight, height, and arm circumference,
whereas the latter may try to establish chest/head ratio, weight/
height ratio or weight/head circumference ratio. The growth retardation is no doubt a great influence on the brain size, and
several authors have indicated a strong correlation between short
stature and reduced intellectual levels.[107,108,111] These workers
assume that the short people as a group are less intelligent than
the tall people. The smaller mean head circumference in the
malnourished subjects may mean that the brain has reached
maturity at a suboptimal size. Social conditions may affect the
difference in the I.Q., but the difference in the head circumference
that is sometimes evident in malnourished and healthy children
as shown by Stoch and Smythe [120] is definitely a result of malnutrition and has nothing to do with the effects of environmental
deprivation.

The question whether or not the growth stunting during the
preschool years under the influence of bad nutrition is made up
by good nutrition during the later adolescent years is not satisfactorily answered. Read [101] made a strong plea for an internation-
ally coordinated research program for the collection of physical
growth data in order to provide a yardstick for the effects of
nutrition improvement programs. Certain instances clearly show
that optimum nutrition in the preschool years not only leads to
satisfactory growth but also helps to attain the genetic potential
for growth. The nutritional improvement of some groups (e.g.
Negroes in U.S.) or countries (e.g. Japan) has led to significant
increases in physical growth, and these communities have a new
generation of taller people compared to their parents.[69,83]

In most instances a lag in neuro-integrative capacity or intersensory functioning reflects in retarded growth in terms of height.
Cravioto and Delicardie [35] studied the intersensory performance of
rural and urban children with different heights for chronological

age and found significant differences in the intersensory integrative skills of these children in the two groups. Although a
large number of taller rural children had the same height as the
large number of urban children with smaller height pattern, the
differences in the neuro-integrative ability was evident in the two
groups, clearly marking out the social setting. It must be stressed,
however, that habitat alone cannot be marked out as an indication
of intersensory integrative organization. The very tall heights
observed in the industrialized countries compared to those men
in the underdeveloped world may have been determined more by
genetic factors and generation after generation of nutritional
differences. At the same time, very short children are also those
who most likely suffered greater privation compared to their
taller counterparts. These children, at an early stage, might have
entered an altered trajectory with respect to mental development,
resulting in neuro-integrative inadequacy, inability to go through
the formal educational process, and subnormal adaptive functioning.[113]

RETARDED MENTAL DEVELOPMENT AS RELATED TO THE AGE OF THE PERSON

A case has often been made that the nervous system is relatively
insensitive to nutritional deficiencies or starvation. Whereas this
may be true of episodes of small duration, malnutrition for prolonged periods of time is likely to affect the central nervous
system adversely. Among the adults, episodes of severe malnutrition may result in apathy, nervousness, confusion, and forget-
fulness, which may be completely cured on rehabilitation.
However, if such a severe degree of malnutrition is imposed on
an infant during its period of maximum brain growth, such as
in the early postnatal life, the effects on the CNS may not only be
drastic but also irreversible, and the impairment may not be
rectified on rehabilitation. After all, the general metabolism is
not different from the cerebral metabolism, and if growth retardation could result from lack of protein in the diet, the brain
may also share the shortages along with other organs.

Discussing the mental development in a normal baby getting
adequate nutrition, Coursin [24] described

the performance of the newborn is primarily reflex. This stage is followed with a gradual orderly appearance of new capacities for neuromuscular activity, socialization, behavior and mentation. The infant's abilities to respond coincide well with maturational process and clinical evidence of his normal central nervous system development. During the early formative years, the brain sequentially acquires each new specific function and integrates the process into its total pattern of performance and experience. Experimental evidence suggests that the timing of this overall procedure is of utmost importance. Each new function makes its appearance chronologically at a "critical period" in the total ongoing pattern and is apparently maximally operant at that time.[109]

If the child does not get adequate nutrition, this sequence of development is likely to be altered and may result in the limitation of specific ability. Coursin [24] believed that a good deal of mischief is already done before any changes are demonstrable clinically. Psychological data clearly demonstrates that significant functional retardation is the result of malnutrition during the early part of infancy, especially during the first six months of postnatal life, in which physical and biochemical damage directly relates to retardation in mental development.

The severity of consequences of malnutrition depends on its timing in relation to the vulnerable period of brain growth. In the human species, such a period is prenatal, whereas in a number of commonly used experimental animals, it is postnatal. Rat's growth is mainly postnatal, and an episode of malnutrition in the postnatal life will be as detrimental to normal mental development as prenatal deprivation in humans. Rajalakshmi [97] reported that the offspring of rats poorly fed during pregnancy and well fed during lactation fare much better than those who were born of healthy mothers but poorly fed during lactation. In humans, it will probably be reverse, and the effects of severe maternal deprivation which will effect the prenatal brain growth of the fetus will be more drastic. It may be that even the worst depleted mother may provide some protection to the baby, and the latter may be able to gain some nourishment at the mother's expense. The lactating ability of such a woman which is essential for the baby in the early postnatal life may, however, be seriously limited. It could exert a significant influence on the course of postnatal development of the baby. If this baby is not given adequate and well-balanced foods in the postweaning period, the period of lag in mental development could be greatly lengthened, thereby making the tragic consequences of nutritional deprivation more grim.

The signs of malnutrition, especially protein malnutrition, are not as well marked in the adult as they are in the children during their preschool years because of the large demands on protein to cope with the genetically based growth potential in the latter. Experimental evidence exists that malnutrition not only hinders the full growth of physical stature but also affects the brain function, and these abnormalities in nervous system may persist even if physical disabilities have disappeared.[12] Apparently malnutrition in these children has impaired the normal processes of cellular maturation and nervous system development. It is believed that these children are 10 to 25 percent below the normal controls in their intellectual, psychological, and neuromuscular capacities. The common symptoms described by a number of workers which reflect the mental condition of the malnourished children are apathy, listlessness, irritability, and general misery. In these conditions, the involvement of the nervous system is very clear, and according to Platt [94] when some of these children die, it should be taken as a CNS death, even though clear neurological signs are not present. Winick [129] summarized the functional changes in the developing brains of the malnourished animals and humans (Table IV). The results are strikingly similar to those of other authors who have described coarse tremors, jerky movements, motor system involvement, and diminished or absent deep reflexes.[72-74,124] These changes are more evident when a program of rehabilitation is started. Wayburne explained that during the early part of recovery, "The tremors effect the face, tongue, neck, abdominal muscles and limbs, particularly the hands and fingers, and may be asymmetrical. Respiration may be jerky, feeding is difficult, reflexes are increased and the patient may be unable to sit up." [126]

When an episode of malnutrition is experienced in adult life, all evidences seem to show that the effects produced are com-

TABLE IV
FUNCTIONAL CHANGES IN THE DEVELOPING BRAINS OF
MALNOURISHED SUBJECTS (Winick 1970)

Functional Changes	Animals	Humans
Neurologic symptoms	Transient; tremors, hobble skirt, gait, convulsions	Transient; apathy, lethargy, or hyperirritability
EEG	Increased slow wave activity (transient)	
Behavioral	Decreased "exploratory" behavior	Exaggerated response to certain stimuli
	Poor ability to extinguish a response	Poor ability to extinguish a response
Intellectual	Difficulty in maze learning	Decrease in cognitive and perceptual development*

* Malnutrition has not been entirely isolated as the sole cause of these changes.

pletely reversible on rehabilitation. A severe episode of malnutrition in an adult individual or even the adolescents, when the brain development has been completed, may not effect the learning ability permanently. Physically the brain in such individuals is not reduced in size or restricted in weight under the effect of severe malnutrition, even at a time when the other tissues of the body have given up and the individual is in a state of hypoglycemic coma characteristic of the late stages of malnutrition.[59,60] During World War II, the French school teachers constantly complained of less attention on the part of the pupils, less capacity to learn, instability with lessons, and duties not well done, obviously because of very much reduced quantities of food available to these adolescents. Finally, when these persons were rehabilitated on sufficient quantities of food, all complaints ceased.

In their classical experiments dealing with the biology of human starvation, Keys *et al.*[75] controlled the food intake for a prolonged period of time in a number of subjects. During this period, physical as well as mental activity was carefully monitored. In a condition of severe starvation, the accuracy of intelligence was somewhat retarded, although the established intelligence remained relatively unchanged. On rehabilitation, all the physical and mental symptoms completely disappeared.

Profound nervous system effects can be brought about by specific deficiencies in the diet of B vitamins (thiamine, riboflavin, niacin) . However, all the symptoms disappear when this dietary deficiency is corrected.[24]

MALNUTRITION AND BEHAVIORAL DISTURBANCES

The subject of malnutrition in early childhood and its impact on the behavioral development is extremely important, but in spite of that, so far only speculative judgments have been made, which may or may not be strictly correct.[56a] However, most of the studies do point out to the general direction that malnutrition in infancy, even if corrected at a later date, leaves a deficit in mental development which could lead to subsequent behavioral impairment. In human situations, the all important factor of environment is always there interacting either with nutritional standards or the incidence of sickness or genetic endowments.

Maternal protein malnutrition, especially in the last stages of pregnancy, affects the development of nervous system of the fetus which results in later behavioral impairment. Similar results are produced on early postnatal malnutrition. These periods (late prenatal and early postnatal) are considered the critical or vulnerable periods of brain growth. A number of studies show evidence of such a critical period in life, in which severe degrees of malnutrition affects not only the mental development in an adverse manner but also leads to permanent behavioral disturbances. It may be safe to assume that the earlier in life the episode of malnutrition begins, the more lasting the effect it has on the behavioral development of the individual.[21,40,62,82,119] The critical period is associated with rapid brain growth and protein synthesis.[35] The nonavailability of protein in the diet or simply the nonavailability of milk during this period could alter the brain composition and mental behavior.[4,9,13,39,48]

There is ample evidence that malnutrition results in severe behavioral abnormalities and results in low psychomotor development. However, in spite of the positive indications, it has not been firmly established that behavioral abnormalities and retarded psychological development lead to lowered intelligence and delayed learning behavior.[2] An obvious impairment could be due to altered motivation or apathy in learning induced by hunger rather than altered capacity. Persistent undernutrition leaves its ugly mark not only on the body but also on the mind and personality.[74a,80] In children suffering from kwashiorkor or marasmus, psychological disturbances are the most prominent, and the same is true of animals subjected to experimental malnutrition. As Zimmerman and Strobell [131] pointed out, malnourished monkeys show retarded curiosity, manipulation and social motivation, while severely ill human children lose all the normal curiosity and desire for exploration that is natural in a young child.

The malnourished state superimposes on the individual certain behavioral disturbances, which could be solely attributed to the absence of sufficient quantity of well-balanced food. It is difficult in the human cases to define a particular abnormality in behavior due to malnutrition, but experimental data in the animals show clearly that such behavioral disturbances under the impact of malnutrition do affect the overall performance of the animal.[130a] These conclusions could be extrapolated to human conditions to a certain extent. Taking some important examples, a number of prominent workers have observed in rats that malnutrition results in the retardation of neurons to develop as defined by decreased spontaneous exploratory activity and increased emotionality. These symptoms don't seem to disappear on rehabilitation* with certain exceptions.[85,99] In the malnourished animals, the learning performance and activity patterns are adversely affected, particularly under the impact of protein malnutrition, which is the most common form of dietary deficiency. Puromycin administered in a particular area of cerebral cortex inhibits protein synthesis and results in loss of memory.[51] Protein deprivation resulting in non-availability of amino acids for protein synthesis may have a similar effect, although the protein concentration of brain tissue has not been found to change with undernutrition.[98,130]

Another fact that may be relevant here is the emotional and psychological disturbance that a kwashiorkor patient may suffer during the period he is separated from the mother for the purpose of treatment in a hospital—such a behaviorally disturbed child may not only respond well to the treatment but also show per-

---

* See references 20, 54–56, 63, 64, 79, 86, 114, 115

sistent behavioral abnormalities after he is physically rehabilitated.

In humans, besides nutrition, environmental and other factors could be potent in altering the mental development or behavioral pattern of the subject, and the response of the individual may vary from person to person. Read [101] suggested that it is highly desirable to have direct measures of brain function in individuals who have been well fed or malnourished so as to pinpoint a critical developmental period as well as specific behavioral changes attributable to these brain changes. Barnes and other investigators rightly pointed out that multidisciplinary approach is needed to understand objectively and subjectively the influence of malnutrition on growth interference during the vulnerable period of maximum brain growth and on the behavioral development of the organism and to sort out the effects of poor or enriched environment on the morphology and biochemistry of the brain as well as on intellectual functioning.[6,8,55,56,67] Recent research publications indicate that a start in the right direction has already been made. The need now is to push forward such a program. A recent Conference attended by the author on the Early Nutritional and Environmental Influences Upon Behavioral Development [22] held in Seattle, Washington, on December 6 and 7, 1971, has made a significant contribution in the area of behavioral disturbances caused by nutrition as well as environment. This conference brought together a multidisciplinary group of scientists for informal interaction, thereby opening a channel of communication among them, which could go a long way in attacking the problem in a concerted manner.

MALNUTRITION AND RETARDED INTELLECTUAL FUNCTIONING—SOME OBSERVATIONAL AND EXPERIMENTAL STUDIES

Depending on the severity of malnutrition, the effect on the nervous system may range from slight behavioral and mental changes to psychiatric disorders, dementia, and convulsions.[24] Change of mental state in severe malnutrition reflects, in general, dullness of intellect, capriciousness of appetite, irritability, apathy, stupor, coma, and possibly death. The mental changes are more pronounced in kwashiorkor than in marasmus.[57] Most commonly and consistently found changes are tremors, athetoid movements and disturbance in gait. It is interesting that such disturbances in humans have been associated with disturbances in the basal ganglia.[118]

Cravioto and his collaborators [35,38] measured the performance of numerous preschool children suffering from severe degrees of protein-calorie malnutrition by Gesell's psychological test and found that all of them showed lower scores and deficits in adaptive, motor language, and personal social behavior as compared to matched controls of the same ethnic groups. Such deficits continued to be present after rehabilitation, especially in those children who suffered from malnutrition during the period of their first six months. These workers found significantly lower intersensory performance of malnourished children. Not only do they suffer physical growth retardation resulting in very short statures, but they are handicapped mentally as well. They believed that such short-statured children are also more prone to school failures, which are attributed to their inability to master primary school subjects. Cabak and Najdanvic [14] examined thoroughly, employing various testing procedures, seven to 14-year-old children who suffered severe malnutrition between four and 24 months of age and found that their mental development was significantly low (I.Q. mean 88), and their intellectual functioning was far lower than the control children coming from low socioeconomic classes. A longitudinal study of 992 children, whose birth weight was less than 2,500 gm, revealed significant mental retardation at approximately four, seven, and nine years of age when I.Q. was used as an index of psychological impairment. These subjects also experienced difficulty in comprehension and perceptual-motor functioning.[127] The effect of low birth weight is more pronounced in arithmetic than in reading.

Visual, heptic, and kinesthetic integration are important parameters which remain unaffected, to a great extent, by sociocultural conditions and hence could give a better idea of the effect of protein-calorie malnutrition. Eichenwald and Fry [50] showed that

> children subjected to chronic but moderate degrees of malnutrition, as reflected by their heights, exhibit major functional lags in the de-

velopment of this capacity. The ability to integrate visual with heptic, heptic with kinesthetic and visual with kinesthetic stimuli is undoubtedly involved in most learning experiences which depend on the ability to integrate patterned information.

Stoch and Smythe [120] presented at the International Conference on Malnutrition, Learning and Behavior held at Cambridge, Massachusetts, in 1967, the results of 11 years of study of psychological and intellectual performance on a group of 20 infants who were severely malnourished during infancy. Matched controls were provided from the local population. The learning ability of these malnourished children in the formal educational set up was extremely poor and lagged much behind the average of all other children of that area. In a test of cognition, the group which was malnourished showed a markedly poor grasp of the concept of time. The studies reviewed here as well as others seem to warrant the conclusion that it is only severe cases of malnutrition in the early infancy where the results in terms of retarded mental development and intellectual functioning are quite clear, and may prove to be permanent and irreversible, even under optimal conditions of nutrition at a later age. The children who go through mild or moderate degrees of malnutrition, either as brief episodes or in chronic form for longer periods, seem to recover from the impairment. When given stimulating environment conditions (socioeconomic, psychological as well as emotional), these children become normal in every respect and may never be distinguished from the average of the population in terms of learning and socializing ability, academic achievement, or behavior. Stoch and Smythe [121] suggested that a severe form of marasmus, when the child is not only deprived of proteins but may also be cannibalizing on his body for calories, has a more dramatic effect on the learning and behavior of the child than does kwashiorkor. This may be due to the fact that kwashiorkor is a disease of weaning and generally develops in the second and third year of life. By that time, the major brain growth has already been completed. The marasmus, on the other hand, could develop at any time of life. If it happens to develop in the early postnatal life due to maternal lactation failure or other reasons, it could effectively arrest normal brain growth. "Long standing marasmus and a superimposed kwashiorkor would have the most devastating result in permanent brain damage, but children with this combination usually do not survive unless brought promptly to hospital or clinic." [113]

Rajalakshmi and Ramakrishnan [100] compared 24 children (2 cases of marasmus and 22 cases of kwashiorkor) suffering from severe malnutrition with 20 children who were grossly underweight, chronically undernourished, and belonged to the same socioeconomic group as the severely malnourished ones. Among the latter, the children showed prominent signs of apathy. Seven of them showed a median I.Q. of 54; 15 others whose condition was not as severe showed a median I.Q. of 71, whereas the two marasmic cases had an average I.Q. of 82. When these scores are compared to the chronically undernourished controls, they are quite significant. The 20 control cases showed a median I.Q. of 99.

Mönckeberg [84] described detailed observations on 14 severely marasmic children who had been malnourished since the first month of their life due to certain social and economic conditions. These children were fully treated and rehabilitated in the hospital, and their health progress was followed up closely for a period of about six years. A well-balanced diet after discharge

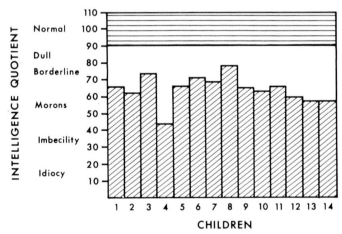

Figure 14. Intelligence quotients of 14 children with marasmic malnutrition in infancy, hospitalized until recovery and observed thereafter at the ages of 3 to 6 years.[84]

from the hospital was assured as far as possible by free supplies of milk to families as well as by frequent visits and physical examinations. At the time of testing these children (3 to 6 years old) for intelligence, they showed all the signs of normal weights and clinical recovery (normal levels of hematocrit, hemoglobin, total protein, and albumin). The I.Q. scores of these children have been given in Figure 14. These results show that the average I.Q. scores of these children was 62, which is lower than the average of the area even for the lowest socioeconomic groups, and none of them scored higher than 76. Figure 15 shows the results of the Gessel test. This figure clearly shows only one child of the whole group was able to reach the limits in all four areas: motor, adaptive, language, and personal-social. Of all the variables, language development was the most seriously affected. These results are fairly conclusive in showing that brain damage in infancy due to severe degree of malnutrition is permanent at least up to the sixth year of life, despite improving nutritional conditions. From these observations, it seems that the effects of early marasmus may be similar to those produced by certain congenital metabolic defects, such as phenylketoneuria, galactosemia.[84]

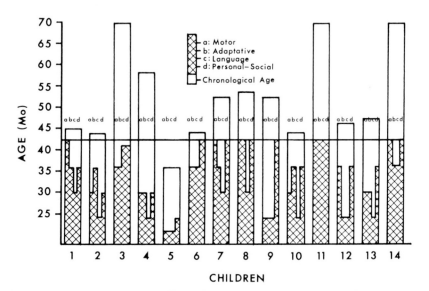

Figure 15. Gesell test of 14 malnourished children after nutritional recovery.[84]

The results of most of the studies appear to convince us that malnutrition in early life profoundly affects the mental development and intellectual functioning of the child; a word of caution may be necessary. Rosenthal [106] has made a big contribution in presenting a detailed discussion on the experimental effects in behavioral research and the effects of expectancy. Romney [105] described one of Rosenthal's experiments in which a group of children were given an I.Q. test, after which they were randomly arranged into two groups—experimental and control. Rosenthal treated the group in the following manner. He gave the experimental group to a teacher and told him, "I think these are the students who will learn more in this class," and three months later he gave the I.Q. test again. Now, those students who were not on the list gained an average of nine points, and those who were on the list gained about 18 to 20 points, which is one half of a standard deviation greater than the mean of the control group. This was a highly stable effect in the first grade, quite stable at the second and third grade levels, but no longer detectable during the fourth, fifth, and sixth grades. The implication of this is that in these experiments, serious thought must be given to the control groups to be sure that they don't, in fact, come up with an artifact due to simple experimenter expectancy.

The malnourished animals, like the humans, fail to achieve simple developmental landmarks and exhibit pronounced deficits in their learning ability. The results of a few important studies show that baby pigs weaned at three months and subsequently fed a diet containing 3% protein for a period of 8 weeks showed signs similar to those observed in cases of human kwashiorkor.[55,56] Experimental work on rats over a period of two generations has been carried out by Cowley and Griesel [27,29] with respect to their prenatal and postnatal effects and emotionality. The rats fed on low-protein diets were mated with normal males by these workers and the mother and the progeny maintained on low-protein diets. These authors concluded that

> A low protein diet fed to one generation of rats affects the growth and development of the next generation; this seems to be due, at least in part, to a deficiency in the nutrients received from the mother during the fetal period. In rehabilitating low protein rats more than

one generation may have to be fed on a high plane of nutrition
before all the effects of the low protein diet are overcome.

Experimental work on dogs also shows that the malnourished
bitches on reaching adulthood produce smaller and fewer pups
compared to the normal mothers, even if both the groups are
mated to healthy dogs. The pups of the malnourished mother
show more pronounced abnormalities and may even experience
convulsive seizures. The congenitally malnourished pups do not
ever recover completely, even if they are given diets of high
protein value from weaning onwards.[96] According to Platt and
Stewart,[96] the rehabilitated dogs in their adult life often have
short legs and always remain somewhat apprehensive and mix
less well than the normal dogs.

If the malnourished state is not severe enough, particularly
in the critical stages of brain growth which vary from species to
species, the undernourished animals in spite of developmental
retardation to some degree are able to undertake complex learning
tasks which may be considered in the normal range.[4,56] Stretching
these observations from the animal kingdom to the human, it
may be believed that most people who suffered mild, moderate,
or even somewhat severe degrees of undernutrition in their early
years do function within the normal range of complex human
learning behavior. In mice as well as pigs, several authors have
reported normal performance in undernourished and rehabilitated
animals with respect to visual discrimination learning,[6,67] which
warrants a conclusion that an undernourished state, where the
degree of malnutrition is not of a very severe degree, does not
affect adversely the complex learning behavior.

The effects of early malnutrition are much more pronounced in
the male as compared to the female. No logical explanation is
available at this time. The detailed studies of Frankova *et al.*[55,56]
on rats also showed that malnutrition affected the males and females in the same direction but to a lesser extent in the females.

NUTRITIONAL STATUS, MENTAL DEVELOPMENT, AND HEREDITY

Genetics and heredity play important roles in the personality,
behavioral development, and physiological makeup of an indi-

vidual. It also determines to a great extent an individual's or even a population's tolerance to the level of food that is made available for prolonged periods of time.[1] In those areas where food deficits are chronic and undernutrition is an accepted way of life over generations, the malnourished population probably has a more physiological tolerance, which is reinforced by their genetic make-up, compared to a population that has not been subjected to episodes of malnutrition. Although there is no confirmed proof, it is probable that there is genetically based variation in physiological adjustment which prevents so much mental damage in populations all over the world living on barely subsistent diets.

No one can deny that genetics plays some role in the determination of physical size as well as intellect, but there are certain limitations to this role. Probably genetics determines the upper limits that the individual can attain.[66] It is probably essential to have well-balanced nutrition and reasonably stimulating environment to reach this optimum growth potential. However, if any of these factors are detrimental, it will prevent the individual from fulfilling his genetic destiny. These days, there are only very rare instances where mental retardation can be traced to genetic causes, yet the institutions dealing with the mentally retarded are full and have more patients than they are equipped to handle.

Most of the children suffering from malnutrition, particularly in its severe form, come from homes where social and economic pressures are strong enough to restrict adequate stimulation for mental development. Studying the adaptive and motor behavior during rehabilitation from kwashiorkor, Cravioto and Robles[38] pointed out that the preschool children of the same age but having different nutritional states experience different motor development. Mönckeberg[84] concluded that "early malnutrition tends to restrict expression of the genetic potential for development, both physical and psychological. Socio-economic factors also strongly affect mental development and cannot be separated satisfactorily from nutritional influences."

Under experimental conditions, pigs born of healthy mothers but given low-protein diets from the second and third weeks of age are listless, apathetic, and show behavioral abnormalities, such as disturbed gait and incoordinated movements of the hind legs.[95] Barnes *et al.*[6] found in such malnourished pigs a relatively poor ability in coordinated avoidance procedures. Investigating the long-term effects of protein or protein-calorie malnutrition, the experimental evidence clearly suggests that the effects are transferred to the next generation. They produce smaller-sized offsprings, comparable to human "small for date" babies, which show emotional deficiencies and retarded intelligence. Such an effect is carried on through the next generation as well.[25-28] Generation after generation of undernutrition and malnutrition would also markedly affect these social and economic groups of people and may predispose their children genetically to lesser levels of mental performance. Some important studies on the state of development or motor and adaptive behavior of the full-term and prematurely born neonates have been carried out in Africa and South America.[36,41,58] These studies show strong evidence of motor precocity and adaptive organization when taking the United States' standards as control values.

It may be an interesting observation that the effects of over-nutrition may be similar to those of undernutrition [112,113] and may be due to delayed neuromotor development.[54] It is possible that "in the overnourished animals, motor development does not keep pace with abnormal body weight increases." [100]

INTERACTION OF MALNUTRITION AND THE SURROUNDING ENVIRONMENT

If undernutrition were to affect the psychomotor growth as prominently as the physical growth, it will be easy to account for the backwardness of underprivileged people living in the culture of poverty, but it is dangerous to simplify this problem in these terms. To date it has been very difficult to differentiate between the effects of malnutrition and those of genetic endowment, social status, parental care, or a combination of these factors. Child raising practices and levels of parental care could significantly influence the nutritional status as well as the psychological development. Children from homes where parental care is deficient may show a conspicuous lack of motivation and resourcefulness so necessary to make up one's genetic potential. The absence of these qualities could result in a major loss of learning time, which may not be compensated for in later life.

> Children at high risk of malnutrition tend to cluster in the lowest social and economic segment of the population, and the fact that these segments tend also to have poor housing, higher infection rates, lower levels of educational achievement, greater degrees of attachment to traditional pattern of child care, and in general live in circumstances which are less conducive for the development of technologic and educational competence.[33]

A number of longitudinal studies have been carried out keeping the environmental factors almost constant in the experimental and control groups (although it is virtually impossible because during rehabilitation the experimenter inadvertently enriches the environment along with better food and sanitary conditions). All these studies, whether they are in the area of intersensory integrative competence or strict behavioral development or intellectual performance, point towards deficits in their development and incomplete recovery on nutritional rehabilitation.* Similar conclusions have been arrived at on experimental animals, and the reader is referred to the extensive work of Barnes and his collaborators.[2,4,6] Some important studies have been conducted recently in which a serious attempt has been made to control the environmental factors. Such studies are bringing to light more and more convincing evidence that severe malnutrition during the first year of life makes a definite contribution to a long-lasting retardation in mental development.[2] At the same time, the classical work of Skeels [116,117] in orphanages has proved that given adequate nutrition, poor environmental conditions alone are sufficient to produce mental retardation. From other studies, it is becoming apparent that there are many similarities between long-term effects that are due to environmental or social deprivations and those that are due to early nutrition deprivations.[3] It is the apathy caused either by nutritional abuse or by the environmental deprivation that makes a child disinterested in his environments. It makes it difficult for him to learn in the classroom and makes it difficult for him to acquire the substance of his culture that

---

* See references 14, 35, 38, 42, 43, 46, 47, 52, 61, 110

puts him on a behavioral plane from which he cannot profit through casual observation and learning opportunities that are offered to him in the course of daily life.[10] The impact of environmental influences on human development will be discussed in some detail in the next chapter. It is becoming more and more apparent, however, that there are many similarities between long-term effects that are due to environmental or social deprivations and those due to early nutritional deprivations.[3] Malnutrition alone or poor environment alone cannot produce the picture often observed in mentally retarded human children, and the battle to end this human misery cannot be successfully waged without an understanding of the right perspective.

SHORT-TERM AND LONG-TERM EFFECTS OF MALNUTRITION

Malnutrition and Nature of Injury to the Nervous System

It is hard at this stage to comment with a degree of certainty on the nature of changes brought about by nutritional deprivation, whether they be of a temporary nature or their effects leave some permanent scars on the personality of the individual even after rehabilitation. The point can be forcefully argued both ways and a lot of multidisciplinary research work is needed in this area. Nutritionists, psychologists, biochemists, clinicians, and investigators from other medical fields have to integrate their findings so that a whole picture may emerge, and at the same time, the effects of a particular manipulation (nutritional or environmental) may be singled out.

We must turn our attention to the time and duration in life at which a severe episode of malnutrition develops, in order to judge the nature of the injury. The earlier in life the malnutrition begins, the most lasting are the consequences. A number of studies have suggested a strong association between the age of onset of malnutrition and the persistence of the residual effects on mental performance.[7,117a,b] Cravioto and Robles [37,38] believed that the rate of recovery between 15 and 41 months of age greatly depends on the severity of malnutrition and the initial lag in mental development in infancy. It is evident that a large number of brain constituents show a high degree of metabolic stability, and once laid down during the period of maximum brain growth, many of the components of the nervous system persist there throughout life.[45,47a,b,c] According to Dobbing [45]

> Since most of the metabolically stable material resides in the myelin
> sheaths, which form a large proportion of the dry weight of the tissue,
> the apparent 'sparing' of the brain by undernutrition could be largely
> due to the resistance of such material to any form of change. If this be
> so, it will be only during the period when myelin constituents are
> being actively synthesized within the brain at the time of its maximum
> growth, that they are likely to be susceptible to undernutrition, and it
> may be, that comparatively small restriction at this time could have
> quite large effects that could even be permanent.

This observation has been challenged by Donald Cheek,[19] who doubts if clear cut evidence has been presented that prenatal or early postnatal protein deficiency can permanently damage the intelligence, particularly if adequate nutrition is given at a later date. This is a little bit too early to pass judgments on either side of the argument, particularly in view of the fact that in human situations it is rare to find a simple case of protein malnutrition without other accompanying factors, such as poor sociocultural environment, infections, hypoxia.

The mental and motor performance of infants who had suffered from marasmus in the early infancy, but were rehabilitated before two years of age, were compared to siblings of similar age, but who did not have any serious medical history of illness. It was found in this study [67] that, "17 of the 19 children who had been malnourished had severe mental and motor retardation despite apparent somatic recovery. In these infants, the lag in many test items was equivalent to eight or more months of life." [33] A similar study in Indonesia to evaluate the mental development in relation to early malnutrition using Goodenough and Wechsler techniques was undertaken on five to 12-year-old children by Pek *et al.*[93] These workers found that the children who had nutritionally suffered between two and four years showed significantly low intelligence scores compared to those who were healthy during this period. Cravioto *et al.*[34] also undertook a detailed study of the mental performance of school children who suffered from some degree of protein-calorie malnutrition in their early preschool years. Siblings of similar socioeconomic groups who did not show any apparent malnutrition syndrome in the corresponding ages were selected as controls. A familiar pattern of conclusions emerged from these detailed investigations. The children malnourished in their early years consistently scored low in a number of psychological tests, e.g. Wechsler Intelligence Scale for children, recognition of geometric forms, analysis of forms, auditory-visual integrative ability. The intersensory development and the auditory-visual integrative abilities of these children are markedly reduced.[11] Cravioto and other investigators have made remarkable contribution to the understanding of neuro-integrative abilities of the children who suffer from protein malnutrition in their critical preschool years.[11a,33a] Cravioto [33] concluded that "mental retardation could occur at mild to moderate degrees of protein-calorie malnutrition associated with stunted growth and is not limited to the extremely severe cases represented by kwashiorkor and marasmus." On the basis of results obtained from a number of studies, Cravioto firmly believed that

> the existence of an association between protein-calorie malnutrition in infancy and retardation in mental development has been established beyond reasonable doubt. It can also be stated that there is a high probability that this lag in mental development may have long lasting consequences if severe malnutrition is experienced at a very early age in the life of the child.

A very interesting observation has been recorded by Rajalakshmi and her associates.[100] A clear explanation of it is not possible at this time nor has one been given by the authors. The glutamic acid seems to have a beneficial effect on the intellectual functioning of the mentally retarded children and appears to correct the deficiences of cerebral enzymes.

Is the Physical and Mental Injury Reversible?

It is extremely difficult to find a satisfactory answer to this tricky question on the reversibility or irreversibility of the effects of nutritional deprivations in early childhood. Observational and experimental data reveal that the children who suffer from severe malnutrition earlier than six months are the ones who do not improve on serial testing even after 220 days of treatment. This is in contrast to the older group of the same socioeconomic classes who were admitted to the hospital at a later date. The recovery of these children in terms of response to the same testing procedure as described above is much more satisfactory. The latter increased their I.Q.s significantly with rehabilitation. The timing of malnutrition, rather than the nutritional state, may be of greater importance in determining whether or not the deleterious effects of malnutrition are reversible.[76,129] Early malnutrition, if it is allowed to effect neuronal development, may overcome the partial resistance of the central nervous system, impair its growth, and result in permanent intellectual damage which cannot be readjusted in later life.[16] There is clear evidence that the malnourished children may never catch up with the other children in intelligence.[84]

The rehabilitated children who suffered earlier from kwashiorkor are at best marginal cases that have recovered from the consequences of nutritional inadequacies. A number of studies based on intelligence tests have been carried out by a number of workers.[89-92] The items chosen to test the mental ability include, besides the conventional procedures, reasoning, organization of knowledge, memory, different perceptual processes, comprehension, and arithmetic tests. Considerable difference was observed in the youngest age groups. The results showed that the experimental children were more retarded in their perceptual and abstract ability than in their memory and verbal ability. The experimental children also scored more poorly in their performance of the intersensory tests than did the control children. Their errors were most marked in the visual-heptic test.[92] Chandra[18] rightly stressed the importance of prolonged longitudinal studies of the children who suffer from kwashiorkor in order to obtain meaningful data and the relationship of malnutrition to mental development. It is only through longitudinal studies that an insight into the question of reversibility of mental handicaps caused by malnutrition can be obtained. It is extremely important to know whether a complete recovery follows the restoration of an adequate diet.[44] Dickerson *et al.*[44] observed that in the rehabilitated pigs, a three and one-half-year-old animal was the equivalent of a normal two-year-old with respect to the brain as this was accompanied by a significant deficit in the concentration of cholesterol. Barnes and associates [4] suggested that a permanent injury to the nervous system or mental development ensued if the animals were subjected to severe preweaning and postweaning deficiences. Novakova [86-88] stressed the importance of disturbed emotionality as well as behavioral abnormalities under the impact of early deprivation. According to Novakova, even if nutritional deprivation does not affect the physical or mental development of the brain at a later date, early deprivation could leave permanent scars on the personality which affects the general attitude, emotionality, and behavioral pattern.

Human personality is a complex entity and may not be affected by one simple variable. Permanent psychological or mental retardation is a result of a number of complex factors, which vary in degree and intensity from person to person depending on the geographical location and circumstances. But very seldom has permanent mental retardation been observed where only one factor was evident. Some reports stressing the permanent nature of injury to mental functioning because of malnutrition in early life, fail to mention the other factors in detail except for a brief mention that the subjects belong to the lower socioeconomic strata of that society. Nor is any mention made of the psychological makeup of the mother, her background, and her ability to mother the child effectively. Rajalakshmi and Ramakrishnan [100] cited an example of two Chinese girls who suffered from a severe degree of malnutrition in their early childhood. These girls were adopted by a Dutch physician who provided not only good food but also a stimulating environment, giving the children a sense of security and belongingness. At present, these girls are having highly successful careers in Holland.

These studies make it extremely difficult to arrive at any firm conclusion regarding the nature of the injury to the nervous system attributable to the effect of malnutrition in early life. The author, in collaboration with Dr. Z. Olkowski, has a research project in progress, in which under controlled experimental conditions the effects of simple protein deficiency on the nervous system during the prenatal, postnatal, and prenatal-postnatal life of subhuman primates are being studied. These primates, being taxonomically closer to humans, may provide some meaningful data. There are some very important questions to be asked. First of all, what is the role that undernutrition or malnutrition plays in mental development? And secondly, what is the level of malnutrition at which the nervous system is functionally effected.[103] Are we more concerned with extreme degrees of malnutrition in early infancy, preschool years, and adolescent life or mild to moderate forms of chronic malnutrition which afflict more than 60 percent of children in the underdeveloped world containing two thirds of the world population? The experimental studies are also important in isolating the effects of nutritional manipulation from those of environmental manipulation on the physiology and biochemistry of the nervous system. The behavioral pattern of the subhuman primates, although not as complex as humans, may provide a better opportunity to extrapolate the results to humans in a somewhat more meaningful manner. In the author's opinion, every feasible method should be applied to save the future generations from unnecessary mental and functional retardation.

NEED FOR COMPREHENSIVE RESEARCH

Need for Culture Free Testing

It is an extremely difficult matter to pass judgments on the effects of malnutrition on mental development by administering certain tests that are not only insensitive but are not culture free. More sensitive mental tests need to be devised which could be conveniently modified to suit particular populations and sufficiently sensitive to differentiate between well-nourished and poorly nourished populations. These tests "must give full consideration to socio-cultural patterns of the population, such as parental expectations, early influences, child rearing practices, social stimulation, system of values, and others of lesser importance." [15] Cultural variation in different populations always poses a difficult problem for the scientists eager to find the impact of either nutrition or environment on the mental capacity or learning ability. Vernon [125] pointed out that so far there is no unbiased test which could compare the mental development or learning ability of populations which are widely different culturally as well as nutritionally.

Most of the testing devices used in the measurement of I.Q. scores are oriented towards the Western culture, and it is extremely hard to modify them to make them culture free for use in other cultures, especially the Eastern and African ones. Furthermore, the intelligence tests are reliable in a sense of getting scores and measurements of an individual's function and are highly dependent on a program of formal schooling, which is always imparted in a culturally defined manner. In a study of the lower class and upper class children in Central America with respect to three sensory systems, i.e. touch, vision and kinesthesis, Cravioto [31,32] noted that the upperclass urban children proved to be significantly more advanced than the rural children in intersensory integrative abilities.

It has been emphasized that the available tools for testing the mental development or intellectual capacity with certain variables are far from satisfactory.[17] New suitable tests need to be devised which should take into consideration not only the cultural differences but also regional-linguistic variations, rural-urban differences, and differences in the level of literacy and education. The necessity to devise methods to test the I.Q.s of populations in an objective manner is being felt more and more as we gain a better understanding and appreciation of the role played by environmental factors with or without the deleterious effects of malnutrition. The I.Q. tests at present work to the disadvantage of the poor population because they are set to the standards of the middle classes. By these standards, the poor populations are implicated in having a very large number of mentally retarded persons. Also the present tests fail to give proper recognition to the environmental causes of retardation.[2]

Need for Prolonged Longitudinal Studies

Since mental development in a human society is not determined by malnutrition alone but by a complex set of environmental situation aggravated by poor diets, the effect on the central nervous systems because of severe nutritional deficiency can be determined only by prospective, longitudinal, ecologically oriented study of children at risk with appropriately selected control subjects.[34] This is particularly true when one wishes to assess the consequences of the early nutritional deprivation on the mental development or intellectual ability of the person in question. A proper assessment of the impairment of the functions may not be possible at the time of the dietary insult because of other accompanying factors under which the child is raised, such as sickness caused by various infections or apathy caused by depressed social circumstances. Cravioto [33] emphasized that the importance of longitudinal studies

> relates not only to their possibilities of providing an answer to the important question of impairment of mental competence by malnutrition; the identification of the underlying patterns of psychological malfunctioning due to infection, and to social disadvantage could make possible anticipation of children's developmental courses and help to establish curricular and other educational opportunities which will result in optimal progress.

CONCLUSIONS AND PERSPECTIVES

Undernutrition during infancy not only retards physical and morphological brain growth but also predisposes the individual to attain less than optimum level of intellectual functioning and personality development. For a great majority of children in the underdeveloped world, retardation of physical growth as a result of undernutrition and further degradation of physical and mental health due to recurrent infections because of unsanitary surroundings, is a fact of existence. Coincidentally, this is also the area which is overpopulated with more than two thirds of the human population. The effects of malnutrition on the performance of the individual are generally a result of interference in the normal process of brain development during its peak period of growth, which results in permanent reduction of brain size and defective intellectual development. They may also operate indirectly through (1) loss of learning time, (2) interference with learning during critical periods of development, or (3) through changes in the individual's motivation and personality.[23] The field of the relationship of nutrition to central nervous system development and intellectual achievement is full of potentialities. There is enormous scope for work on the incidence, the extent, and reversibility of mental handicap caused by malnutrition.[18]

There is overwhelming evidence that severe malnutrition during the early years of life, especially the first two years, leads to retarded brain growth, permanent reduction in brain size, and defective intellectual development. Malnutrition has, therefore, been rightly blamed as one of the main causes of mental retardation.[30] The marasmic condition may have more deleterious effects on the mental development and learning potentialities than the kwashiorkor. There are good reasons for such a conclusion. Marasmus develops in the early period, generally before one year of age, and this is the time when the brain is still growing and needs adequate nutrition to grow to the optimum size. During this period, nutritional deprivation leads to drastic morphological and biochemical changes in the brain which are responsible for retarded mental development. Experiments on animals also show that malnutrition during the period of optimal growth leaves permanent marks on intellectual functioning. Such a deficit may never be overcome, even on dietary rehabilitation. Kwashiorkor, on the other hand, develops in the second and third year of life, when brain growth is less active. Scrimshaw and Gordon [113] pointed out that a combination of early marasmus and kwashiorkor in the later years would have the most devastating results in producing permanent brain damage and corresponding mental retardation. In most instances, however, such children do not survive. Trowell *et al.*[123] as early as 1954 pointed out that nothing is known about the completeness of recovery from severe kwashiorkor, and despite the enormous amount of literature, this is still true, especially in the area of mental development. Attention may be drawn to the reports on the inability of the rehabilitated children to learn a language as well as the matched controls.[14] Factors affecting the eventual "intelligence" are manifold and interacting, and no one factor could be singled out. Malnutrition during periods of brain growth could damage the physical and biochemical character of the brain, but poor environment during the same period or later in life could lead to psychological impairment, which in the end has the same impact on the individual intellectual capacity. Coursin [24] described it in an excellent manner:

> the integral roles of nutrition in the biochemistry of the brain with its physiologic function and clinical performance are gradually becoming better understood. New concepts of the molecular basis of intelligence, learning, memory and behavior are being formulated to provide a framework for operation of these complex interrelationships. It is apparent that the intimate involvement of nutrition in these mechanisms makes it important both as an experimental and therapeutic tool.

For a better understanding of the subject, it may be appropriate here to reiterate the conclusions arrived at by two prominent workers after their detailed studies for over a decade on the association of nutritional and mental development and the effect of malnutrition on behavioral patterns. Richardson [102] pointed out that

> (1) for a population of underprivileged children, measurements are obtained of size and mental functioning. A positive association is found between smaller size and poorer mental functioning. (2) There is evidence that children who live in environments in which nutrition is poor are smaller than children who live in areas in which it is good. It is then inferred that differences in height- and weight-for-age within the population studied reflect differences in nutrition. (3) The positive association between size and mental ability is then restated as an association between level of early nutrition and later mental ability.
> (4) A casual relationship is then inferred between poor nutrition and impaired mental ability.

Barnes [2] put more forcefully the relationship between malnutrition and mental development and arrived at the following conclusions:

> First, it is probable that severe protein-caloric malnutrition in the infant can have long-lasting effects upon behavioral development. Retarded intellectual development can be one of the characteristics affected by this early, severe malnutrition. Second, malnutrition of the very severe type just mentioned is only rarely seen in the United States and at this time there is no basis for attempting to predict the possible consequences to mental development of the milder conditions of poor nutrition that are prevalent in our country. Third, it is probable that the behavioral changes that will be most prominent in individuals who were severely malnourished in early life will reflect

changes in emotionality and elevated response levels to aversive stimuli. Fourth, behavioral changes seen in animals that were malnourished in early life appear to be identical to the changes that result from early social isolation. Social and nutritional deprivations undoubtedly interact so as to modify the resulting behavioral characteristics. Therefore, it would seem highly inappropriate to introduce a type of intervention that would attempt to correct one form of deprivation but not the other.

Overeating produces results not dissimilar from undernutrition. It is a fact that the human systems are not built to function efficiently in a state of chronic undernutrition, nor do they thrive on a perpetual state of overnutrition. So far, there is no experimental evidence that overnutrition affects the intellectual development and growth, although some workers have strong suspicions about it. Suchman [122] emphasized that if the underdeveloped countries are nutritionally deprived, the affluent ones are nutritionally depraved. Overnutrition and consequent obesity are a major cause of a number of metabolic diseases, and an association between too much of a good thing (meats, eggs, and butter) and cardiovascular disorders is well established.

A better and deeper knowledge of the relationship between malnutrition (undernutrition or overnutrition in certain nutrients accompanied by lack of other nutrients) in early life and mental development is needed before we can blame dietary abuse as the main villain in retarding intellectual functioning of the infants, and this should form the basis of action to remedy the situation. Once the process of brain involvement and function in relation to nutrition is precisely understood, it may even be possible to increase the normal accepted levels of ability in humans. The presentation of Lat *et al.*,[77] Frankova,[53,54] and Novakova [86,87] point out that it is experimentally possible. Coursin [24] remarked that "the progressive increase in the rate of maturation, physical size and performance seen in man during the past several generations has been impressive and may well be indicative of coincidental advances in his central nervous system."

REFERENCES

1. Allen, G.: In N. S. Scrimshaw and J. E. Gordon (Eds.) : *Nutrition, Learning and Behavior.* Cambridge, MIT Press (1968) .

2. Barnes, R. H.: *Fed. Proc., 30:*1929 (1971).
3. Barnes, R. H.: Personal Communication.
4. Barnes, R. H., Cunnold, S. R., Zimmerman, R. R., *et al.: J. Nutr., 89:* 399 (1966).
5. Barnes, R. H., Moore, A. U., Reid, I. M., and Pond, W. G.: *J. Am. Diet. Assoc., 51:*34 (1967).
6. Barnes, R. H., Neely, C. S., Kwamp, E., Labadan, B. A., and Frankova, S.: *J. Nutr., 96:*467 (1968).
7. Barnes, R. H., Moore, A. V., Reid, I. M., and Pond, W. G.: In N. S. Scrimshaw and J. E. Gordon (Eds.): *Malnutrition, Learning and Behavior.* Cambridge, MIT Press (1968).
8. Bennett, E. L., Rosenzweig, M. R., and Diamond, M. C.: *Science, 163:* 825 (1969).
9. Benton, J. W., Moser, H. W., Dodge, P. R., and Carr, S.: *Pediatrics, 38:*801 (1966).
10. Birch, H. G.: In N. S. Scrimshaw and J. E. Gordon (Eds.): *Malnutrition, Learning and Behavior.* Cambridge, MIT Press (1968).
11. Birch, H. G. and Cravioto, J.: PHS Publication 1692, Washington, D. C. (1968).
11a. Brockman, L. M. and Ricciuti, H. N.: *Develop. Psychol., 4:*312 (1971).
12. Brown, R. E.: *East Afr. Med. J., 42:*584 (1965).
13. Brozek, J. and Vaes, A.: *Vitam. Horm. 19:*43 (1961).
14. Cabak, V. and Najdanvic, R.: *Arch. Dis. Child. 40:*532 (1965).
15. Canosa, C. A.: In N. S. Scrimshaw and J. E. Gordon (Eds.): *Malnutrition, Learning and Behavior.* Cambridge, MIT Press (1968).
16. Carothers, J. C.: *The African Mind in Health & Disease.* W.H.O. Monograph Series (1953).
17. Champakam, M. A., Srikantia, S. G., and Gopalan, C.: *Am. J. Clin. Nutr., 21:*844–852 (1968).
18. Chandra, C.: *Indian J. Pediatr., 35:*70 (1968).
19. Cheek, D.: Medical Tribune Report, May 1971.
20. Chow, B. F., Blackwell, R. Q., and Sherwin, R. W.: *Borden's Rev. Nutr., Res., 29:*26 (1968).
21. Chow, B. and Lee, C. J.: *J. Nutr., 82:*10 (1964).
22. Conference on Early Nutritional and Environmental Influences upon Behavioral Development, Co-Sponsored by U. S. Dept. of Agriculture and Battelle Memorial Research Institute, December 6, 7, 1971, Seattle, Washington.
23. Coursin, D. B.: *Fed. Proc., 26:*134 (1967).
24. Coursin, D. B.: In M. G. Wohl and R. S. Goodhart (Eds.): *Modern Nutrition in Health and Disease.* Philadelphia, Lea & Febiger (1968).
25. Cowley, J. J. and Criesel, R. D.: *J. Genet Psychol., 95:*187–201 (1959).
26. Cowley, J. J. and Criesel, R. D.: *Psych. Afr., 9:*216 (1961).

27. Cowley, J. J. and Griesel, R. D.: *J. Genet. Psychol., 103:*233 (1963).
28. Cowley, J. J. and Griesel, R. D.: *J. Genet. Pshchol., 104:*89–98 (1964).
29. Cowley, J. J. and Griesel, R. D.: *Anim. Behav., 14:*506–517 (1966).
30. Crane, L. C. and Stern, J.: *Pathology of Mental Retardation.* London, Churchill (1967).
31. Cravioto, J.: *Am. J. Clin. Nutr., 11:*484–492 (1962).
32. Cravioto, J.: In *Pre-school Child Malnutrition:* NAS–NRC Publ. 1282, Washington, Academy of Science (1966).
33. Cravioto, J.: In P. Gyorgy and O. L. Kline (Eds.): *Malnutrition is a Problem of Ecology.* Basel, S. Karger (1970).
33a. Cravioto, J.: Paper delivered at Int Cong. National Development on Planning. Cambridge, Mass. Oct., (1971).
34. Cravioto, J. and Delicardie, E. R.: In N. S. Scrimshaw and J. E. Gordon (Eds.): *Malnutrition, Learning and Behavior.* Cambridge, MIT Press, (1968).
35. Cravioto, J., Delicardie, E. R., and Birch, H. G.: *Pediatrics, 38* (2):319 (1966).
36. Cravioto, J., Delicardie, E. R., Montiel, R., and Birch, H. G.: *Biol. Neonate, 11:*151 (1967).
37. Cravioto, J. and DeLicardie, E. R.: In N. S. Scrimshaw and J. E. Gordon (Eds.). *Malnutrition, Learning and Behavior.* Cambridge, MIT Press (1968).
38. Cravioto, J. and Robles, B.: *Am. J. Orthopsychiatry, 35:*449–464. (1965).
39. Culley, W. and Mertz, E.: *Fed. Proc., 25:*674 (1966).
40. Dean, R. F. A.: *Modern Problem of Pediatrics.* Basel, S. Karger (1960), Vol. 5.
41. Delicardie, E. R., Birch, H. G., and Cravioto, J.: Proceedings Reunion Reglamentaris Asociacian de Investigacias Pediatrica, Cuautha, Mor. (1966).
42. Dickerson, J. W. T. and Dobbing, J.: *Proc. R. Soc. Lond., 166B:*384–395 (1967a).
43. Dickerson, J. W. T. and Dobbing, J.: *Proc. Nutr. Soc. 26:*5 (1967b).
44. Dickerson, J. W. T. and Jarvis, J.: *Proc. Nutr. Soc., 27:*4A–5A (1970).
45. Dobbing, J.: Medical Tribune Report, May 2, 1966.
46. Dobbing, J.: In N. S. Scrimshaw and J. E. Gordon (Eds.): *Malnutrition, Learning and Behavior.* Cambridge, MIT Press (1968).
47. Dobbing, J.: Personal communication quoted by Drillien (1970).
47a. Dobbing, J.: In *Handbook of Neurochemistry,* A. Lajtha (ed.) New York, Plenum Press, (1971).
47b. Dobbing, J. and Sands, J.: *Brain Res. 17:*115 (1970).
47c. Dobbing, J. and Sands, J.: *Nature* (Lond.) *226:*639 (1970).
48. Dobbing, J. and Widdowson, E.: *Brain, 88:*357 (1965).

49. Edozien, J. C.: In P. Gyorgy and O. L. Kline (Eds.) : *Malnutrition in a Problem of Ecology.* Basel, S. Karger (1970) .
50. Eichenwald, H. P. and Fry, P. C.: *Science, 163*:644 (1969) .
50a. Elias, M. F.: *Behavioral consequences of malnutrition in infancy: A review of human studies.* Personal communication (1972) .
51. Flexner, J. B., Flexner, L. B., dela Haba, G., and Roberts, R. B.: *J. Neurochem., 12*:535 (1965) .
52. Fox, M. W.: *Brain Res., 2*:3–20 (1966) .
53. Frankova, S.: Proceedings VII International Congress of Nutrition, Hamburg, Germany (1966) .
54. Frankova, S.: In N. S. Scrimshaw and J. E. Gordon (Eds.) : *Malnutrition, Learning and Behavior.* Cambridge, MIT Press (1968) .
55. Frankova, S. and Barnes, R. H.: *J. Nutr., 96*:477 (1968a) .
56. Frankova, S. and Barnes, R. H.: *J Nutr., 96*:485 (1968b) .
56a. Frisch, R. E.: *Am. J. Clin. Nutr., 23*:189 (1970) .
57. Garrow, J. S.: *Lancet, 2*:643–645 (1967) .
58. Geber, M. and Dean, R. F. A.: *Pediatrics, 20*:1055 (1957) .
59. Gounelle, H.: In N. S. Scrimshaw and J. E. Gordon (Eds.) : *Malnutrition, Learning and Behavior.* Cambridge, MIT Press (1968) .
60. Gounelle, H. and Marche, J.: *Occup. Med., 1*:48 (1946) .
61. Graham, G. G.: *Fed. Proc., 26*:139–143 (1967) .
62. Graham, G. G., Cordano, A., Baertl, J. M., Morales, E.: In *Preschool Child Malnutrition: Primary Deterrent to Human Progress.* Washington National Academy of Sciences (1966) .
63. Guthrie, H. A.: *Physiol. Behav. 3*:619 (1968) .
64. Guthrie, H. A. and Brown, M. L.: *J. Nutr., 94*:419 (1968) .
65. Guzman, M. A.: In N. S. Scrimshaw and J. E. Gordon (Eds.) : *Malnutrition, Learning and Behavior.* Cambridge, MIT Press (1968) .
66. Holley, W. L., Rosenbaum, A. L., and Churchill, J. A.: Proceedings of Pan-American Health Organization (1969) .
67. Howard, E. and Granoff, D. M.: *J. Nutr., 95*:111 (1968) .
68. *Hunger is a Problem.* Agricultural Marketing, Washington, USA Consumer and Marketing Service (1969) , vol. 14, p. 3.
69. Insull, W., Oiso, T., and Tsuchiya, K.: *Am. J. Clin. Nutr., 21*:753 (1968) .
70. Jelliffe, D. B.: In P. Gyorgy and O. L. Kline (Eds.) : *Malnutrition is a Problem of Ecology.* Basel and New York S. Karger (1970) .
71. Jelliffe, D. B. and Jelliffe, E. F. P.: In N. S. Scrimshaw and J. E. Gordon (Eds.) : *Malnutrition, Learning and Behavior.* Cambridge, MIT Press (1968) .
72. Kahn, E.: *Arch. Dis. Child., 29*:256–261 (1954) .
73. Hahn, E.: *Cent. Afr. J. Med., 3*:398–400 (1957) .
74. Kahn, E. and Falcke, H. C.: *J. Pediatr. 49*:37–45 (1956) .
74a. Kallen, D. J.: JAMA *215*:94 (1971) .

75. Keys, A., Brozek, J. Henschel, A., *et al.: The Biology of Human Starvation*. Minneapolis, Minnesota Press (1950), vols. 1 and 2.
76. Kugelmass, I. N., Poull, L. E., and Samuel, E. L.: *Am. J. Med. Sci., 208*:631 (1944).
77. Lat, J., Widdowson, E. M., and McCance, R. A.: *Proc. R. Soc. Lond., 153*:347 (1960).
78. Livingston, S. K.: *J. Nutr. Educ. 3*:18 (1971).
79. Lowe, C. U.: Committee of Nutrition of American Academy of Pediatrics. Before the Committee on Agriculture, House of Representatives (1969).
80. Lowenburg, M. E., Todhunter, E. N., Wilson, E. D., Feeney, N. C., and Savage, J. R.: *Food and Man*. New York, John Wiley & Sons (1968).
81. Scrimshaw, N. S. and Gordon, J. E. (Eds.): *Malnutrition, Learning and Behavior*. Cambridge, MIT Press (1968).
82. McCance, R. A.: *Lancet, 2*:671 (1962).
83. Mitchell, H. S.: *J. Am. Diet. Assoc. 44*:165 (1964).
84. Mönckeberg, F.: In N. S. Scrimshaw and J. E. Gordon (Eds.): *Malnutrition, Learning and Behavior*. Cambridge, MIT Press (1968).
85. Myslivecek, J., Chaloupka, Z., Hassmannova, J., *et al.*: L. Jilek and S. Trojan (Eds.): *Onthogenesis of Brain*. Prague, Charles University (1968).
86. Novakova, V.: *Physiol. Behav., 1*:219 (1966a).
87. Novakova, V.: *Science, 171*:475–476 (1966b).
88. Novakova, V., Koldovsky, O., Hahn, P. and Krecek, J.: In *Health and Nutrition*. Proceedings VII International Congress of Nutrition, London, Pergamon Press (1967), vol. 1.
89. *Nutr. Rev., 23*:65 (1965).
90. *Nutr. Rev., 25*:334 (1967).
91. *Nutr. Rev., 26*:111 (1968).
92. *Nutr. Rev., 27*:46 (1969).
93. Pek, H. L., Tyook, T. H., Oery, H. J., and Lauw, T .G.: *Am. J. Clin. Nutr., 20*:1290 (1967).
94. Platt, B. S.: In J. Folch-Pi (Ed.): *Chemical Pathology of Nervous System*. London, Pergamon Press (1961).
95. Platt, B. S., Pampiglione, G., and Stewart, R. J. C.: *Dev. Med. Child. Neurol., 7*:9–26 (1965).
96. Platt, B. S. and Stewart, R. J. C.: *Dev. Med. Child. Neurol., 10*:3 (1968).
97. Rajalakshmi, R.: In N. S. Scrimshaw and J. E. Gordon (Eds.): *Malnutrition, Learning and Behavior*. Cambridge, MIT Press (1968).
98. Rajalakshmi, R., Ali, S. Z., and Ramakrishnan, C. V.: *J. Neurochem., 14*:29 (1967).

99. Rajalakshmi, R. and Ramakrishman, C. V.: *Nutrition, Learning Performance and Brain Biochemistry.* Terminal report of PL 480 project FG–In–176. Washington U. S. Dept. of Agriculture, (1969).
100. Rajalakshmi, R. and Ramakrishnan, C. V.: In G. H. Bourne (Ed.): *World Review Nutrition and Dietetics.* vol. 14. Basel, S. Karger (1971).
101. Read, M. S.: In P. Gyorgy and O. L. Kline (Eds.): *Malnutrition is a Problem of Ecology.* Basel, S. Karger (1970).
102. Richardson, S. A.: In N. S. Scrimshaw and J. E. Gordon (Eds.): *Malnutrition, Learning and Behavior.* Cambridge, MIT Press (1968).
103. Riecken, H. W.: In N. S. Scrimshaw and J. E. Gordon (Eds.): *Malnutrition, Learning and Behavior.* Cambridge, MIT Press (1968).
104. Robles, B., Cravioto, J. Rivera, L., *et al.*: Reunion Mexican Society for Pediatric Research, Cuernavaca, Mor. (1959).
105. Romney, A. K.: In N. S. Scrimshaw and J. E. Gordon (Eds.): *Malnutrition, Learning and Behavior.* Cambridge, MIT Press (1968).
106. Rosenthal, R.: *Experimental Effects in Behavioral Research.* New York, Appleton-Century-Crafts (1966).
107. Schreider, E.: *Biotypologie, 17:*21–37 (1956).
108. Scott, J. A.: *Br. J. Proc. Soc. Med., 16:*165–173 (1962).
109. Scott, J. P.: *Soc. Res. Child Dev., 28:*1 (1963).
110. Scott, J. P.: *Am. Rev. Psychol., 18:*1–40 (1967).
111. Scott, E. M., Illsley, R., and Thomson, A. R.: *J. Obstet. Gynaecol. Br. Commonw., 63:*338–343 (1956).
112. Scrimshaw, N. S.: In N. S. Scrimshaw and J. E. Gordon (Eds.): *Malnutrition, Learning and Behavior.* Cambridge, MIT Press (1968).
113. Scrimshaw, N. S. and Gordon, J. E. (Eds.): *Malnutrition, Learning and Behavior.* Cambridge, MIT Press (1968).
114. Seitz, P. F. D.: *Am. J. Psychiatry, 110:*916 (1954).
115. Simonson, M., Sherwin, R. W., Anilane, J. K., Jw, W. Y., and Chow, B. F.: *J. Nutr., 98:*18 (1969).
116. Skeels, H. M.: *Child Dev., 31:*3 (1966).
117. Skeels, H. M., Updegraff, R., Wellman, B. L., and Williams, H. M.: *Univ. Iowa Studies in Child Welfare, 15:*10 (1938).
117a. Smart, J. L. *Psychiatr Neurol Neurochir, 74:*443 (1971).
117b. Smart, J. L. and Dobbing, J. *Brain Res. 33:*303 (1971).
118. Stewart, R. J. C. and Platt, B. S.: In N. S. Scrimshaw and J. E. Gordon (Eds.): *Malnutrition, Learning and Behavior.* Cambridge, MIT Press (1968).
119. Stoch, M. B. and Smythe, P. M.: *Arch. Dis. Child., 38:*546 (1963).
120. Stoch, M. B. and Smythe, P. M.: *S. Afr. Med. J., 41:*1027–1030 (1967).
121. Stoch, M. B. and Smythe, P. M.: In N. S. Scrimshaw and J. E. Gordon (Eds.): *Malnutrition, Learning and Behavior.* Cambridge, MIT Press (1968).

122. Suchman, E. A.: In N. S. Scrimshaw and J. E. Gordon (Eds.) : *Malnutrition, Learning and Behavior.* Cambridge, MIT Press (1968).
123. Trowell, H. C., Davies, J. N. P., and Dean, R. F. A.: *Kwashiorkor.* London, Arnold (1954).
124. Udani, P. M.: *Indian J. Child. Health, 11:*498–501 (1962).
125. Vernon, P. E.: In N. S. Scrimshaw and J. E. Gordon (Eds.) : *Malnutrition, Learning and Behavior.* Cambridge, MIT Press (1968).
126. Wayburne, S.: In R. A. McCance and E. M. Widdowson (Eds.) : *Calorie Deficiencies and Protein Deficiencies.,* Boston, Little, Brown and Company (1968).
127. Wiener, G.: *J. Spec. Ed., 2:*237 (1968).
128. Winick, M.: *Pediatr. Res. 2:*352 (1968).
129. Winick, M.: *Med. Clin. North Am., 54:*1413 (1970).
130. Winick, M. and Noble, A.: *J. Nutr., 89:*300 (1966).
130a. Yatkin, U. S.; and McLaren, D. S. *J. Ment. Defic. Res.* 14:25 (1970).
131. Zimmerman, R. and Strobell, D.: Proceedings of the 77th Annual Convention, APA (1969).

Chapter IV

ENVIRONMENTAL INFLUENCES IN HUMAN DEVELOPMENT

THE BEHAVIOR AND mental development of children malnourished in early life has beeen studied retrospectively and prospectively. These studies indicate striking mental deficiencies in these children.[72] However, in human situations, it is always extremely difficult to isolate the effects produced by bad nutrition from those for which the quality of the surrounding environment can be held responsible. It is rare to find malnourished children who are not also culturally and socially deprived. Invariably the malnourished children come from poor backgrounds, low socioeconomic conditions, and a deprived atmosphere. Malnutrition in combination with poor environment predisposes a child to a period of behavioral unresponsiveness. A strange sense of apathy and indifference towards the surroundings dominates the behavioral pattern of the child, with the result that he wastes a certain period of his life in which he would lose a great deal of learning, and produces in him marked retardation in language, adaptive personal, social, and psychological behavior. Malnutrition merely has a catalyzing or accelerating effect. The apathy provoked by dull environment, which does not allow a healthy interaction of physical, biological, and social factors, provokes more apathy and results in reduced adult-child interaction. If this trend continues, the child shows significant developmental lags, and the psychologist then pronounces him mentally retarded and significantly backward in intellectual performance.

It is evident that a fuller understanding of the environment, in order to assess the precise relationship between malnutrition and mental development, requires detailed knowledge of such variables of the sociocultural features as family composition, socialization processes, customs, beliefs, economic factors, patterns of communications, migration, secular and introduced changes.[12]

Rajalakshmi and Ramakrishnan remarked that a number of variables which include heredity, perceptual environment, emotional status as well as nutritional state act simply or in combination and influence the psychological development of the person.[52] Other variables affecting psychological development include such factors as illiteracy, faulty methods of child care or rearing, social attitudes and values, and above all, broken homes and lack of responsibility on the part of the parents. These factors in single or multiple combination could significantly add to the sufferings of a child and affect his mental development and intellectual functioning at a later stage.

Although social and cultural factors are important variables, the incidence of infectious diseases in the areas where malnutrition is omnipresent must not be relegated to the background. A thorough study of the incidence of infectious diseases will bring about a better understanding of the relationship between nutrition, learning, and behavior and the role played by certain cultural aspects in perpetuating malnutrition and lower levels of learning generation after generation. Jelliffe and Jelliffe[32] stressed this point and believed that "the fullest details are required of dietary and cultural practices, especially those that tend to limit protein intake in early childhood or to have psychologically traumatic consequences."

In order to develop a better understanding of the impairment of mental ability one has to weigh thoroughly the part played by inadequate or unbalanced diets during the critical years of growth as well as the socioeconomic and cultural environments surrounding the child. To ignore the impact of either one of them is bound to be misleading.

A study of the factors conditioning malnutrition in widely separated geographical regions of the earth reveals that there is a particular setting (cultural or social) under which malnutrition generally thrives. This setting generally involves illiteracy, low income, low cultural level, low intellectual performance, bad sanitary conditions, and deep-rooted cultural, racial, or religious prejudices.[44] It is futile to fight malnutrition in these areas without a deep insight into this complex socioeconomic religio-cultural setting.

As discussed in the previous chapter, there are strong indications that inadequate nutrition during the critical period of physical growth and brain development leads to poorer mental performance compared to those who get better diets, all other factors being the same in both the groups. There are also equally strong indications that even if two groups of children during the early years of life get well-balanced diets and one group is exposed to very poor environments, the latter is bound to show emotional instability, apathy, and lack of mental agility. Richardson [55] rightly pointed out that so much stress is being laid on nutrition as a factor in mental development that the social, environmental, obstetrical, and genetic factors are being ignored. This is not to minimize the importance of nutrition but to emphasize that the bad nutrition in most instances is forced by socioeconomic conditions and cultural prejudices perpetuated by ignorance, and all these must be tackled simultaneously in order to improve the situation.

Except under controlled conditions under which animals are subjected to experimental manipulations, such as a specific type of malnutrition, the undernutrition and malnutrition states in the human populations do not occur alone. They exist "as a part of a constellation of social, economic, public health and medical factors which may also influence growth, disease patterns, learning ability and behavioral patterns."[54] The social and ecologic factors are equally important to perpetuate the states of malnutrition along with diet, first because they significantly influence the choice of items of the daily diet. Secondly, one community may suffer malnutrition more than the other, eating similar diets, because of varying standards of hygiene and incidence of infectious diseases.

It is important, therefore, to devise studies by which we could distinguish the stress caused by malnutrition vis-a-vis other environmental factors such as the quality of parental affection, infant coddling, language training, peer group adjustments,[1] and other socio-cultural ways of life of the family to which the child belongs. "A true evaluation of the significance of nutrition will come from looking at it in a comparative setting, with its importance judged in relation to other conceivably relevant intervening variables." [1]

The biggest obstacle in studying the human population is the difficulty of finding a matched control to the experimental subject. It is invariably the case that malnourished children come from poor backgrounds, low socioeconomic conditions, and a deprived atmosphere. Even the most carefully matched controls would not make it any easier to isolate the results produced by nutritional deprivation and environmental deprivation. Certainly the complex socioeconomic degradation of individuals and communities produce retarded development even when adequate nutrition is available. The question that remains unanswered is the degree.

INSEPARABILITY OF NUTRITIONAL STATUS AND ENVIRONMENTAL FACTORS

In human situations, both the dietary and environmental influences are so intertwined that it is difficult to assess or distinguish the effects of one from the other. One does not find malnourished children in the well-to-do families, who not only give good nutrition but also provide a stimulating environment for a fuller growth. At the same time it is an overstatement to say that inadequate nutrition causes retarded mental development. Is it not possible that bad nutrition contributes more to retarded physical growth so that the children are of smaller stature according to their chronological age, whereas the poor environment contributes heavily to the retarded mental growth in the absence of adequate visual and emotional stimulation.

Psychological upsets and emotional disturbances are often the reason for personality retardation, which may develop into clinical manifestations of kwashiorkor. The kwashiorkor patients function poorly, and their level of mental development is poorer compared to healthier children of the same area because they have been weaned on starchy foods which are grossly inadequate in protein content. Lack of proteins and calories is an important reason for retarded mental development, but a number of field studies also emphasize that the psychological disturbances and a sense of insecurity and emotional instability created by separation from the mother, due to the arrival of a new baby, is equally important in creating retarded intellectual functioning. In general, the condition of the child deteriorates if he is sent away from the mother to some relative, as is done in some parts of Africa. Such a child exhibits a typical clinical picture of severe apathy and disturbed EEG patterns.[25,48] It may be emphasized though that during the period of nutritional rehabilitation, the environmental stimulation acts as an added stimulus for recovery, whereas the poor, unstimulating environment acts conversely. The children whose mothers showed the greatest interest and solicitude and develop very warm and comforting relationships so as to create a sense of emotional stability are the ones who recover faster and better during nutritional rehabilitation.

The chances of mental retardation because of bad nutrition are indeed great. However, the poor environment in the lower classes acts to modify the growth and development of the central nervous system and because of the general apathy causes the individual to lose the motivation to learn from his daily experiences? It may be presumed that it is the poor socioeconomic conditions that set the stage for malnutrition, which may determine the intersensory development and the smaller stature of the individual. Cravioto and Delicardie [17] put forth two schemes of things. In one, malnutrition is assumed as the immediate underlying process responsible for shorter stature and neuro-integrative capacity, whereas in the other, the social condition of an impoverished environment leads to poor intersensory functioning. It may be safer to assume that a combination of both, i.e. social factors and malnutrition, influences the intersensory integration independently and also interacts with each other to produce the same result.[64,65]

This is generally true that emotionally disturbed children are apathetic to learning situations and lose their valuable time that never goes by again and in turn are at a permanent disadvantage. But the important questions so far remain unanswered. Riecken [56] asked

> are we interested in apathy in the school room which makes it difficult for a child to learn, or indeed apathy outside of the school room which may make it difficult for the child to acquire the substance of his culture, or which may cause him not to profit from casual observational learning opportunities that occur in the course of daily life?

Ketcham and associates [35,36] concluded that

> the interrelationship between children's school performance and their social and emotional problems must now be re-examined. It may be that clinical psychologists and psychiatrists have in the past oversold the schools on the frequency of a casual interrelationship. Consequently, the conclusion was prematurely reached that, since many severely neurotic and psychotic children have severe school behavior and learning problems, most of the less severe but nevertheless troublesome school problems exhibited by children can be traced to a social or emotional origin.

Although the effect of dietary abuse and the deleterious effects produced by bad environment cannot be separated, the following study carried out in India clearly illustrates that if the children are raised under stimulating environments, where they are treated with affection, care, and tender love, a dietary abuse, at least to a certain extent, does not affect the mental development adversely.

Longitudinal studies were carried on chronically malnourished children whose body weight was 60 to 70 percent of their expected weight for chronological age. The home environment of these children gave them security, a sense of belongingness, and there was no frustration or anger in their lives. They did not have any toys, but they also could play with all kinds of cans, including kitchen utensils or old magazines or books. The parents, although illiterate, had affectionate relationships with each other. These children when tested for I.Q. were surprisingly as alert and intelligent as their age mates belonging to upper classes. In this case it is evident that dietary abuse reflected only in growth retardation in terms of their physical size but did not affect the mental development.[52]

SOCIOECONOMIC AND CULTURAL FACTORS IN INFLUENCING CHILD'S DEVELOPMENT

Parental Background and Child's Development

Granted, the level of nutrition plays a significant role in the all-round development of the child, but it is equally clear that the family environment and the type of stimulation it provides during infancy is equally a deciding factor in influencing the intellectual growth.[8] For both practical and ethical reasons, it is extremely im-

portant, therefore, to study malnutrition in human, uncomplicated by social and cultural factors, which is an integral part of the
environment surrounding the growth of the baby. The environmental effect on the child would include impact of the parents to
whom these children are born.

> Poor social and poor nutritional factors exist in environments in
> which there are higher reproductive risks for women during pregnancy
> and delivery, higher infant mortality, higher risks of infection, includ-
> ing intestinal parasites, and poorer hygiene—all may provide, directly
> or indirectly, biologic insults to a child's central nervous system and
> result in impaired mental ability. These additional factors must be
> accounted for and ruled out before the casual role of poor nutrition
> in impaired mental development can be clearly established.[55]

The educational status of the parents not only plays an important role in determining the economic level of the family but also
in determining the nutritional status of the family.[41] Parents who
are less educated and suffer economic hardships tend to reject their
children, leaving them without love, food, and other essentials.[23]
In such families where children do not get adequate food, love,
and security, the incidence of mental deficiency may be three to
five times more than those who are poor but feel a sense of security and belongingness.[30] This may mean that psychological and
social deprivation could have a stronger impact on intellectual
performance than the debilitating effect of malnutrition.

In a detailed study of the effect of a variety of social factors that
influence the intersensory development of the child, Cravioto and
Delicardie [17] found out, " (1) no significant association of neuro-
integrative function with financial status, with house facilities,
with proportion of total income, or with the total expenditure on
food; (2) a weak inverse correlation with father's education; and
(3) no correlation with conditions of personal cleanliness." There
was, however, a significant association between the mental development of the child and the maternal attitudes, social background,
and educational background of the mother.

When we talk of environment in the strict sense of the word, an
enriched or a poor environment makes significant contributions to
the mental development of the child. A child from a privileged
class environment may prove quite poor, when in spite of material

opulence the child is deprived of maternal love and is exposed to emotional tension between the members of his family. As an example, these are homes where alcoholism, illegitimacy, and divorced parents are the rule. Such a child may in terms of mental development experience as much poor environment as an offspring of lower social class parents who does not get any valuable exposure to the world through toys or other stimulating media. The point that needs to be emphasized here is that it is not merely the socioeconomic status of the family but the quality of the parent's mental makeup that makes the most important difference in a child's environment.

Malnutrition and poor environments are inseparably interlinked. A study of malnourished children reveals at the first glance their connections with a low socioeconomic group and belonging to parents who are barely educated, of poor intelligence, and who are unable to make the best of their income to provide for the nutritional or medical needs of children. The children are subjected to the influences of alcoholism, illegitimacy, and broken homes. They in turn develop equally poor intelligence and levels of education. Platt and Stewart [50] rightly remarked that "in these circumstances, it is extremely difficult to differentiate between the effects of genetic endowment, social status, lack of parental care, malnutrition and the various combinations of these factors."

Maternal Attitude and Learning Behavior of the Child

The impact of environment does not necessarily start after reaching the certain age when interaction with adults begins, but it exerts its influence through the mother from conception to fetal life and continues into postnatal period until maturity.

The person who influences the immediate environment of the child and who greatly determines the course of emotional and behavioral development of the child is the mother. The mother with her tender touch imparts a sense of security and emotional stability from the earliest period of infancy, and the child, from this secure citadel, can explore his environment with confidence and is able to move about with a sense of dignity and belongingness. A correlation between maternal attitude and school performance of the child has been indicated by a number of field studies.[49] If the maternal attitude towards the child is negative, it is as though the whole world is hostile towards the child in question, and this affects the emotionality and personality of a child similarly. A number of workers believe that the majority of the mothers of malnourished children are in fact "rejecting mothers." Yankauer *et al.*[73] pointed out that it is these kinds of rejecting mothers who do not seek any prenatal care, and this attitude may be considered an outward manifestation of the rejection of pregnancy and a loss of the sense of personal dignity and worth. According to Yankauer, "these women possessed traits that implied an unstable, irresponsible and unsuccessful family life, out of wedlock births, welfare dependency, abnormal mobility, and excessive fertility. These traits, associated with low economic status result in poor living habits and inadequate nutrition." [53]

In early years of life, the environment of the child is determined by the manner in which the mother and close relatives handle the baby. In turn, malnutrition in this age would also affect the mother's feelings towards the baby. Birch [9] observed that underfed children are less responsive and so are less satisfying to their mothers. Mothers often lose interest in such children. It would mean that malnutrition and environment interact at an age as early as a few months. The undernourished children due to less handling are deprived of early sensory stimulation that is essential for the development of the normal intellect.

The background of the mother in a sense of *her* own background greatly influences the growth pattern of the baby. If the today's mother had an unsatisfactory childhood, if she suffered from nutritional deprivation, grew under least stimulating environment, and failed to get any formal education, she has developed a certain behavioral attitude that she is bound to impart to her baby, which most certainly will lead to inadequate infant care. The field experience of a number of workers showed that malnourished children are frequently the offsprings of mothers who as children had gone through a period of nutritional abuse. In Latin American countries, Cravioto [15] found that the children who showed poor growth during the first six months of life had mothers whose educational backgrounds were very poor compared to mothers whose children grew well. Commenting on the influence of the educational and cultural levels of the parents on the motivation and aspirations for learning in the child, Birch [8] pointed out that

> When the educational level of the parents is low and cultural attachment is to either a parochial or a highly localized indigenous culture, the likelihood is markedly reduced that the child will have appropriately directed motivations and aspirations for the kinds of learning that make for good "intelligence" in advanced societies. Such factors, when associated with the phenomenon of malnutrition, may well produce a confounded product in which it is difficult indeed to separate familial and environmental effects in a general sense from malnutritional effects.

An illiterate mother does not question the traditional methods of child care, even if the child is visibly effected,[69] and does not have the background to provide a stimulating environment. The educated mother, on the other hand, not only shows respect for new ideas of child raising but also exerts a positive socializing influence. Some workers have even reported a strong association between the I.Q. of the mothers and that of the children.[7,33] Even in the absence of toys and books, the mother may encourage the child to play with kitchen utensils or other articles and provide a varied and interestingly stimulating experience. Such a mother, by constant attention and talking, can greatly help in language development and other facets of the child's personality.

Maternal education, in a sense of fuller realization of maternal role in child rearing, becomes very significant in the nutritional care of the infant and the determination of his I.Q. level. The offsprings of the mother with poorer educational background are always at a great disadvantage from those whose mothers have better social standing and education. As mentioned earlier, the malnourished children are in certain respects rejected by their mothers who themselves did not experience emotional stability, security, education, and acceptance by the poor environment under which they were raised. In order to understand the full impact of environment as a vital force in the continuation of malnutrition in certain sections of the society, one has to go deeper into the psychological makeup of the mothers over a number of generations. The above discussion confirms the findings of several field studies which have concluded that the malnourished children are the offsprings of mothers who are equally malnourished and had been so in their early childhood through the adolescent period, and today's female infants of these mothers are the least equipped nutritionally to become mothers at a later date. If these have been the circumstances during the past number of generations, it may very well explain the existence of a larger number of poor functioning people in the poor classes and may accumulate over the generations "an abundant gene pool that may contribute to the production of an inordinately large number of intellectually defective children." [8] Richardson,[55] while discussing the influence of social environment and nutritional factors on mental ability, emphasized that the intellectual performance of the child depends on the premarital social class of the mother and the kind of relationship that she develops with the child. That is precisely the reason why emotionally deprived children raised in orphanages generally suffer from a certain degree of mental retardation. An objective analysis of human situation reveals clearly that the mental impairment is a result of material poverty and cultural and genetic backwardness. The former perpetuates nutritional deficiencies, whereas the latter reflects an unhealthy environment and generation after generation of inheritable features of intellectual incompetence.[8]

Socioeconomic and Cultural Setting and Child's Development

Hunger causes changes in social behavior and distracts people from their attempts to continue their cultural and other interests. Preoccupation with food induces a negative approach to things.[43] Although the social class to which an individual belongs should not determine the environment and dietary standards in which he is raised; unfortunately this is true to a certain extent. The children belonging to parents of the lower socioeconomic classes suffer from certain handicaps besides nutrition, which the children of the upper socioeconomic groups do not. For example, the former tend to have poor housing, lower levels of formal education, higher incidence of infectious disease, greater attachment to outmoded patterns of child care, and obsolete concepts on health and disease. These people, in general, live in circumstances which are less conducive to the development of technological and educational competence. Moreover, the effects of these circumstances may continue from one generation to another and suggest a familial or hereditary process.[17,29] These handicaps are mainly responsible for the major clustering of the malnourished children in lower classes. In the upper classes, the malnutrition is mainly due to ignorance of the parents of the dietary needs of the growing child, but the latter is generally raised in a sound stimulating environment.

Unless it is a case of gross malnutrition, the mental performance of a child cannot be judged at an early age because it is only in the later period that the adverse effects of socioeconomic retardation can be identified,[39] and this has proved a very thorny problem for the investigators. One of the most formidable tasks that faces a psychologist these days is to separate the effect of each from a concordance of nutritional deprivation and cultural deprivation. Psychologists traditionally have been concerned with social and psychological problems caused by socioeconomic and cultural deprivations, but the problem of ever increasing hunger, scarcity of food has fired the imagination of not only psychologists but scientists in other areas of human health and welfare to investigate the role of nutritional variables in the growth and development of children. There is growing evidence that in the economically depressed population, the children with retarded motor development come from homes where economic and social pressures restrict adequate stimulation for mental development.[10,44]

The deleterious effects of poor cultural setting which work to the child's disadvantage have been shown in a number of studies, particularly from orphanages where children show poor performance. In better circumstances and in the hands of affectionate parents, these children would have blossomed into physically healthy, mentally vigorous and alert young men and women. In defining the state of malnutrition, one has to take into account the whole constellation of socioeconomic, cultural and ecologic factors, besides nutrition, as it has become obvious that the high frequency of mentally retarded children in the socioeconomically depressed classes is not merely the consequence of malnutrition.[44] Despair resulting from lower socioeconomic status and poverty, which immensely contributes to dietary abuse and malnutrition, expresses itself in feelings of powerlessness, meaninglessness, anomie, and isolation.[31] The individuals caught in this trap feel powerless to influence the workings of the society, fail to understand their place in society, and therefore tend to be cynical, fatalistic and isolated. Ireland [31] emphasized that their behavior is a result of deprived alienated condition and is characterized by four distinctive themes: fatalism, orientation to the present, authoritarianism, and concreteness.

In some of the developing countries, the socioeconomic and cultural condition for certain communities or groups are such that malnutrition is a lifelong process and probably has been present for generations, with consequent physiological adaptations. In the lives of these unfortunate people there is no such thing as rehabilitation after a certain period of malnutrition.[14] This situation is in contrast to the experimental studies on animals, where the period of deprivation is followed by rehabilitation on a well-balanced diet. Under the circumstances, it becomes difficult to find a bridge between the research results obtained from animals and human populations. In general, the investigations on the experimental animals indicate positively that early malnutrition and undernutrition can affect their learning and behavior.

Cravioto [15] compared the school performance of short and tall children from upper and lower income families in Mexico City. He observed that the height of the shorter children from poor families was limited by poor nutrition rather than hereditary potential. The poorer the nutrition, the shorter the height of the child, and it is those poorly nourished, small-sized children that most often encounter difficulty in learning to read and write. Robinow [57] extensively studied growth and development of children of different socioeconomic groups and concluded that the relationship between growth failure, head size, and intelligence is not always as close as might be expected. He described a child whose home environment was not favorable and who at the same time suffered extreme degree of growth retardation due to congenital hydronephrosis and chronic uremia. This child, in spite of the handicaps, scored 82 on the Binet I.Q. test, which, although commensurate with his environmental deprivation, reflects a good level of mental development in spite of the extreme degree of physical retardation.

The environmental factors, besides the commonly listed socioeconomic and cultural variables, which could affect the child's performance on any test scale, should include an understanding of the parental I.Q., emotional security, schooling, training at home, birth order, family size, physical illness.[13] A number of studies on the relationship between cultural and socioeconomic status and intelligence or the child's performance at school relative to home environment [19,24,46] have clearly demonstrated that primary or secondary malnutrition is an intermediate link in the chain with socio-environment conditions on the one hand and impaired behavioral functioning on the other. Such a relationship becomes quite evident when we study the child-rearing practices in different social groups, for example, the parental values and parent-child relationship among the families where parents are unskilled and less educated compared to those who are highly skilled professional people.[37,38]

Only a few decades back, the racial difference in the growth of the Negro and white children in the United States was quite evident, the former being lighter and shorter than the latter. In recent years, when social changes have brought about favorable environmental conditions for the blacks, such differences are becoming negligible. Detailed studies of some workers indicate that the Negro infants are as large and grow at the same rate as the comparable white infants of the same economic level.[50,68] When all infants are given equal conditions in their intrauterine as well as postnatal life, it is likely that the so-called racial characteristics between blacks, browns, yellows, and whites will disappear.

There is another category of behavioral difference often seen among the urban and rural population in all countries that cannot be attributed to the standards of nutrition or due to any cultural pattern. It may be that because of the very mode of their life or environmental conditions determined by their interaction with cunning urbanites, businessmen, or government officials, the country people are believed to be dull, unresponsive, unintelligent, and apathetic, and hence one may presume that it is due to their poor nutritional standard in the early years of their life in combination with the unstimulating dull environment of the countryside.[1] This is a complex problem and judgment cannot be passed from superficial observations. Adams expressed that such a behavior is more of an adaptive mechanism rather than any nutritional deficiency syndrome, which is considered a sure way to guard against exploitation by outsiders. "Children are taught, of course, not to be expressive, simply because over the years adults have learnt that the surest way to survive is to reduce communication with outsiders to a minimum." [1]

QUALITY OF CHILD'S ENVIRONMENT IN RELATION TO PHYSICAL AND MENTAL GROWTH

There is no doubt that a combination of poor diets and poor environments produces conditions that are quite ideal for retarded development, physical as well as mental. Malnutrition reduces the activity level of the organism, instills in him a sense of apathy towards his surroundings and his desire to explore his environment. The diet and environment play an important role in the realization of full genetic potential as well as physical and mental development. A child subjected to dietary abuse and poor environment cannot reach his full genetic stature. The apathy introduced by poor environment affects the sensory responsiveness, which affects the chemical environment of the nervous system and the emotional state of the individual. One cannot, therefore, minimize or underestimate the role played by environment on the physical and mental growth of the child. A number of studies have shown that even when a child is getting adequate nutrition, his physical and mental growth may be retarded if his environments are poor. Commenting on mental contentment and physical growth, Widdowson [70] observed significant differences in children raised in orphanages under authoritarian supervision or with affectionate mothering, in spite of the fact that both the groups were getting similar diets. A number of other studies have also shown that the infants raised in poor environments show retarded learning ability compared to those raised affectionately and under better social and cultural environments, the nutrition factor being the same in both the groups.

An enriched or a poor environment could have a great impact on the intelligence level of two members getting equally balanced diets. Simultaneously, two children raised in different social environments may differ dramatically in their intellectual scores.[54] According to Read,[54] in order to make a proper assessment of the mental performance of a child, it is important to look into three important factors:

1. Nutrition or dietary pattern—balanced or unbalanced diet in adequate or inadequate quantities.

2. Social and cultural environment—whether or not it is conducive for achieving maximum growth potential.

3. Pattern of disease occurrence—whether it is congenital or due to unsanitary surroundings.

The last one is relatively simple to correct, although it involves tremendous effort, capital investment, and improvement of public health services. The social and cultural environments, if they are not conducive for adequate growth, are, however, much harder to correct.

As it is with nutrition, there is a critical period of life when emotional disturbance could prove more detrimental to child's mental development. During this critical period the poor environments predispose a child to emotional deprivation and affect his mental development. It has been observed that children admitted to orphanages at the age of one or two years or less are more emotionally disturbed and show lower performance at a later age than those who were admitted at the age of three or four years or older, in spite of the same dietary pattern in both groups.[52]

It may be pertinent here to summarize the results of two extremely significant studies conducted by Dr. Skeels on the same subjects about 26 years apart. The first study [66] conducted during the 1930s described the conditions of an orphanage nursery, where babies are provided with nourishing food adequate for promoting normal physical growth, but no attention was paid to their environment.

These babies were under the supervision of overworked and indifferent staff and had little human interaction, person to person relationships, or toys, or any other form of visual stimulation. The whole situation could be considered ideal for an experiment where the subjects are given adequate food but very poor environment. Most of the children raised under these conditions showed I.Q. below the average. Their academic achievements were extremely poor, and few crossed the third grade, and a significant number had to be admitted to the institutions for mentally retarded. So much for those who stayed for a long period of time under these poor environments. Dr. Skeels conducted a novel experiment and transferred 13 children under three years old as house guests in an institution of mentally retarded. Before leaving, these children had an I.Q. range from 35 to 89. At the new institute the children were given an enriched environment. The staff spent a good deal of time with them, and they were given a good deal of love and opportunity for playing. According to Dr. Skeels, the birth, medical histories, and family background of these children and of those who stayed back in the parent orphanage were similar. After a period of four to five years, these children were tesetd for their I.Q., and Skeels discovered that they had made gains of 7 to 58 points. In contrast the children in the parent orphanage had lost 9 to 45 points during the same period. Twenty-one years later Dr. Skeels [67] traced most of these subjects who were then adults. Skeels found that the subjects who had been given enriched environments in the mental institute had proved to be a group of well-adjusted people. Most of them had a minimum of high school diploma and were self-supporting. This is in sharp contrast to the subjects raised in the parent orphanage with poor environment, who were either mentally retarded or showed grossly deficient mental performance.

Rajalakshmi and Ramakrishnan [51] reported the results of an unplanned experiment in India. They provided a balanced lunch program along with play activities at school to a group of children, who benefitted from improved food as well as environmental stimulation. A few children, however, did not eat at the school but came to play. The I.Q. scores of these children indicate that the children who came to play and those who played and ate lunch were higher than the control group who did not participate in these activities. The effect of environmental stimulation is, therefore, clear. The investigation of Rajalakshmi and associates on the lower and upper classes in India showed a consistent difference in favor of the upper class with regard to weight, height, educational attainments, and I.Q. scores. Nutrition alone cannot be singled out as a reason for this difference. Heredity and environment must have played an important role in creating this difference.

Extreme cases of kwashiorkor showed mental retardation for which diet is always blamed. But is it not possible that along with diet the psychological depression created by poor surroundings was equally responsible for creating mental apathy. Chronic undernutrition, where environmental conditions are somewhat better, may not produce such a depressive psychosis and prevent further degeneration into severe cases of clinical kwashiorkor. Furthermore, hospitals in the underdeveloped countries generally do not provide enriched environment. They are more close to orphanages, where the needs of the children are met by duty-conscious, overworked staff, who do not have the time or inclination to develop personal affectionate relationships with these children. A long stay in the hospital could also prove to be a contributing factor in influencing the psychological and mental development of the patients. There are millions of children in the underdeveloped countries who suffer chronic undernutrition, and yet they seem to function normally in their adult life. It may be assumed, therefore, that undernutrition to a certain extent does not affect the mental development.

> It would appear that when nutritional deficiency exceeds certain critical limits, intelligence is affected but we may not be justified thereby in assuming some sort of linear relationship between nutrition and intelligence. The latter would be analogous to assuming that since an elastic string snaps when it is stretched hard, it must snap a little when it is stretched a little. The job of the nutritionist is to identify the critical levels which cause the string to snap clearly. Practical nutritional measures must aim at maintaining dietary standards well above these dangerous levels.[52]

Most of the time it is difficult to separate conditions which provide bad food to a child in his growing years and conditions which deprive him of a source of enriched environment conducive to maximum learning. Experimental evidence on humans that malnutrition alone is a cause of impaired mental ability has not been conclusively presented so far, although some evidence, such as Skeels [66] work discussed above, does convince us that even in the presence of good nutrition, a child's behavioral and mental development may be greatly disturbed because of poor environment.

An improved nutrition will improve the mental development of the child, but the combination of suitable diet and stimulating environment is the only way by which a child retarded in early childhood may recover to some extent with respect to its intellectual functioning. Without adequate diet and good environment the dead may be more fortunate than the survivors, who are permanently disabled and have to face this hostile world with insufficient mental equipment.

ROLE OF INFECTIONS IN DETERMINING THE CHILD'S ENVIRONMENT

Infection plays a significant part in dramatizing the impairment that dietary abuse causes. Scrimshaw [63] pointed out that in developing countries the children of the lower socioeconomic groups suffer so much and so frequently from diarrhea, respiratory infections, and other communicable diseases that the body cannot benefit from the poor diets that they get, and these children suffer further metabolic losses of protein and other essential nutrients. Scrimshaw rightly emphasized that

> the children in developing countries are ill so much of their early life and at such frequent intervals that growth and development are impaired more than would be predicted from their food intakes when they are not sick. Each episode of infectious disease reduces appetite, causes added metabolic loss of protein and other essential nutrients, and most important, perhaps, the mother gives the child a more liquid and less nourishing diet. Diarrhea, frequently augmented by purgatives, worsens the problem by reducing absorption of nutrients from the gastrointestinal tract. While some reduction in diarrheal disease burden is known to result from improved nutrition alone, this is not enough to counteract the high incidence and serious effects of infectious disease.[63]

It is because of these serious episodes that the rate of infant mortality during the first year of life in most developing countries is quite high compared to the industrialized countries, where the children are less susceptible to infections because of sanitary surroundings and adequate nutrition.

Judging infant mortality rates as an index of malnutrition and poverty, Lowe [42] stated before a congressional committee that among the average white population of the United States the infant mortality rate is 1 to 6 percent of the live births. This compares to 5% infant mortality among the poor black communities and is as high as 10 percent in the black rural slums, which means that 10 percent of all the children born in these slums die within the first year of their life. In these situations, it is difficult to assess the burden of infection and the role of malnutrition in the emergence of the final picture. The nutritional disorders cannot be studied independently from other elements which closely interact with it. The presence of malnutrition exaggerates the processes of infections because of the depleted systems and inability of the organism to fight infection. As a part of the environmental setting, a pattern of series of infections superimposed on a malnourished child takes him to the downward path much faster. A few of the most important environmental influences that preset the child to recurring infections are poor housing, overcrowding, inadequate water supply, poor socioeconomic circumstances, low educational standards, or specific cultural taboos. [28]

The interesting monograph on the incidence of infection by Scrimshaw *et al.* [65] brings to light sufficient data which clearly demonstrates

(1) that infections are more readily acquired by malnourished children; (2) that the development of the immune response to infection is absent, inadequate or depressed in malnourished children; and (3) that infectious disease has far more serious general systemic consequences for malnourished than for well-nourished children. Thus, malnutrition can result in an organism with markedly increased vulnerability to infectious disease. Such disease, if generalized, may have both general and specific effects on the course of nervous system growth and, in fact, produce central nervous system damage.

It is, therefore, most important, when considering the consequences of malnutrition for intellectual growth, that one takes into account the exaggerated effects of infectious diseases occurring in malnourished children. The standard of nutrition may be a decisive factor, although inevitably bound to the social, economic, and cultural characteristics of a population. However, preventive and curative services could be doomed to failure, unless serious consideration is given to these interlocking influences.[28]

The incidence of infections and infectious diseases are a direct reflection of the socio-cultural setup of the community in which a particular child is raised. Social customs not only create conditions to check or perpetuate certain infections but also influence its handling when it is there, for example, the dangerous social practice of purging after an episode of diarrhea or a misplaced treatment. Eichenwald,[20] Fry,[21] Eisenberg,[22] Birch and Cravioto,[11] and other prominent workers have made extensive observations on the role of infection in mental development under different socio-economic conditions. Eichenwald and Fry [21] stressed that infectious diseases cause nervous system damage either by acting in a direct or in an indirect manner. In the former category, some infections are readily recognizable as causing disease processes with significant changes in structure and function of the nervous system. Indirectly, a middle ear infection, so common in children, may remain unattended and lead to learning impairment. Such a person would be seriously handicapped in mental development because of impaired input of information from outside due to impaired hearing.

The incidence of permanent neuronal damage because of infections is quite high in the overpopulated underdeveloped countries, but the cases of mental damage due to infection in the United States are not rare either. Infections leading to impairment in spite of highly advanced human knowledge in preventive medicine is an unnecessary waste and must be given serious attention. It is crystal clear that a close relationship exists between the level of nutrition and incidence of infections, and one could not control one without a satisfactory solution of the other.

POPULATION PRESSURES AND ENVIRONMENTAL QUALITY

The problem of malnutrition and the resulting retarded human development has been aggravated during the last two to three decades by two major factors. The first is overpopulation and unabated growth of populations in the industrially underdeveloped countries of Asia, Africa, and South America as a direct result of improved medical services leading to declining death rates in childhood and sharply reducing the infant mortality. The second main reason for the degradation of the environmental quality is increasing pollution of our natural resources and environment, resulting in profound changes in our society as well as culture. It is clear that standards of nutrition of a population have to be viewed in terms of numbers as well as social, economic, cultural and political stability. We should have the ability to handle the various aspects of human development in proportion to the numbers without letting them threaten all human progress, as it has tended to do in the overcrowded Asia. Too much heavy burden on the earth or its resources is bound to have repercussions in the development of the human species with respect to its physical growth and mental development, generating the kind of social pressures that will not respond favorably to massive injection of nutrition in an effort to improve the dietary standards of the community.

Overpopulation pollutes the environment and indirectly adds to human misery. When we compare a sparsely populated country and an overpopulated one, extreme differences in the frequency of death and physical and mental disability become at once evident. Although there is no detailed study pointing to a direct relationship, the infant mortality rate in the overpopulated countries is a direct reflection of the strain on the surrounding environment to sustain bigger populations. While comparing highly industrialized nations with underdeveloped ones, which incidently are very much overpopulated, Scrimshaw [63] showed that

> infant mortality in an industrialized country is primarily a function of the first month of life; in greatest extent the first week of life. The deaths of the first 28 days are about twice those during the next 11 months. In developing countries, that relationship is reversed, with more deaths in the postneonatal period than in the first four weeks. Furthermore, the situation extends into subsequent years, with the result that the second-year death rate, instead of a common seven percent of infant mortality, in some countries is as much as three-fourths of the infant rate.

The rate at which human population is growing is adding each day several hundred thousand babies in the already large pool of poverty ridden malnourished children who are exposed to under-nutrition, recurrent infections and unstimulating environments. A number of them die and the survivors are doomed to a life long retardation in physical growth and mental development. More and more evidence is accumulating that a child who survives after severe episodes of malnutrition is seriously handicapped.[71] Cravi-oto *et al.*[16,18] believed that such a child is a link in a vicious cycle started in the family in which he is born, which sets into motion a self-perpetuating and continuous period of suffering from genera-tion to generation. Winick[71] has expressed this cycle in a beautiful manner:

> The malnourished infant growing up in poverty is unable to acquire the skills to deal with the complexities of modern society. The result is that he remains poor for the rest of his life and his children are born into the same social and economic conditions. The family does not have the resources to adequately nourish the new infant. He in turn becomes seriously malnourished and if able to survive, is handi-capped in such a way as to prevent him from extricating himself from the plight of his parents. Thus, a condition of poverty is perpetuated and will pass from one generation to the next. The genetic endow-ment is presumably normal, but the environment prevents achieve-ment of the genetic potential. This analysis suggests that there already exists a pool of people who have been so handicapped, and that this pool is increasing in almost geometric proportions with the present day population explosion.

Scrimshaw has rightly warned that the future of the developing countries, which house two thirds of the human population, de-pends on improving the technological competence of the people which could produce more food as well as healthy environments. "Investments in other aspects of development, including schools and teachers, will be reduced in value if the generations of the future are being damaged now in mind and body." [62] By present neglect, we are simply exaggerating the problems of the future.[43] Even if the individual does not suffer a big loss in his intellectual capacity, accumulatingly in a nation where malnutrition is com-mon the effects could be disastrous. This could mean an adverse effect on the general enterprise of the population and on their re-sponsiveness to opportunities for advancement or change.[47] Exist-ing conditions in the underdeveloped countries as well as in some segments of the U.S. society make it impossible, therefore, to isolate malnutrition from other consequences of socioeconomic and cultural poverty and how much each factor is responsible for producing retarded development.[71]

IMPORTANCE OF FIELD STUDIES ON THE ROLE OF ENVIRONMENT IN BEHAVIORAL DEVELOPMENT

Observational Studies on Human Populations

It is important that longitudinal semi-experimental and observational field studies be undertaken in human children in those areas where malnutrition is an endemic problem. Field assessment of nutritional status in relation to the surrounding environmental factors is liable to give a more accurate picture of the role of either variable (environment or nutrition) on the growth and development of the human child. Canosa [12] emphasized that long-term prospective field studies must be taken seriously and planned painstakingly and an effort be made to end the present incompetent methods of measurements, particularly those used to correlate malnutrition and mental ability during the first two years of life. These methods at present don't have any predictive value.

Adams [1] stressed the importance of objective field studies in the area of environment and malnutrition, although he also believed that it is somewhat illogical to conduct such studies on the persons only up to eight or ten years of age. To him, it is important to have a long-term evaluation of those adults, along with their social and cultural behavior, who have suffered nutritional insults as infants. Most of the observations point out, however, that mental deficiency or mental confusion caused by severe nutritional deficiencies after 13 years of age are markedly less pronounced compared to the earlier years; yet there is no justification to consider later periods as superfluous and stop the study. Adams [1] believed that "failure to obtain a full answer to the ultimate consequences of influences which cause such concern is scientifically irresponsible."

In human situations, the environmental conditions, which constitute an interplay of social, cultural and infective factors, and the quality and quantity of diet can be assessed in their proper perspective only by undertaking long-term longitudinal studies.

Traditions, superstitions, and poor recreational facilities play very detrimental roles besides such factors as poor intake, large families, overcrowding, poor sanitation, ignorance, recurrent infections, and poor management of infections. Jelliffe and Jelliffe [32] suggested that more meaningful data can be collected by starting such studies on the newborn which have the additional advantage of recording correct anthropometric measurements. However, if these studies are meant to establish the effects of malnutrition on intellectual performance, they may fail to be conclusive if they do not consider the role of multiplicity of factors such as psychological and social deprivation, education of the parents, motivation, and external stimuli.[62] When longitudinal studies on kwashiorkor patients are carried out, generally controls who do not have a history of hospitalization for malnutrition are selected from the same socioeconomic groups. It is questionable if these children are the matched controls, because they are probably as much malnourished as the experimental subjects except that so far they do not show certain clinical symptoms. The comparison of these two groups could give misleading results. The problem of the choice of controls is exceedingly difficult in the longitudinal studies because one must study similar populations in which nutrition or environment is the only variable.[72]

It is evident that the type of environment affects the learning performance of the children, and that the children brought up under depressed environments show subnormal intelligence even with the best diet. Under experimental conditions, certain animals show not only a disturbed behavior but also retarded learning performance, brain weight, and the activity of certain enzymes such as cholinesterase and acetylcholinesterase. Rosenzweig,[58-60] Altman and co-workers [2] observed that such animals raised in depressed environmental conditions show dramatic improvements in behavior as well as in the area of the neocortex and number of glial cells when they are exposed to enriched and stimulating environment even for a period of two hours a day.

Experimental Studies on Animals

It is always a difficult question to isolate the effects on the mental development produced by malnutrition from those resulting from the interaction of environmental and cultural factors. Animal studies are the only sources from which to collect any meaningful data in the field of nutrition and behavioral development, and the results may be extrapolated to humans, although in the latter the environmental complexities are much more difficult to analyze. To the extent that the interplay between the social and nutritional factors in humans as determinants of behavior characteristics are extremely complex, the animal studies may not be of much use, Barnes *et al.*[4,6] extrapolated certain hypotheses from the animal studies which may be summarized as follows: food restriction in early years restricts behavioral characteristics to looking for food rather than exploratory behavior. Long-lasting behavior disturbances are set in motion by severe deprivations in early life, and they may continue to show retarded learning behavior both in complex problem solving and in test situations relevant to drive, even if the animals are rehabilitated at a later date. However, physical growth retardation or body stunting seems to have no relationship with the extent of behavioral changes due to early nutritional deprivation.

It is not easy to extrapolate the results to humans, especially when data on anatomical and chemical changes cannot be obtained on the human brain. Experimentally the animals show considerable impairment in their learning ability after feeding them protein-deficient diets, but it is not valid to apply this data straight way to human conditions. Studies with rats show that such deprivations result in permanent learning behavior abnormalities.[26,27] In a very important investigative effort in primates on the effects of malnutrition, Zimmerman and Strobell [74] found out that the gross apathy towards the environment seen in the malnourished monkeys is very similar to that of a poverty culture child. The interest in the surroundings and hence any benefit from interacting with the surrounding environment is greatly diminished and retarded. The quality of social development is a direct result of malnutrition. Zimmerman and Strobell concluded that

> the effects of a low protein diet are not simple and interact with the development of other motivational systems in the infant monkey. The normally curious, playful, manipulating infant monkey undoubtedly

learns a great deal about his environment and this appears during the extended play periods that are characteristic of the free-roaming Macaque. The low protein diet appears to definitely retard social interaction and it would suggest, therefore, retard social development.

Experimental studies on animals, especially primates, being closer taxonomically to humans, are essential for obvious reasons because well-controlled conditions could be created in which the effect of malnutrition could be studied separately from that of the environment on the subsequent behavior and learning ability of the organism. In these studies it is also important to have a multidisciplinary approach, i.e. a combination clinical, nutritional, behavioral, biochemical, and cytochemical studies. These studies should be combined with the most sensitive possible testing procedures which could differentiate between a state of good health, undernutrition, and malnutrition not only when the latter has significantly affected the mental development, but even in its earlier stages when the body starts making physiological adjustments to lower food intake.

NUTRITIONAL AND ENVIRONMENTAL POVERTY AND ITS IMPACT ON HUMAN SOCIETY

In the course of human development, nutrition, whether adequate or inadequate, balanced in all nutrients or unbalanced, is only one aspect of the environment. The environment in all its complexity has an overwhelming influence on the life of all bio-behavioral organisms and could very well be a deciding factor in their destiny on this planet. Environment is a biological resultant of complex social, cultural, and economic factors.[3] Read [54] put it extremely well that the man

> must recognize that nutrition, medicine, public health, economics, social environment, cultural patterns and the broad spectrum of factors influencing human development are inexorably intertwined. In this context, nutrition may well be less of a discrete science than it is a crossroad well traveled on the way to converting research findings into solutions for improving the quality of human life.

We have to ask certain questions and find answers for them. Are the better fed populations mentally and behaviorally more stable than those who do not get adequate quantities of food in their early years of life, or as Adams [1] asked, Should we expect that

a population favorably fed will, as adults, show greater discrima-
tion in voting, decision making, be more likely to lead happy lives,
or have a lower or higher incidence of suicide and functional psychological disorders? Genetic endowments play some part, but the
environmental factors, such as poverty, ignorant and illiterate
parents, overcrowding, a high prevalence of infectious disease,
poor learning opportunities and several others, may prove more
effective in influencing the psychological as well as intellectual
development.[40] At this point, it may be a matter of great controversy how much genetic endowments play a role in creating
poor environmental conditions, which along with lower levels of
nutrition play a significant part in general retardation of individuals or communities. The remarks of Birch [8] are quite pertinent
and may be quoted here. Birch believed that

> low social status is associated with familial, hereditary, or genetic
> characteristics of intellectual inferiority. In short, that among the poor
> there is an abundant gene pool that may contribute to the production
> of an inordinately large number of intellectually defective children.
> Although evidence for the existence of such a pool is, indeed, sparse
> and inferential, the possibility of its presence has been a point of view
> argued sufficiently often, and with sufficient force, to warrant serious
> concern. If, in fact, a high familial rate of retardation exists among
> the poor and this high familial rate is associated with social incompe-
> tence, which in its turn results in increased risk for malnutrition,
> one could be confronted with a body of data showing mental back-
> wardness to be significantly associated with nutritional inadequacy
> when in reality both could be reflecting familial and inheritable
> features of intellectual incompetence.

The areas of the world in which the pattern of infantile and
adult malnutrition is a fact of existence, the major contributing
causes are those which show a characteristic culture of poverty,
such as low wages, mass scale unemployment, discrimination based
on sex, color, or creed, and the resulting feelings of inferiority and
deprivation, illiteracy, and social and cultural customs detrimental
to health.[3] Correction of conditions which perpetuate malnutrition is of extreme importance. The corrective measures may include increasing the output of traditional foods of the community
and introducing them to new foods which help to make their
diets qualitatively balanced in all the nutrients needed for good

health. These corrective measures will greatly help to improve the health of the community and reduce the chance of mental impairment among the children. This approach, although ideal to look at, reveals on a closer analysis that it is likely to touch only the periphery of the problem. In Chile, the experiment of providing free milk failed miserably, and providing large quantities of food to the needy families did not drop the infant mortality rate even 1 percent.[45] An attempt has to be made to correct those environments which breed poverty and malnutrition. Enlarged public health facilities are needed to control the spread of recurrent infections, but above all is needed the nutrition education which should cover all aspects of social and cultural life of the community. Improving nutritional standards of the children may improve the mental development to some extent, but it is only when the environments are improved that it will have any lasting impact. It has to be recognized, therefore, that the prevention of malnutrition cannot be taken up solely on the basis of conventional procedures; for example, adequate care of pregnant mothers to allow satisfactory prenatal growth of the baby, pouring tons of dry milk and other foodstuffs into areas of poverty where children suffer the most in their postnatal life, or even improving the health services to fight infections. The greatest need is the education of the parents in developing the right concept of child care and nutritional needs of pregnant mothers; the need for hygienic sanitary dwellings, the need for providing rich sociocultural experiences to the child, and above all the necessity to produce only as many children as can be properly taken care of. This would give the child a sense of belonging, emotional stability, and security, so necessary for the development of right behavioral patterns.

We have to tackle the social problems with as much vigor as making available extra quantities of high-quality food. For example, which customs or practices influence feeding patterns in breast feeding, or supplementation of breast milk, time and manner of weaning, or the selection and preparation of foods and the allocation of food resources in the family? How do feeding practices change when the child is perceived as being sick, and what are perceived as symptoms of sickness?[55] Kallen[34] rightly emphasized the interdependence of social structure, nutrition, and family behavior, including child training factors as well as intellectual and social behavior. Nutrition, although important, is only secondary to enriched environment to produce children with well-balanced personalities. The problem of prevention of malnutrition is not a problem of nutrition alone but has social, cultural, and environmental implications, and its solutions need considerable attention in the areas of education and development of technology for the exploitation of vast natural resources lying idle in the midst of those who suffer from malnutrition.

Results from experiments on highly evolved animals, such as primates, whose behavioral development is very much affected by the environmental quality, reveal a pattern not dissimilar from the human. Zimmerman and Strobell [74] showed that protein malnutrition induces indifference to the environment with the result that the animal does not interact with the environment and loses the opportunity to learn. A malnourished animal shows retarded curiosity, manipulation as well as social motivation, which compared to the healthy ones would put them at a serious disadvantage in their normally competitive society. It is well known that the human species is much more competitive than the highly evolved animals, and the struggle for the existence among human population is more intense in a certain sense. If the findings on animals are stretched to apply to the human society, it will have wide implication with regard to the future of human civilization when it is imagined that at present two thirds of the human population live in those areas where undernutrition is the fact of existence and good nutrition is a big luxury. Unfortunately, these are also the areas where infections are rampant due to unsanitary conditions and nonavailability of uncontaminated baby food, especially milk. At the same time, the minds of the people are riddled with ignorance and cultural supersitions which provide a very poor environment to a growing baby. The child does not have the motivation to interact with the environment due to poor nutrition, and the environment itself is so poor as to provide no stimulating experience. The result is a combination of poor food and poor environment which affect the all-round development of the child and in turn the future prospects of the human society.

REFERENCES

1. Adams, R. N.: In N. S. Scrimshaw and J. E. Gordon (Eds.): *Malnutrition, Learning and Behavior*. Cambridge, MIT Press, (1968).
2. Altman, J. and Das, G. D.: *Nature, 204:*1161 (1964).
3. Barnes, R. H.: *Fed. Proc. 30:*1429 (1971).
4. Barnes, R. H., Cunnold, S. R., Zimmermann, R. R., *et al.: J. Nutr., 89:* 399–410 (1966).
5. Barnes, R. H., Moore, A. U., Reid, I. M., and Pond, W. G.: *J. Am. Diet. Assoc., 51:*34 (1967).
6. Barnes, R. H., Moore, A. U., Reid, I. M., and Pond, W. G.: In N. S. Scrimshaw and J. E. Gordon (Eds.): *Malnutrition, Learning and Behavior*. Cambridge, MIT Press (1968).
7. Bayley, N.: *Children, 5:*129 (1958).
8. Birch, H. G.: In N. S. Scrimshaw and J. E. Gordon (Eds.): *Malnutrition, Learning and Behavior*. Cambridge, MIT Press (1968).
9. Birch, H. G.: Gainesville *SUN*, Report by J. Randal, November 26, 1970.
10. Birch, H. G. and Belmont, L.: *Percept. Mot. Skills, 20:*295 (1965).
11. Birch, H. G. and Cravioto, J.: Proceedings of a Conference on Prevention of Mental Retardation through Control of Infectious Disease. Washington, PHS Publ. 1692, (1968).
12. Canosa, C. A.: In N. S. Scrimshaw and J. E. Gordon (Eds.): *Malnutrition, Learning and Behavior*. Cambridge, MIT Press (1968).
13. Chandra, R. K.: *Indian J. Pediatr., 35:*70 (1968).
14. Coursin, D. B.: In N. S. Scrimshaw and J. E. Gordon (Eds.): *Malnutrition, Learning and Behavior*. Cambridge, MIT Press (1968).
15. Cravioto, J.: In *Preschool Child Malnutrition*. NAS–NRC Publ. 1282, Washington Academy of Sciences (1966).
16. Cravioto, J.: In P. Gyorgy and O. L. Kline (Eds.): *Malnutrition is a Problem of Ecology*. Basel, S. Karger (1970).
17. Cravioto, J. and De Licardie, E. R.: In N. S. Scrimshaw and J. E. Gordon (Eds.): *Malnutrition, Learning and Behavior*. Cambridge, MIT Press (1968).
18. Cravioto, J., Pinero, C., Arroyo, M., and Alcalde, E.: Symposium, Swedish Nutrition Foundation (1968).
19. Douglas, J. W. B.: In *Home and School*. London, McGibbon and Kee (1964).
20. Eichenwald, H. F.: In N. S. Scrimshaw and J. E. Gordon (Eds.): *Malnutrition, Learning and Behavior*. Cambridge, MIT Press (1968).
21. Eichenwald, H. F. and Fry, P. C.: *Science, 163:*644 (1968).

22. Eisenberg, L.: Proceedings of a Conference on Prevention of Mental Retardation through Control of Infectious Disease. Washington, PHS Publ. 1692 (1968).
23. Egan, M. C.: *Children, 16:*67 (1969).
24. Ells, K. and Davis, A.: In *Intelligence and Cultural Differences.* Chicago, University of Chicago Press (1951).
25. Engel, R.: *Electroencephalogr. Clin. Neurophysiol., 8:*489–500 (1956).
26. Frankova, S. and Barnes, R. H.: *J. Nutr., 96:*477 (1968a).
27. Frankova, S. and Barnes, R. H.: *J. Nutr., 96:*485 (1968b).
28. Hansen, J. D. L., Wittman, W., Moudie, A. D., and Fellingham, S. A.: In N. S. Scrimshaw and J. E. Gordon (Eds.): *Malnutrition, Learning and Behavior.* Cambridge, MIT Press (1968).
29. Hsuch, A. M., Augustine, C. E., and Chow, B. F.: *J. Nutr., 91:*195 (1967).
30. *Hunger is a Problem.* Agricultural Marketing, Washington, USDA Consumer and Marketing Service, (1969), vol. 14, p. 3.
31. Ireland, L. M.: *Low-Income Life Styles.* Washington, U. S. Dept. of Health, Education, and Welfare. (1967).
32. Jelliffe, D. B. and Jelliffe, E. F. P.: In N. S. Scrimshaw and J. E. Gordon (Eds.): *Malnutrition, Learning and Behavior.* Cambridge, MIT Press (1968).
33. Kagan, J. and Moss, H. A.: *Child. Dev., 30:*325 (1959).
34. Kallen, D. J.: In N. S. Scrimshaw and J. E. Gordon (Eds.): *Malnutrition, Learning and Behavior.* Cambridge, MIT Press (1968).
35. Ketcham, W. A.: In N. S. Scrimshaw and J. E. Gordon (Eds.): *Malnutrition, Learning and Behavior.* Cambridge, MIT Press (1968).
36. Ketcham, W. A. and Morse, W. C.: Cooperative Research Project No. 1286, Child Development Laboratories, University of Michigan, Ann Arbor (1965).
37. Kohn, M. L.: *Am. J. Soc., 64:*337 (1959).
38. Kohn, M. L.: *Am. J. Soc., 68:*471 (1963).
39. Knoblock, H. and Pasamanick, B.: *Am. J. Dis. Child., 106:*43–51 (1963).
40. Latham, M. C., McGandy, R. P., McCann, M. B., and Stare, F. J.: In *Scope Manual on Nutrition.* Kalamazoo, Upjohn (1970).
41. Livingston, S. K.: *J. Nutr. Educ., 3:*18 (1971).
42. Lowe, C. U.: Committee of Nutrition, American Academy of Pediatrics Before the Committee on Agriculture, House of Representatives (1969).
43. Lowenberg, M. E., Todhunter, E. N., Wilson, E. D., Feeney, N. C., and Savage, J. R.: In *Food and Man.* New York, John Wiley & Sons (1968).
44. Mockeberg, F.: In P. Gyorgy and O. L. Kline (Eds.): *Malnutrition is a Problem of Ecology.* Basel, S. Karger (1970).
45. National Health Service of Chile (1967).
46. Neff, W. S.: *Psychol. Bull., 35:*727 (1938).

47. *Nutr. Rev., 27:*301 (1969).
48. Nelson, G. K.: *Electroencephalogr. Clin. Neurophysiol., 11:*73–84 (1959a).
49. Olmedo, Z. M., Urdapilleta, D., Ramos–Galvan, R., and Lubeski, M.: *Bol. Med. Hosp. Infantil.* (Mex.), *24:*43 (1967).
50. Platt, B. S. and Stewart, R. J. C.: In G. H. Bourne (Ed.): *World Review Nutrition.* Basel, S. Karger (1971), vol. 13.
51. Rajalakshmi, R. and Ramakrishnan, C. V.: Terminal Report of P1480 Project FG–In–176. Baroda University, Baroda, India (1969a).
52. Rajalakshmi, R. and Ramakrishnan, C. V.: In G. H. Bourne (Ed.): *World Review Nutrition and Dietetics.* Basel, S. Karger, vol. 14 (1971).
53. Ramos–Galvan, R.: In N. S. Scrimshaw and J. E. Gordon (Eds.): *Malnutrition, Learning and Behavior.* Cambridge, MIT Press (1968).
54. Read, M. S.: In P. Gyorgy and O. L. Kline (Eds.): *Malnutrition is a Problem of Ecology.* Basel, S. Karger (1970).
55. Richardson, S. A.: In N. S. Scrimshaw and J. E. Gordon (Eds.): *Malnutrition, Learning and Behavior.* Cambridge, MIT Press (1968).
56. Riecken, H. W.: In N. S. Scrimshaw and J. E. Gordon (Eds.): *Malnutrition, Learning and Behavior.* Cambridge, MIT Press (1968).
57. Robinow, M.: In N. S. Scrimshaw and J. E. Gordon (Eds.); *Malnutrition, Learning and Behavior.* Cambridge, MIT Press (1968).
58. Rosenzweig, M. R. and Bennett, E. L.: *Dev. Psychol., 2:*87 (1969).
59. Rosenzweig, M. R., Bennett, E. L., Diamond, M. C., *et al.: Brain Res., 14:*427 (1969).
60. Rosenzweig, M. R., Love, W., and Bennett, E. L.: *Physiol. Behav., 3:*819 (1968).
61. Scott, R. B., Carbozo, W. W., Smith, G., and DeLilly, M. R.: *J. Pediatr., 37:*885 (1950).
62. Scrimshaw, N. S.: *Am. J. Clin. Nutr., 20:*493 (1967).
63. Scrimshaw, N. S.: In N. S. Scrimshaw and J. E. Gordon (Eds.): *Malnutrition, Learning and Behavior.* Cambridge, MIT Press (1968).
64. Scrimshaw, N. S. and Gordon, J. E. (Eds.): *Malnutrition, Learning and Behavior.* Cambridge, MIT Press (1968).
65. Scrimshaw, N. S., Taylor, C. E., and Gordon, J. E.: In *Interaction of Nutrition and Infection.* W.H.O. Monograph, Geneva (1968).
66. Skeels, H. M., Updegraff, R., Wellman, B. L., and Williams, H. M.: *Univ. Iowa Studies Child Welfare, 15:*10 (1938).
67. Skeels, H. M.: *Child. Dev., 31:*3 (1966).
68. Stuart, H. C. and Stevenson, S. S.: In *Nelson Text Book of Pediatrics,* 7th ed. Philadelphia, W. B. Saunders (1959).

69. Trowell, H. C., Davies, J. N. P., and Dean, R. F. A.: *Kwashiorkor.* London, Arnold (1954).

70. Widdowson, E. M.: *Lancet, 260:*B16–18 (1951).

71. Winick, M.: *J. Pediatr., 74:*667–679 (1969).

72. Winick, M.: *Med. Clin. North Am., 54:*1413 (1970).

73. Yankauer, A., Goss, K. G., and Romero, S. M.: *Am. J. Public Health, 43:*1001 (1953).

74. Zimmerman, R. and Strobell, D.: Proceedings 77th Annual Convention, APA (1969).

Chapter V

MATERNAL MALNUTRITION—EFFECT ON THE GROWING FETUS AND NEONATE

In AREAS OF THE WORLD where protein-calorie malnutrition is an endemic problem, women do not get diets during pregnancy which are in any way different from those received during their pregravidic state. A prolonged lack of a well-balanced diet during pregnancy could affect the fetus at a very critical state of its growth. If this pattern of maternal malnutrition is continued into the postnatal life of the infant, the mother may not lactate adequately, and in the absence of extra supplementary food, the infant may suffer a double deprivation (pre and postnatal). This may have severe consequences for the physical and mental growth and the intellectual functioning of the infant. A report [163] of a WHO expert committee in 1965 commented on maternal nutrition and concluded that,

> Reports from many parts of the world have illustrated a general association between low birth weights, high foetal and infant mortality, and diets of poor nutritive value; and it seems reasonable to conclude that undernutrition and malnutrition among mothers, especially in the developing countries contribute towards impaired maternal, foetal and infant health and vitality.

Studies have indicated that a child born to a severely malnourished mother may catch up to a great extent in physical growth with adequate diet, but the impairment of the nervous system may be irreversible and leave the individual permanently damaged with respect to intellectual functioning. Beargie *et al.*[12] showed that the small for date newborn lags behind its development compared to its control. Winick and Noble [170] provided very meaningful data from the study of rats and showed that "catch up" growth may be unlikely in cases where growth failure has taken place quite early during development. The fetal

166

organs during development have a certain criteria of growth
priority. The brain, for obvious reasons, has the highest priority,
but if the maternal diet is grossly inadequate, it is likely to
affect the brain growth and the mental development of the child
as well. Cabak and Najdanvic [21] measured the intelligence and
physical growth of children who suffered postnatal malnutrition and followed their progress to the age of 16 years. Out of
36 children under study, 18 had I.Q.s within normal limits (91 to
94), 12 were stupid with I.Q.s between 71 and 90, and the re-
maining six showed I.Q.s less than 70. In this sample no child
showed an I.Q. greater than 110. This is a very unlikely outcome,
and if a random sample of 36 normal healthy children is picked
up from a street, such percentages may not be obtained. In
such a large sample size, some of them will definitely show an
I.Q. higher than 110. Cabak and Najdanvic [21] concluded that these
Serbian children, malnourished in early life, had normal physical characteristics but subnormal mental capacity. That the
amount of available protein in the maternal diet, particularly
during gestation, greatly influences the growth and development of the offspring has also been recently shown by Hsuch [66]
in his studies on rats.

Numerous studies have given conclusive evidence that the
ability of a woman to nurture a healthy fetus (physically, physiologically, and mentally) depends to a great extent on her
own nutritional state, not only during pregnancy but during her
whole preconceptual life. Good nutrition results from lifelong
habits of good diet. Too often the preconceptional health of the
mother is ignored and all the concern is concentrated on her
dietary intake during pregnancy. For example, a woman who
had adequate and well-balanced food before her pregnancy can
have an inadequate diet during her pregnancy and still have
enough reserves to satisfy all the nutritional demands of the
fetus. The baby born to such a mother will, in all likelihood, be
in the normal range of birth weight. On the other hand, a
woman whose diet has been poor in the preconceptual state and
has not been adequately provided for during pregnancy may
have a hard time in meeting fully the demands of the growing

fetus, even at the expense of her own tissue reserves. Even if such a woman is successful in giving birth to a baby in the normal range of birth weight, she may have extreme difficulties in establishing adequate lactation and thereby may hurt the baby in the postnatal stage. Thomson [140] made extensive field studies and concluded that small unhealthy women give birth to premature children five times as often as tall healthy women. Similarly, Tompkin and Wiehl [148] showed that women whose height at the beginning of their pregnancy is below the mean of their social group have a much higher incidence of prematurely born children. As with underweight and undernourished women, obese women with or without diabetes tend to give birth to larger babies who have an abnormal body composition including increased fat. The infants of diabetic mothers may have hyperinsulinism with associated hypoglycemia and damage to the central nervous system.[70] The above observations support the findings of an extensive study made earlier by Burke and collaborators [20] in Boston. These workers divided the neonates during their first two weeks of life into two groups. The first contained infants who were rated excellent physically and functionally by pediatricians, whereas the second group consisted of infants who were rated poor, physically or functionally. Fifty-six percent of the mothers of the first group of infants had excellent diets, 35 percent fair, and 9 percent poor diets during pregnancy. Amongst the mothers of the second group of infants, 79 percent had very poor diets, 18 percent fair, and only 3 percent good. These findings showed a direct relationship between maternal nutrition and the physical and physiological well-being of the infant. They are in agreement with the findings of some other workers who, after extensive research work, concluded [105,106,133] that nutritional deficiencies are shared by mother and offspring. Higher nutritional states of the mother during pregnancy not only give greater protection to the fetus, but the mother's diet, even 15 to 20 years before parturition, may have an effect on the vitality of the offspring. During the recent years, the obstetric practice in the U.S. tends to discourage too much weight gain, obviously for good reasons. But the faulty dietary practices of mothers anxious to maintain their figure contribute to large number of low birth weight infants and to high perinatal and infant mortality rates.[81]

MATERNAL NUTRITION AND STRESS OF PREGNANCY

Maternal nutrition is one of the most important factors which not only affects the successful completion of pregnancy but is important in the process of organogenesis as well as the growth of the fetus. Growth, beginning with conception, requires dietary essentials to a greater extent than does maintenance because pregnancy is not a process of fetal growth superimposed on the ordinary metabolism of the mother. It is accompanied by extensive changes in maternal metabolism as well as dietary needs.[163] Although in its earliest stages the fertilized egg carries some nutrient material, it has to depend on a constant supply of nutrients from the mother for its growth and development. The interrelationship of the mother and her growing fetus and the extent to which the fetus depends on the maternal diet are problems that need more elaborate investigation. It is certain, however, that under the impact of fetal growth, metabolic alteration in the mother's body results in greater stress and consequently increases her nutritional requirements. "The orderly sequence of fetal development and growth, the mechanisms for nourishment of the fetus, the storage of nutrients in anticipation of labor and delivery, and the development of the mammary glands represent a level of anabolism unequaled in any other time of life." [115] Gopalan [53] believed that the important question is: how does the state of maternal nutrition affect the coming pregnancy and the condition of the infant at birth and during the neonatal period?

A woman who has been poorly nourished in pregravidic state is much more subject to the complications of pregnancy, including toxemia, hypertension, anemia, and premature birth.[115] In a paper submitted to the WHO by the expert Committee on Maternal and Child Health, Venkatachalam [152] revealed the results of a survey of low socioeconomic pregnant women in South India. These women, according to this survey, underwent the nutritional stress of pregnancy without any nutritional improvement either prior to or after conception and showed gross signs of protein-calorie malnutrition. The women, subsisting on approximately 1,408 calories and 38 gm of protein daily, showed a high percentage of premature termination of pregnancy. Venkatachalam[152] reported that in this group, 20 percent of all pregnancies terminated in abortion, miscarriage, or stillbirth. Experimental studies on rats showed that when the dietary protein level is reduced to less than 5 percent during pregnancy the incidence of fetal resorptions is as high as 70 to 100 percent.[96] The survey of Venkatachalam revealed that the subjects, with a few exceptions, were unaware of the increased food needs during pregnancy, and a few actually believed that food restriction would facilitate normal delivery. Using the birth weight set by the World Health Organization [162] (below 2,500 gm birth weight) as the definition of prematurity, one third of the infants born to these mothers were premature. A normal weight gain during pregnancy is generally around 25 percent of the initial pregravidic weight. Indian women of poor socioeconomic status gained around 6 kg during pregnancy, starting with an initial weight of 42 kg. In the area of India where the Venkatachalam survey was taken, neonatal mortality contributed heavily to the deaths occurring during infancy, and 73 percent of all deaths within one month of age were a direct result of "debility and prematurity." Venkatachalam suggested that whereas the small-sized underweight infants may manage to mature physiologically and functionally, they do not have nutritional reserves of their own, and any nutritional neglect makes them candidates for nutritional deficiency syndromes, such as kwashiorkor and marasmus. There is, however, no direct correlation between maternal deprivation or birth weight of an infant and the development of kwashiorkor or marasmus, since kwashiorkor under one year of age has been rarely reported. Infants develop Kwashiorkor generally between one and three years of age.

It has been commonly observed in underdeveloped countries that although infants born to protein-malnourished mothers are most often low in birth weight, they appear to function normally. They survive because the fetus is apparently able to drain at least a minimum of essential nutrients from the mother, and some kind of adaptive mechanism of the mother facilitates the conservation and maximum utilization of the available nutrients for the fetus.[152] The placenta probably plays an important role in this adaptive mechanism because the nutrition of the fetus takes place through this organ. In my laboratory, I am presently studying the placentas of healthy primates and of those in which a protein deficiency has been experimentally created during pregnancy. I hope to answer such questions as: Does the placenta keep a reserve capacity of nutrients irrespective of the diet of the pregnant female; does the difference in size and weight of placenta in healthy and malnourished mothers influence the birth weight of the offspring, and what are the gross morphological and cytochemical indicators of maternal malnutrition?

The preconceptional nutritional status of the mother, particularly during adolescence, is directly related to the stress of pregnancy, as indicated by the birth weight of the infant, its general well-being, its chances of survival, and the lactating ability of the mother. A study of Aykroyd and Hossain [6] in the United Kingdom of immigrant Pakistani women and native women may be somewhat illustrative.

> Both groups were said to have taken full advantage of the maternal and child welfare facilities, and the offspring were bottle fed. The deaths from 1 to 11 months of age were similar, being slightly but not significantly higher in the immigrant group (15.7 compared with 9.3 per 1,000), but the neonatal deaths were 2.4 times greater than the indigenous group. These families were not impoverished. Malnutrition was not present during gestation, and it is probable that the different neonatal death rates are a reflection of the mother's nutritional status during growth and adolescence.

Similar findings have been experimentally produced. Malnourished animals produce immature offspring whose chances of survival are slight.[134] The effect of nutritional deficiency in early life on the reproductive performances of bitches is quite clear.[133] All the offspring of rats maintained on diets with very low protein content during gestation and lactation died before weaning. Such a high mortality rate may be related to deficiency in lactation because 78 percent of the offspring born of normal mothers also died when fostered by malnourished ones.[154] It seems unlikely that lactational deficiency is the sole reason for this mortality rate, because 40 percent of the rats born of malnourished mothers still died when nursed by well-fed mothers, compared to 9 percent of the normal offspring similarly fostered. It appears that the quality and quantity of protein in the maternal diet in the pregravidic as well as gravidic state is a critical factor in determining the health of the progeny, and there is an association between inadequate maternal diet and subsequent poor utilization of food by the progeny.[27]

Recent studies on rats show that malnutrition during gestation caused a decrease in fecundity, and the progeny are smaller than the offspring of the controls. If the undernourishment is continued into lactation period, mortality rate is very high and the surviving pups show severe growth stunting. Payne and Wheeler,[102] however, pointed out that the stress of pregnancy in primates is considerably less than that in nonprimate mammals, so one has to be cautious when generalizing the results of studies on rats and dogs with humans. The progeny of malnourished rats are always underweight by at least 30 percent, even when given good quality foods in ad libitum quantities, whereas in humans, the underweight offsprings of the malnourished mothers catch up in body weight with their more privileged colleagues born of healthy mothers.[27]

An interesting correlation exists between the resumption of menstruation after delivery and nutrition. Some studies[53] indicate that in malnourished mothers, the resumption of regular menstruation takes much longer than in well-nourished mothers. Whether early resumption of menstruation in the well-fed mothers is the result of a good pregravidic or gravidic diet or due to successful lactation is not clear at this time.

LEVEL OF MATERNAL NUTRITION, MATERNAL WEIGHT GAIN AND BIRTH WEIGHT OF THE NEONATE

Maternal Weight Gain

There is a direct relationship between preconceptional maternal health, adequate well-balanced diets during pregnancy and the birth weight, and the physical and physiological well-being of the neonate. A strong positive association exists between the maternal weight gain and the birth weight of the infant.[44] The relationship between maternal health and weight gain during pregnancy, however, is indirect, and many workers have not observed any correlation between the maternal weight gain and the infant's birth weight. Occasionally excessive weight gain during pregnancy can be due to the body's retention of extra water associated with sodium retention. Normal weight gain during pregnancy should be approximately 25 percent of the initial body weight. Out of the total increase in weight, very little is gained in the first trimester, approximately 8 to 10 percent of initial body weight is gained in the second trimester, and 12 to 15 percent in the third trimester. In Asian countries where not only the dietary standards during pregnancy are quite low, but the preconceptional health of young mothers, especially those from the lower socioeconomic strata of the society are poor, and weight gain during pregnancy is relatively low.[153] The total body water of undernourished pregnant women was observed by Venkatachalam and co-workers to be 56 percent between the nine and 14 weeks of gestation. This figure is similar to that for nonpregnant females from the same population. Between the twentieth and twenty-eighth week, the total body water of pregnant females reached about 60 percent, and this figure climbed to 70 percent after 28 weeks. The weight increase in these subjects was greater than would be expected due to the incrase in total-body water. Also these women lost a lot of body fat. Seitchik and Alper [123] showed in studies in the United States that the losses of body fat during pregnancy, when given adequate nutrition, resulted in an increase in lean body tissue. It is not certain whether the fat depletion is a result of undernutrition or the fat is simply utilized in the synthesis of lean body tissue, irrespective of nutritional standard of the mother. Elaborate work is needed in this area.

Birth Weight and Maternal Nutrition

The birth weight of a neonate generally depends on the length of gestation. Children born prior to the completion of full term are usually of lower birth weight compared to those born after full term. However, statistical figures collected all over the world show that a larger number of babies, particularly in the under-developed countries, have a birth weight below 2,500 gm, the criterion for prematurity established in 1950, even when they were full term as determined by the gestation period. Using the standard of 2,500 gms, a survey by Venkatachalam [152] showed that in India 29.3 percent of the babies born in the lower socioeco-nomic group have a low birth weight, 13.8 percent in the high socioeconomic group, and 2 percent in the upper socioeconomic class. In the lower class 9.2 percent neonates were less than 2,000 gms. One third of all babies of this class were born pre-maturely by WHO standards. Udani [150] has similar findings in a sample of 3,270 children in Bombay. Irrespective of the gesta-tion period, babies (whether born prematurely or after full term) less than 2,000 gms in weight suffer a high incidence of illness and mortality. The immature group (having suffered in-trauterine growth retardation) may either die *in utero,* develop hypoglycemia postnatally, or have permanent physical or mental deficits. Drillien [42] in his treatise on the growth and development of the prematurely born infant showed that $4\frac{1}{2}$ to $5\frac{1}{2}$ lb (2,000 gms or more) babies born prematurely gained in height or weight at the same rate as $4\frac{1}{2}$ to $5\frac{1}{2}$ lb babies born at full term. This indicates that a few weeks' prematurity does not differentially affect the rate of growth if the intrauterine fetal growth has been satisfactory.

Retarded prenatal growth has been attributed to a number of factors, such as a genetic factor responsible for a low weight throughout life,[28] placental abnormalities restricting transfer of nutrients to the fetus,[55,86] or poor nutrition of the mother lead-ing to poor storage of fat and perhaps nitrogen in the fetus.[28] Rumbolz and McGoogan [118] attributed a smaller size of the in-fant solely to placental insufficiency, and Wigglesworth [165] believed that changes in the placenta are responsible for low birth weight, hypoglycemia, and mental defects. Other placental stud-ies show that the birth weight of the neonate correlates with the DNA content of the placenta. Placental DNA has also been found to correlate with the collagen, zinc, manganese, and magnesium content of the placenta.[81]

Wigglesworth[165] believed that growth retardation in the fetus is most often the result of maternal malnutrition, although the apparent cause may be different. According to him:

> Poor foetal growth could in theory result from: (1) conditions affecting the nutrient content of the maternal blood or its supply to the placenta, (2) poor development, damage to, or specific abnormalities of the placental membrane affecting transport across the placenta, or (3) disorders of the foetal-placental circulation. Available evidence suggests that foetal nutrition may be impaired at any of these sites.

Genetic endowments are also extremely important factors in determining the size of the offspring, but may not be so important as the maternal nutrition when it comes to the growth of the fetus.[56] A large number of workers agree that maternal malnutrition is a major contributory factor in low birth weight or immaturity.*

There also exists a definite relationship between the quality of the mother's diet during pregnancy, particularly with respect to its protein content, and the length of the baby at birth. Protein supply in the diet appears more important than the number of calories in the maternal food or height of the mother as a determiner of the length of the baby.

> It would appear correct to assume that the amount of total protein in the prenatal diet is a more influential factor in determining the birth length of the infant than either calcium or riboflavin. Since a high phosphorus content is so closely associated with protein-rich foods, it is difficult to determine the effect of phosphorus.[125]

Nutrition of the Fetus

The fertilized egg carries along with it some nutrient material and for the first few days develops in the fallopian tubes. After the ovum is firmly implanted in the uterine mucosa, it feeds on a mixture of uterine secretions and damaged autolyzing cells, including the blood cells.[105] When the placenta develops, it takes upon itself the role of nutrient supply by facilitating exchange between the blood of the mother and that of the embryo. From then on, the embryo and later the fetus is directly

---

* See references 35, 83, 84, 86, 94, 106, 139–146.

dependent on the mother for its nutrition, and as a result fetal growth depends greatly on the quality and quantity of the maternal diet. This growth could continue as far as possible, even at the expense of maternal tissues.[67] The mother has inborn or endocrine-controlled adaptive mechanisms such that the storage of nutrients in the tissues starts long before they are needed by the fetus, and if the mother is short of food during a certain period in her pregnancy, her tissues could be utilized in meeting the growth requirement of the fetus. It is, however, becoming clear that there is a limit to such host-parasite relationship, and the food shortages would be shared by mother and fetus. The growth of the fetus, therefore, depends largely on the nutritional supply of the mother.

The main components of the fetus are water and fat, and as explained by Clements [28] in a full-term fetus, 70 percent of the birth weight and 93 percent of the fat are acquired during the third trimester. The water is held in place by the action of protein and fat. In general, the sequence of fetal nutrition consists of the transfer of maternal plasma amino acids across the placenta, and since the level of plasma amino acid on the fetal side are higher than the maternal, the placenta plays an important role in trapping and storing maternal amino acids and delivering them into fetal blood supply. A woman whose dietary intake is defective, particularly in proteins, will have a very low plasma amino nitrogen, and only very small quantities of amino acids may be available for transfer to the fetus. This could seriously retard its growth, particularly since the fetus is dependent on maternal supply for its entire supply of gamma globulins, some albumin, and some other proteins.[28] In some women, although their protein intake is adequate, the total food intake is not in sufficient quantity, and the fetus may suffer because of conversion of protein for use as energy. Such an undesirable use of proteins for providing energy would decrease the level of maternal plasma amino acids. The fetal growth, and as a consequence the birth weight of the neonate, therefore, depends to a great extent on the quality as well as the quantity of the nutrition of the mother. The undernourished mother, however, undertakes a physiological adaptation for conservation and maximum utilization of the available nutrients in order to safeguard the developing fetus, but she also retains additional proteins, over and above the needed quantity to undergo the stress of pregnancy and normal nutrition of the fetus. This extra protein is stored in the maternal tissues in order to cope with the increased demands of lactation after delivery and to help the fetal tissues meet the additional needs of quick growth during the first few months of life.[28] Experimental studies, however, show that rats whose mothers were given about 50 percent of the required food during the gestation periods not only showed retarded physical growth but also an impaired capacity for the efficient use of proteins in the diet.[27]

Implications of Birth Weight

Venkatachalam [152] observed that virtually none of the small-sized premature babies weighing in the vicinity of 2,000 gms examined by him in India showed any clinical symptoms of prematurity as recognized by physicians or any evidence of functional or physiological immaturity, and he believed that the practice of classifying all infants under 2,500 gms as premature may not be a sound one. However, infants with such a low birth weight are nutritionally deficient in comparison to their healthy counterparts, and unless nursed carefully, will deplete their protein reserves in a short time. Clinical manifestations may then begin to appear and lead to permanent stunting or death. In a survey in India nearly 25 percent of the deaths of low-birth-weight children took place during the first seven days and 38 percent within the first month. A clinical analysis revealed that nearly 73 percent of all deaths were due to "debility and prematurity." [152] The infants included in this survey weighed 2,000 gms or less at birth and were born to mothers whose nutritional status during pregnancy was considered unsatisfactory. This is in contrast to the results obtained from a random sample of women belonging to low socioeconomic groups in India who were admitted to the nutrition ward of a hospital during the last four weeks of gestation due to malnutritional state. During their stay in the hospital they were given an adequately balanced diet, containing nearly 85 gms of protein and over 2,500 calories per day. In addition, they were able to enjoy complete physical rest. The mean birthweight [152] of the babies born to these women was 2986 ± 86 gms.

Birth weight of the infant most often correlates with weight and height of the mother and weight gain during pregnancy. Tompkin and Wiehl [149] believed that women who are underweight for their height and age in the preconceptional period and who do not gain adequate weight during the first and second trimesters are more likely to have lower birth weight babies, premature separations of the placenta, and higher rates of infant morbidity and mortality. It may, however, be misleading to judge the maturity or immaturity of the infant from the birth weight only. Although birth weight does appear to be correlated with maternal preconceptual weight and her nutrition, these correlations are not always consistent,[65] and the present writer is inclined to endorse Thomson's [139-146] concept of quality of babies. The quality of the baby from the physiological point of view may be as variable as the size. A satisfactory nutrition at the onset protects against the adverse effects of an unsatisfactory gain throughout the subsequent early antepartum period.[149] Large infants (1 to 2 lbs above average and postmature) may have adiposity and fare as poorly as those who are underweight to the same degree at birth,[10,11] and big babies with a high birth weight may not physiologically be the best kind to have.

Loss of Weight of the Neonate

Under normal circumstances, irrespective of the nutritional status of the mother or the birth weight of the neonate, babies lose their maximum weight during the second or third day after delivery and regain their weight between the fifth and sixth day. Venkatachalam [152] divided newborns into two groups to study the weight loss of children with different birth weights and their pattern of regaining. The first group of 25 infants had a mean birth weight of 3067 gms (range 2752 to 3519 gms), and the second group of 40 infants had a mean birth weight of 2305 gms (range 1603 to 2710 gms). He found that infants in the first group regained their birth weight during the fifth and sixth day, whereas infants in the second group regained their weight during the fourth and fifth day. This difference was probably a reflection of their weight loss. Whereas infants in the first group (high birth weight) lost 102 gms ± 9.91 gms, infants in the second group (low birth weight) lost only 75.8 gms ± 7.12 gms, which may mean that the loss of weight during the first four days of life is influenced by the birth weight of a particular infant.

Birth Weight and Kwashiorkor

Kwashiorkor has been rarely observed in infants of less than one year of age and is most common in children between one to three years of age. It would be quite interesting to know the birth weight of the kwashiorkor patients so as to investigate if any relationship exists between birth weight and potential development of kwashiorkor at a later stage, and whether maternal malnutrition, leading to low birth weight, contributes in a subsequent period to the development of kwashiorkor in toddlers and preschool children. Varkki *et al.*[151] traced back a series of kwashiorkor patients between one and three years and from their birth weights elucidated that their mean birth weight was 2729 gms and 80 percent of the babies weighed more than 2,500 gms. These workers did not find any correlation between birth weight and age of onset of the disease. Venkatachalam [152] concluded that birth weight or even maternal malnutrition does not contribute directly to the development of protein malnutrition among the children.

Maternal Malnutrition and Growth Retardation of Fetal Tissues

A number of studies have shown that poor maternal malnutrition results in intrauterine growth retardation, and the poor fetal growth is a result of fetal malnutrition and marasmus.[82,94,136] Naeye [82] investigated the anatomic growth retardation of tissues of 11 neonates who died of severe maternal malnutrition at the gestational periods of 36 to 41 weeks. A comparison of different prenatally retarded organs with those of children dying with alimentary malnutrition would give a fair idea of the role of maternal malnutrition in fetal growth retardation. These authors noticed a close resemblance in the manner of organ abnormalities in both groups. In both groups, brain, pancreas, heart, lungs, and kidneys were quite close to their normal weight, whereas the liver and spleen were disproportionately small. The smaller size of these organs was due to a subnormal amount of cytoplasm in their cells. Also, the number of parenchymal cells in the liver, spleen, pancreas, kidney, and adrenal glands were reduced. The close similarity in the manner of anatomic changes in the various tissues retarded prenatally or postnatally clearly shows that these changes are brought about under the influence of malnutrition, whether it is maternal malnutrition creating lack of available nutrients in the fetus or postnatal. Both groups also show organ abnormalities which indicated a disturbance in carbohydrate metabolism and subsequent abnormalities in physical and mental growth. Both groups also showed pituitary abnormalities which explain their growth retardation. Prenatally retarded infants showed brain weights 18 percent less than the postnatally malnourished ones, and some of the prenatally malnourished infants who survived showed an increased incidence of mental subnormality.[7,158]

Clinical and anatomical investigation of the children suffering intrauterine growth retardation suggests a pattern very similar to postnatal protein calorie malnutrition.[23] O'brien *et al.*[99] showed that a large number of neonates born with intrauterine growth retardation (IGR) show asphyxia, which points towards an impaired ability to stand the stress of labor and delivery. Cassady [23] studied in detail the body composition of the neonates born after experiencing IGR, and the reader is referred to this article. He suggested that the initial changes in IGR consist of expansion of the extracellular compartment, particularly the intravascular or plasma volume phase. He demonstrated elevated mean plasma volume (ml/kg) in a number of neonates. Here again the observation of the expansion of extracellular compartment is similar to the one observed in postnatal malnutrition, as is the contraction of cell size due to the reduction of intracellular water and lesser amounts of total body solids.

Growth Retardation and Chromosomal Abnormalities

In cases of intrauterine growth retardation, cytogenetical examination for chromosomal abnormalities is in order. Growth retardation of the fetus is very prominent, particularly in the case of 18 and D_1 trisomy syndromes. The fetuses which show evidence of Down's and Turners' syndromes also fail to grow or thrive, and their chance of *in utero* or postnatal survival are greatly reduced. The reader is referred to a detailed article of Reisman [113] on the subject.

Prominent growth retardation in trisomy 18 results in a markedly reduced birth weight, and on a study of 90 infants with this aberration, Warkany described the mean birth weight as 2183 gms, with half of them having a gestation period of over 40 weeks. The placental size is small, and Hecht [62] reported certain pathological changes, such as patchy fibrosis and focal placental infarctions.

The abnormalities of the sex chromosomes lead to prenatal as well as postnatal growth retardation. The loss of short arm of the X chromosome is directly related to such stunting of growth [113] and leads to dwarfism and other characteristic features of Turner's syndrome.[114] The ovaries are always defective in such cases. The triple X or poly X (XXXX or XXXXX) females do not show any prominent growth retardation, nor do the individuals with Klinefelter's syndrome (47/XXY). However, the males with XXXXY abnormality do show prominent postnatal growth retardation.[113]

The chromosomal abnormalities in the fetus are a prelude to a continuous chain of events which leads to faulty cellular devision and hence an abnormal growth pattern. A high percentage of cases with chromosomal abnormalities leads to abortions, and it is estimated that "90% of the abnormal conceptuses are eliminated as abortuses; the remainder survive as abnormal birth weight and age of onset of the disease. Venkatachalam [152] the infants with 18 trisomy and estimated that 70 percent of the cases survive to one month, 10 percent to a year and 1 percent to ten years. Only a fraction of the people with intra-uterine growth retardation resulting from chromosomal ab-normalities lead a long life.

MATERNAL MALNUTRITION AND ITS EFFECTS ON THE CENTRAL NERVOUS SYSTEM

Brain Growth of the Fetus and Neonate

The brain is greatly susceptible to permanent damage from malnutrition, especially when the fetus is not able to draw suffi-cient nutrient supply from the maternal source during its period of rapid growth in late fetal life or in early postnatal life. It is es-timated that approximately 50 per cent of prenatal brain growth takes place during the last ten weeks of pregnancy, and 50 per cent of postnatal growth takes place during the first year of life. The last ten weeks of gestation are extremely important as far as the intrauterine growth of brain is concerned.

The rate of human brain growth reaches a peak about the fifth fetal month, and the tempo of growth at this level, with re-spect to neural maturation, is maintained until birth. The growth of the fetus is conditioned by the nutritional state of the mother and the quality and quantity of her diet. The maternal malnu-trition may, therefore, interfere with fetal neuronal development. Studies on the animals as well as on humans reveal that there is a critical period during which the brain is growing at the fastest rate, and if this process gets interrupted even for a brief period under the effect of nutritional deprivation, it could produce irre-versible damages.[167,171] The fetus in such a case is bound to have neurologic abnormalities. The placentas belonging to such fe-tuses showing intrauterine growth retardation show fewer number of cells as well as an increased RNA/DNA ratio compared to the controls.[171] The intracellular dynamic equilibrium of RNA and protein as well as the linear development of DNA in the fetus becomes seriously disturbed if the mother is not able to provide at least a bare minimum of nutrients, especially proteins. This observation becomes significantly important in view of the findings that placentas from malnourished populations in Guatemala also showed fewer than normal cells. Winick and Rosso [172] showed in a sample of nine brains from Santiago, Chile, that the marasmic children showed reduced quantities of DNA, RNA, and proteins. In this sample the three infants showed DNA content as low as 40 per cent of the expected. From the anatomical viewpoint it must be stressed that the younger the fetus or infant at the time of experiencing malnutrition, the more marked are the effects on the brain. Platt and Stewart [107] studied the rat brain and found that the brain weight was significantly subnormal if the growth stunting due to malnutrition began at an early age.

Altman and Das [4] used autoradiographic methods in rats in order to assess the kinetics of cell division in the brain and found out that different areas of the brain react differently to protein deprivation. The cerebral cortex reacts mildly; the area adjacent to the third ventricle reacts moderately, whereas the cerebellum and the area adjacent to the lateral ventricle are profoundly affected.[168] Among humans, the cerebral cortex shows its maximum growth during the postnatal period, which therefore implies that neonatal and early postnatal malnutrition could have serious effects on the growth and development of the cerebral cortex.

The DNA content, cell number, and myelination during the critical period of brain growth are significant factors in the mental development, but there is an additional factor that needs more elaborate investigations. It is the period of rapid increase of many enzymes and certain cytological changes such as the first appearance of cell processes and cell bodies. Flexner [48] undertook such studies in the guinea pigs and defined 41 to 45 days gestation period as the most critical period when the activity of certain enzymes belonging to different metabolic cycles increases greatly. These enzyme changes occur at a time when earliest evidences of function are manifest. Davies [36] believed that a corresponding critical period in humans exists between 12 to 16 weeks of gestation age, whereas Dobbing [40] believed that such a critical period may be as late as the third trimester, when the brain is growing at the highest level coinciding with a peak period of increase in brain weight. Irrespective of the timing of this period, a severe degree of maternal malnutrition would hinder the development of enzyme systems which could have profound influence on the mental development of the offspring.

Morphological studies on rats indicate that maternal malnutrition during pregnancy results in offsprings whose brains are not only smaller in size but also have lesser number of cells compared to the healthy infants.[175] A reduction in their number at the time of birth because of maternal malnutrition could have serious consequences in terms of permanent brain neuron deficiency and can irreversibly impair mental development. This quantitative decrease is probably the basis for frequently reported disturbances in behavior of the offsprings of the protein-deprived mothers.[175] Winick and his associates [171,172] commented further that such infants having suffered prenatal malnutrition do not ever recover completely, and even if they are fed adequately in their postnatal life, the cell deficit created during their intrautrine life persists.

Winick [169] reported that in humans the sequence of cellular changes is qualitatively similar to that in rats, i.e., the DNA values and the cell number increase linearly until birth. If during this phase the quantity of available protein is restricted, the brain suffers greatly during the process of the development, and its physical composition is greatly affected, and this in turn leads to impairments in intellectual and neurological performance.

Besides the brain, other fetal organs are even more susceptible to growth retardation as a result of maternal malnutrition or insufficient vascular supply. Nayae [94] compared the weights and organ structure of prenatally retarded children with those of children dying with postnatal alimentary malnutrition. Whereas the other organs were significantly retarded, the brain weights of infants with prenatal retardation were 82 percent of the control weights compared to 73 percent of the control values in infants with alimentary malnutrition. Since anatomical changes are a prelude to changes in mental development or intellectual functioning, prenatal malnutrition of the fetus, inspired by the maternal deprivation or early postnatal deprivation due to inability of the mother to lactate properly, may irrevocably impair the normal functioning ability of the offspring.

Maternal Malnutrition and Retarded Mental Development of the Infant

Both animal and human studies suggest that malnutrition in its critical stage of growth of the nervous system (before birth and early postnatal life) results in a large pool of poorly functioning people who in turn produce children who are destined to contribute to a new generation of malnourished individuals. Especially important is the mental development of the children who are born to malnourished mothers and have suffered intrauterine growth retardation. In these individuals, the retardation of intellectual capacity is a likely consequence.[32,33]

Maternal malnutrition puts certain limits to the protein synthesizing system of the growing fetus, and this could be a dangerous prognosis. It is possible that the deficient turnover of proteins in response to inadequate supply of nutrients may be the reason for the occurrence of mental defects in association with amino acid changes. Studies indicate that the brain is particularly subject to functional derangement by alterations in its metabolic environment, which impairs its normal processes of cellular maturation and development.

It may be hypothesized that maternal malnutrition in the pregravidic and gravidic state greatly reduces the efficiency of the mother to produce an infant with normal birth weight and mental development. Grossly underweight infants do not reach their full physical and mental potential and do not catch up with their counterparts born to healthy mothers, even with a better diet at a later stage.[42] Wiener [164] firmly believed that the effects of low birth weight on mental performance persist even at 12 to 13 years of age. Such children are always at a disadvantage with respect to work efficiency or mental stability. The children of low birth weight (probably caused by poor maternal dietary intake during the critical period of brain growth) always score low on a variety of psychological measures. Drillien [42] showed that the incidence of severe mental, neurological, or physical handicaps increased significantly with decreasing birth weight. He calculated that such mental disturbances were evident only in 1 percent of cases with normal birth weight compared to 64 percent in children with 1250 gm or less birth weight.

Low birth weight may be a result of various factors, such as placental insufficiency, genetic factors, maternal malnutrition. Wigglesworth [165] pointed out that the fetal growth retardation may be due to maternal undernutrition, maternal hypertension and toxemia of pregnancy, reduction in placenta mass due to damage of the placental tissue, or some fetal vascular abnormality. Whatever be the reason, Wigglesworth believed that babies with low birth weight show a high incidence of severe physical and mental handicaps on examination later in childhood.

A low birth weight of around 1,500 gms would be quite a critical factor in putting the neonates to a permanent intellectual disadvantage. With a birth weight of over 1,700 gms or in the vicinity of 2,000 gms there is less of a chance that a child may be severely mentally handicapped. A brief description of some important studies may be in order which show that full-term infants who have suffered intrauterine growth retardation, due to maternal malnutrition or other physiological disturbances, suffer severe mental impairment. Warkany *et al.*[156,158] studied 22 such children for a prolonged period of time and found only five of them within the normal range of intelligence. On the other hand, prematurely born infants of similar birth weight may not show such serious handicaps. Drillien [43] believed that the most conspicuous effect of intrauterine retardation could be a general lowering of intelligence rather than the production of severe handicaps.

A comment about the "small for dates" babies may be in order. A large number of such low birth weight children are born all over the world, and this may or may not be due to the nutritional standard of the mother. Some extranutritional congenital factors may be involved in growth retardation. However, these babies are more prone to neonatal hypoglycemia, which may result in brain damage. Under normal circumstances, the small for date babies may regain their weight within a short period of their postnatal life. The investigations of DeSilva,[125] Rajalakshmi and associates [111] in Ceylon and India show that most of the small for date babies exhibit satisfactory psychological development in spite of the birth weight as low as 1.5 kg. According to them, 11 children with birth weights below 2.4 kgs. fared no worse than 15 children with birth weight between 2.5 to 3 kgs.

Chow [26] emphasized that the intrauterine malnutrition may have equally or even more serious consequences than postnatal and that no adequately controlled longitudinal studies exist in children which will relate maternal malnutrition, especially in the third trimester of pregnancy, to the long-term functional development of children. Experimental studies in this area also indicate that it may not always be right to depend on the birth weight or size to predict the future mental development. Some experimental data shows that "serious metabolic abnormalities can be caused by maternal restriction during gestation even though the size of the progency is little affected." [26]

Lubchenko *et al.*[80] studied ten-year-old children who were born with a birth weight of 1,500 gms or less: 25 children out of this sample of 60 children showed I.Q.s below 90, indicating impairment of their mental capacity; 30 children out of this group also showed abnormalities in their electroencephalograms; 35 children appeared to have normal intelligence, but 20 of them had problems in their progress at school. The results of this study are in contrast to Bossier,[117] who believed that 78 percent of the children with a birth weight of less than 1,500 gms were normal, and that in United States about 16,000 children with a birth weight of less than 1,500 gms survive and grow to adult life every year. Knoblock and Pasamanuch,[74] however, believe that at least 20 percent of them would be mentally defective. Capper,[22] as early as 1928, described a full-term immature infant as a "pathological museum" which "becomes the backward school child and is a potential psychopathic or neuropathic patient and even a potential candidate for the home for imbeciles and idiots." Bacola and co-workers [8] carried out a detailed investigation of low-birth-weight children. Amongst children who weighed between 1,500 to 2,500 gms the intelligence level represented in terms of normal, borderline, and retarded was 65 percent, 27 percent, and 8 percent respectively. Amongst children whose birth weight ranged between 1,250 to 1,500 gms, these percentages of normal, borderline, and retarded were changed to 54 percent, 32 percent, and 14 percent respectively. These percentages, however, took a somewhat serious turn towards the worst when children with less than 1,250 gm birth weight were examined. Bacola *et al.*[8] observed that in this group 41.5 percent were completely retarded, 41.5 percent were borderline cases, and only 17 percent came in the range that could be considered somewhat normal. The work of Cabak and Najdanvic[21] showed in Serbian children that those born of malnourished mothers and undernourished in infancy were found at school age to have normal physical characteristics but subnormal mental capacity.

Stoch and Smythe[135] followed groups of undernourished children and their controls for a period of five years and concluded that intrauterine malnutrition caused by maternal deprivation significantly interfered with brain growth and intellectual capacity.

Warkany[156] stressed the importance of differentiating between full-term and premature infants on an age rather than a weight basis, and Naeye[94] believed that children with low birth weight who have also suffered marked intrauterine growth retardation may be more seriously affected compared to those who were born before the full term but had the same body weight. Douglas,[41] however, found no difference in the I.Q. and performance of children born at full term and those born four weeks prematurely but having the same birth weight, even at the age of 15 years.

In experimental animals, maternal protein deprivation has a significant effect on the offsprings in terms of growth retardation and behavioral abnormalities. In most instances these changes are reversible if well-balanced diets are given in the postnatal life. However, if these animals born to malnourished mothers are further deprived, these abnormalities may be irreversible. Some authors believe that maternal protein deficiency affects the learning performance of the offspring, which persists to the next generation even after rehabilitation.[31] Simonson *et al.*[127] found that maternal deprivation during pregnancy had more pronounced effects than such a dietary abuse during the period of lactation. In the former case, neuromotor development in early life is significantly affected, and the behavioral abnormalities persist in later life. Their observations seem to fit in with other reports that maternal protein deprivation leads to reduction in protein and DNA content,[175] and if the offspring starts his life with lesser number of nerve cells, it is bound to have a permanent disadvantage throughout life,[167,168] and its effects may be manifested in the next generation as well.

In addition to the birth weight, postnatal nutrition, sickness, social status, the mother's educational position in the family, and surrounding environments are important factors in determining the intellectual performance of a low-birth-weight child. Although some difference of achievement among the low-birth-weight may become evident in certain cases, Alm[2] found that the majority had carrying capacities as great, behaved as well, and were promoted as often during military service as those of the control group. Some other studies have indicated that the difference between the performance of low-birth-weight and high-birth-weight children becomes evident even in adolescent and adult life.

A study of twins born with different birth weights but raised under similar conditions could better explain the influence of nutrition on intellectual performance. Drillien,[42] Babson *et al.*,[7] Kaelber and Pogh[72] found significant differences in the intellectual performance of heavier-birth-weight and lighter-birth-weight offspring among the twins. Babson *et al.*[7] studied the growth and development of 16 twin pairs and showed that where there is a marked discrepancy in birth weights, the smaller twin is most likely to be at a great disadvantage in physique and intellect. Platt and Stewart[106] after their comprehensive studies on reversible and irreversible effects of protein-calorie deficiency on the nervous system were fully convinced that, "Children who are markedly undersized, relative to their ethnic background, are unlikely to attain the same level of intelligence as children of the same race but of normal weight at birth."

It cannot be denied that home circumstances, size of the family, and other environmental factors play an important role in determining the intellectual development of the children, but in the case of low-birth-weight children who have suffered intrauterine growth retardation, even a small degree of adverse environment has a profound effect on their mental development. These children are less likely to be selected at school for courses requiring a higher level of academic competence compared to children born heavier but belonging to same social group as the low-birthweight children.

There could be a number of factors during the course of pregnancy which could lead to very low birth weight of the infants, but certainly the inadequate dietary intake of a mother not in good physical condition in the pregravidic state is one of the most important factors. Drillien [42] studied a sample of 112 babies whose birth weight was 1360 gms or less. These babies showed obvious signs of physical and mental handicaps even compared to those children who had the same birth weight but were prematurely expelled due to certain other reasons. Drillien summarized after detailed investigation that

> over one-third of the total group are likely to be ineducable in normal school for reason of physical or mental handicap or both; over one-third are dull children who will probably be retained in normal school but will require special educational treatment, and less than one-third are low average, average, or above average in ability.

Of the 66 such children in the school age only six showed I.Q. scores above 100. Among these children restlessness, poor concentration, and hyperactivity were common problems, and only 30 percent of these children were without significant behavioral disturbances. In this group 43 percent of the children were considered restless with poor concentration. Thirteen percent were described as "insecure, overdependent, lacking confidence and needing constant encouragement." Nineteen percent were described as being "apathetic, solitary, unforthcoming or withdrawn making little contact with teachers or other children and showing little interest or initiative in school activities." Another 13 percent were "excessively timid or nervous or subject to irrational fears," while 9 percent were "aggressive, destructive, deliberately naughty or uncontrollable." All these are the signs of a significantly retarded mental development and abnormal behavior.

MATERNAL MALNUTRITION AND COMPLICATIONS OF PREGNANCY

Toxemia and Eclampsia

Toxemia of pregnancy may not be a direct result of nutritional PCM, but its incidence is high among individuals belonging to the low socioeconomic groups, whose dietary standards during pregnancy are low, in some countries. Among such people a direct relationship between maternal nutrition and toxemia has been recognized.[18,34,45,149] The working group of the committee on maternal nutrition [81] found that the mortality rate due to toxemias of pregnancy varied from 3.8 percent in higher income groups, 5.9 percent in the middle class, and 11.9 percent in low-income group, which appears to be a very significant observation. The pattern of distribution and incidence of toxemia all over the world, however, makes it difficult to ascertain the real cause of prevalent toxemia. Its incidence is quite low in Thailand, Ethiopia, and Central Africa, whereas it is high in India, Ceylon, and Europe. Is it because of any racial difference? Different geography and climate do not seem to be important factors in its incidence because in Fiji, Trinidad, and Panama different races having varying proneness to toxemia live in the same area.[89] Scrimshaw [120] observed that in Panama, the low-income Negroes of West Indies origin had much higher incidence compared to the Panamanians of the same economic status.

The incidence of preeclampsia and toxemias of pregnancy require a careful evaluation before any judgment is made with respect to whether or not malnutrition makes a significant contribution in its causation. Gopalan [53] suggested that the higher incidence of eclampsia in undernourished women is the result of poor obstetric care because among most of the poor people the patients do not go to physicians regularly, and cases of preeclampsia are not spotted in time, and most of them develop into eclampsia. Toxemia of pregnancy in developed countries, characterized by high blood pressure, swelling of ankles, and protein in urine, is generally associated with overweight or rapid gain in weight due to high calorie intake but poor in nutritive quality. It is common among women who gain excessive weights during the second and third trimesters. This may not mean that excessive weight gain is the direct result of toxemia or vice versa. Some workers believe that excessive pregnancy weight gain and toxemia should be largely dissociated. Doctors generally recommend a high protein and 1500 to 1800 calorie diet restricted in sodium to approximately 1000 mg/day,[115] as it is believed that toxemia is a result of retention of salt and water.[19,61,88,97,112] Toxemia may also be observed amongst women who are grossly underweight and fail to gain the minimum required weight during the gravidic period.[53,54,61,161]

Evidence exists that toxemia of pregnancy becomes more apparent in a mother with unbalanced diet pattern (involving protein metabolism, vitamin components such as ascorbic acid, B6) than in those containing well-balanced diets with high protein content. The latter certainly protects against the development of toxemia.* Emotionally stressful conditions [129,130] of the mother or a diabetic condition [132] may also lead to alteration in the metabolism, thereby causing excessive weight gain and increase the chances of toxemia. As suggested by Hillman and Hall,[65] whatever be the reasons, a sudden gain in weight, especially after the twenty-ninth week, should alert the physician towards the possibility of a developing toxemia. One must be careful, however, to distinguish between weight gain due to disposition of fat or weight gain due to water retention.

Hypoglycemia

Most of the underweight children are premature to some degree; however, in some neonates smaller weight may not be a result of immaturity but due to retardation of their intrauterine growth.[55,119] The reason for this retardation may be quite complex, ranging from placental insufficiency to extreme degree of maternal malnutrition. Such children may either die *in utero* or may develop symptomatic hypoglycemia after the first postnatal day.[94,37,174,119] These neonates, in spite of their satisfactory growth patterns, may show in the later stages evident signs of permanent physical and mental retardation.[63,64] Generally, hypogly-

---

* See references 1, 13, 14, 15, 32, 77, 116, 128

cemia in the neonates who have suffered intrauterine growth retardation is evident during the first few days of their birth, but may also develop in some older children with severe malnutrition.[73] The hypoglycemic infants generally go through a series of convulsions, as described by a number of workers.[119,174]

The mechanism for the development of hypoglycemia is not fully understood, but some of the steps leading to it are known. The hypoglycemic infants show a deficiency of hepatic glycogen [124] accompanied by a decrease of cytoplasmic mass of the hepatic cells, probably because of reduced glycogen. Such a deficiency will adversely affect the brain of a neonate which has very little stored glycogen and is totally dependent upon blood glucose and hepatic glycogenolysis for its energy requirements. However, hypoglycemia may not be adequately explained on the basis of glycogen deficiency alone because most neonates develop this condition after the first 24 hours of life, when even the normal infants are not dependent completely on hepatic glycogenolysis.[119,174] Naeye [95] postulated that neonatal hypoglycemia may be due to deficient gluconeogenesis, and the reduced hepatic cell cytoplasm may be associated with retarded development of hepatic enzymes essential for gluconeogenesis. Gluconeogenesis may also be the result of reduced size and presumably reduced function of adrenal cortex,[94] as adrenal corticosteroids stimulate the hepatic synthesis of key enzymes essential for gluconeogenesis.[79] The older malnourished children, who may show signs of hypoglycemia, have decreased output of corticosteroids.[24,92,93,103]

Hypoglycemia in the malnourished neonates may also be caused by hyperinsulinism and increased islet tissue compared to the body weight. Presumably insulin content has been increased in some malnourished neonates.[131] Cornblath [30] discussed at length the symptomatic neonatal hypoglycemia and showed that neonates develop an abnormal degree of hypoglycemia after the administration of leucine or tolbutamide, suggesting again an increased capacity of the body to release insulin.

Anemia

The possibility of anemia due to unbalanced or deficient diets during pregnancy always exists in countries where the general dietary levels are low. During the course of a normal pregnancy, maternal erythropoiesis increases along with the enhanced nutritional requirements to satisfy the needs of the growing products of conception.[109] The several anemias of pregnancy are characterized by different morphological and clinical attributes and must be distinguished from preexisting anemias of specific origin (e.g. sickle cell anemia, thalassemia, mixed hemoglobinopathies) which in most instances are not common during pregnancy. Usually, the physician is concerned with the commonly occurring hypochronic normocytic anemia or pseudoanemia (hemodilution) followed by hemoconcentration in labor and the parturition.[91,108,110,147] As explained by Hillman and Hall,[85] the circulating plasma is increased 20 to 40 percent and circulating hemoglobin about half that figure in the majority of untreated cases. The reaction to plasma volume is quite significant as related to the number of red cells even without any recognizable nutritional deficiency. Macrocytic anemias are common, not only in Asia and South Africa where the dietary standards are low,[38,53,54,76,173] but they are not uncommon in the U.K.[51,126] and some populations in the U.S.,[65] though in the advanced countries it does not pose any major health problems.

The prevalent iron deficiency anemia during pregnancy or puerperium is a result of low storage iron, low dietary iron intake, and greatly increased demands for iron for maternal hemoglobin synthesis.[109] The possible effects of anemias during the gravidic state on the hematological status of the infant at birth and during the neonatal period become very important. Gopalan [53] cited the work of Shanker who made a survey of 400 pregnant women in South India. Twenty percent of the women showed hemoglobin levels less than 10 gm% in the first trimester, and over 50 percent of the women had such values in the second and third trimesters, which clearly shows the advisability of routine iron administration throughout the prenatal period. It is well established that the iron requirements are considerably increased during pregnancy, whereas the iron stores of most women are very small. The woman must have ample reserves when increased absorption prevails in the third trimester, and the growing fetus reinforces its iron stores for use in early postnatal life. An infant under normal circumstances takes enough iron from the mother so that it does not need iron supplements for a number of months. Among the infants born to mothers in the above survey, Shanker found that hemoglobin values decrease from about 18 to 20 gm% at birth to about 10 gm% by about the third month. Further deterioration was observed during the next weeks, until by the sixth month the average was about 8.5 gm%. This may indicate that the anemic infant born to malnourished mothers may be due to inadequate stores of fetal iron reflecting the unsatisfactory state of maternal nutrition with regard to iron during pregnancy or even the preconceptional state and may not be affected by postnatal feeding. Such a conclusion is reinforced by a study of Bhavani *et al.*,[17] who found no difference in iron content of the milk of malnourished mothers and healthy ones, and there was no correlation between the hemoglobin levels of the nursing mothers and the iron content of their milk. Also the speed with which infants born to malnourished mothers develop anemia is highly suggestive of inadequate or defective iron storage during fetal development.[53]

There is a great disagreement among physicians as to the advisability of giving routine iron supplements throughout the prenatal period. Since it is clinically very difficult to distinguish between normal and abnormal features of maternal health, it may be practical to give regularly small doses of iron to all pregnant women. The effectiveness of available iron is also enhanced by certain salts (molybdenum and cobalt,[100] ascorbic acid, folic acid) .

In some countries (particularly India) , pregnant women are under some kind of impulse to eat clay, which may be harmful in the sense that it hinders the utilization of available iron.[46,98] The folic acid metabolism is also altered during pregnancy, and pregnant women show an increased rate of clearance of intravenously injected folic acid in the third trimester as compared to the nonpregnant controls.[65] As discussed by these authors, "Folic acid is recommended with increasing frequency, not only in the less common megaloblastic, macrocytic anemia, but also as a routine adjunct to iron in the treatment and prevention of the more usual hypochronic anemias."[3,16,50,60] Folic acid also appears beneficial in the hemolytic anemias associated with the hemoglobinopathies and has been credited with prevention of other fetal and maternal complications.[16,50] Total requirements have been estimated as close to $300\mu g$/day.[96] Protein supplements may enhance folate effectiveness in instances where severe dietary limitation prevails.

Macrocytic anemias [25,101] are also generally improved by vitamin B_{12}. Human blood B_{12} levels may not be so important as folic acid in the prevention of anemia, and Laurace and Klipstein[75] believe that it is the folate deficiency that most often seems responsible for antepartum megaloblastic anemia. Our knowledge with respect to the precise role of hematopoietic substance must be improved in order to completely overcome the uncertainty of having to deal with some degree of anemia among pregnant women all over the world, irrespective of their dietary patterns.

Congenital Malformations

Congenital malformations in the offsprings of mammals can be induced by maternal dietary deficiencies.[53,155,156] Although no proof of congenital anomalies in humans has been obtained which could be directly linked to maternal nutritional deficiencies, a correlation can nevertheless be drawn indicating that malnourished mothers are more susceptible to malformations in the fetuses as compared to those who are well fed. The animal studies should, however, be accepted with great caution because the comparative period of organogenesis in humans is short and is followed by long periods of fetal growth during which time the damaged fetuses are generally aborted. This hypothesis is borne by the fact the incidence of abortions, stillbirths, and miscarriages is much more among women whose nutritional status is poor compared to healthy mothers.

In human and animal studies a number of workers are convinced that malnutrition, notably deficiency states, is responsible for the etiology of these aberrations.[59,121,122] Some of them, however, blame pharmaceutical agents for these anomalies. A United Kingdom study confirmed a greater frequency of anomalies among the offspring of the low socioeconomic groups.[5,29] Additional evidence that genetic factors are responsible for less than 10 percent of the prevalent malformations,[23,78,89,90,113,115] has further highlighted the importance of nutrition and that a well-balanced diet during the pregravidic or gravidic state may be helpful to reduce the incidence of these untoward incidents. For example, endemic cretinism in the infant may be a direct result of iodine deficiency in the maternal diet because in Switzerland, eradication of endemic cretinism has been achieved through iodization of salt and general dietary improvements, and this may be taken as evidence of the possible effect of maternal diet on the physical and mental makeup of the infant.[53] As Hillman and Hall [65] put it: "in the advanced or economically well-off countries the not infrequent occurrence of malnutrition and, particularly, of metabolic stress associated with hyperemesis among women must also be considered in attempts to equate nutrition with social status."

Increased deficiency of malformation in children born to diabetic mothers also points to the fact that maternal physiology, stress, and nutrition are of paramount importance in the formation or avoidance of congenital malformations.[138]

HEMOGLOBIN, SERUM PROTEINS, AND VITAMIN A VALUES OF PREGNANT WOMEN AND NEONATES

Hemoglobin

Venkatachalam [152] conducted an elaborate survey of hemoglobin content of pregnant mothers and the neonates, particularly in the low socioeconomic groups in India. This study reveals that in most cases, women in their early periods of pregnancy had hemoglobin values over 10 gm/100 ml. In the latter half of the gravidic period, however, the hemoglobin values fell down significantly, and according to some Indian workers, 20 percent of all of the subjects suffered from anemia to some degree. "While nearly one quarter of the subjects in the third trimester had hemoglobin value of less than 10 grams, only 2% and 16% showed values of less than 10 grams in the first and second trimester respectively." [152] Venkatachalam felt that anemia during the third trimester is more prevalent than indicated by the survey, and another examination of 198 women, randomly selected, showed that 56 percent of them had hemoglobin values of less than 10 gms, which may be considered a value representing anemia. The newborns on the other hand have rarely been observed to be anemic, and a study of 50 infants showed their hemoglobin value at an average of 17.6/100. The high hemoglobin level does not, however, indicate the iron reserves of the neonate in the liver and may not prove an effective protection against the development of anemia because of lack of iron.

Serum Proteins

In a sample of Indian women of low socioeconomic groups, Venkatachalam [152] carried out an examination of serum proteins of nonpregnant and pregnant women and showed a decline in the albumin concentration with advancing pregnancy. Significant hypoalbuminemia was observed in this survey even amongst the nonpregnant women, suggesting protein deficiency. A comparison of total serum proteins of neonates and their mothers revealed 5.55 gm/100 ml $\pm$ 0.124 and 6.25 gm/100 ml $\pm$ 0.073 of value respectively. The serum albumin values were 3.13 gm/100 ml $\pm$ 0.072 gm and 2.96 gm/100 ml $\pm$ 0.056 respectively, showing a significant correlation between neonatal and maternal values.[71] It is clear that maternal hypoalbuminemia is reflected in the neonatal blood.

Vitamin A

The mean carotene levels amongst the pregnant females were 99.0 IU/100 ml in the neonate. The mean values of serum vitamin A were 104.3 international units (IU), 67.2 IU, 88.2 IU per/100 ml in first, second, and third trimesters respectively in the women of low socioeconomic group under study. The neonates contained 84.2 IU/100 ml of serum vitamin A.[152] If the mother's diet during the last trimester is supplemented with sufficient vitamin A, the nutritional status of the neonate with respect to vitamin A is significantly improved, and these infants, because of better hepatic storage of vitamin A, do not suffer from a deficiency syndrome as observed in the infants of mothers whose diets were not supplemented. The vitamin A content of the colostrum even among malnourished mothers is as high as 600 IU/100 ml, and if nursing is started soon after birth, the neonate is assured of good hepatic storage of this vitamin during the first three days, because the concentration in milk declines during the subsequent period to about 70 IU/100 ml. It is a good practice in certain countries to start nursing the baby soon after birth so that the valuable colostrum is not wasted.

MALNOURISHED MOTHER AND LACTATION

The maternal nutrition in the preconceptional and gravidic state generally influences the quality as well as the quantity of milk made available to the infant. Severe malnutrition of the mother may be reflected in a low amount of protein in the milk as well as the quantity. It appears that undernutrition in childhood and adolescence impairs the development of mammary tissue [57] and may result in inadequate lactation (Fig. 16). In the qualitative sense, a mother provided with a well-balanced diet would provide milk of better quality, although it shows an overall consistency in its analysis, irrespective of the maternal diet. A single dose of vitamin A doubled its quantity in the milk in 12 hrs but fell to its previous value in 48 hrs.[137] Other vitamins, such as vitamin C in the milk, are also in proportion to its availability in maternal diet.[39] Even if additional quantities are not eaten by the mother, a certain amount of it is always present in the milk irrespective of the maternal diet. Deodhar et al.[39] found in India that women of low nutritional status secreted 14 mg vitamin C in milk and were taking only 1.5 mg in their diet. Dietary supplementation of riboflavin and thiamine also led to a subsequent increase in their concentration in the milk. The undernourished mothers also supplied normal range of important minerals in the milk, such as calcium and iron.[17] This is quite interesting in view of the fact that these

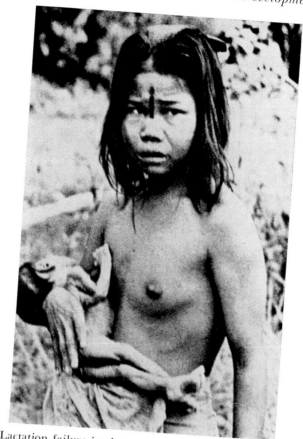

Figure 16. Lactation failure in the mother resulting in nutritional marasmus in the infant.[71a]

women hardly take 300 mg of calcium per day and are generally anemic. According to Bhavani *et al.*,[17] supplementation of the diet with extra calcium or iron did not increase their concentration in the milk. Analytical studies indicate that the milk from the undernourished mothers is quite satisfactory to facilitate adequate growth of the child, provided it is available in adequate quantities. The concentration of vitamins is low in the milk of undernourished mothers compared to those women getting better diets during lactation, but not so low as to jeopardize the survival of the infant. Quantitatively, several studies have indicated that undernourished women of low socioeconomic groups put out 400 to 600 gm of milk daily for periods extending to over a year.[53]

An interesting observation of Illingsworth and Kilpatrick [68] may be maintained here. They showed that drinking water in amounts beyond the natural inclination of thirst impairs lactation, which may be due to an inhibitory effect on posterior pituitary secretion because of waterlogging.

The concentration of protein in the milk, although greatly dependent on the amount of protein in the maternal diet, does not vary too much between samples taken from undernourished and well-nourished mothers, provided the undernourished mother gets at least 45 to 60 gm of protein daily. During lactation, the protein needs are certainly greatly enhanced. An average adult male, weighing 159 lb, will need approximately 70 gm of protein per day, whereas a lactating female weighing 128 lb will need 98 gm of protein daily.[87]

Gopalan [53] referred to an interesting correlation between undernourished and well-fed mothers with respect to the resumption of menstruation and believed that it may be related to the extent of success in lactation. The undernourished mothers took a much longer period, compared to the well-fed ones, in resuming regular menstruation after delivery. The present author could not find any recent study on this subject. It seems important, however, that a woman should maintain better nutritional standards during pregnancy as well as through a period of lactation.

REFERENCES

1. Alfonso, J. F. and DeAlvarez, R. R.: *Am. J. Obstet. & Gynecol., 86:*815 (1963).
2. Alm, I.: *Acta. Paediatr.* (Uppsula), Suppl. 94 (1953).
3. Alperin, J. B., Hutchinson, H. T., and Levin, W. C.: *Arch. Intern. Med., 117:*684 (1966).
4. Altman, J. and Das, G. D.: *J. Comp. Neurol., 126:*337 (1966).
5. Anderson, W. J. R., Baird, D., and Thomson, A. M.: *Lancet, 1:*1304, (1958).
6. Aykroyd, W. R. and Hossoin, M. A.: *Br. Med. J., 1:*42–43 (1967).
7. Babson, S. G., Kangas, J., Young, N., and Bramhell, J. L.: *Pediatrics, 33:*327–333 (1964).

8. Bacola, E., Behrle, F. C., DeSchweinitz, L., Miller, H. C., and Mira, M.: *Am. J. Dis. Child., 112*:359–368; 369–379 (1966a,b) .

9. Barnes, R. H.: *Fed. Proc., 30*:1929 (1971) .

10. Baumgartner, L.: *Bull. W.H.O., 26*:175 (196) .

11. Baumgartner, L., Bessin, V., Wegman, M. E., and Parker, S. L.: *Pediatrics, 6*:329 (1950) .

12. Beargie, R. A., James, V. L., and Green, J. W.: *Pediatr. Clin. North Am., 17*:159 (1970) .

13. Beaton, G. H.: *Fed. Proc., 20* (Suppl. 7, Pt. 3) :196 (1961) .

14. Beaton, G. H. and Arroyane, G.: *Fed. Proc., 22*:608 (1963) .

15. Beaton, G. H., Arroyane, G., and Flores, M.: *Am. J. Clin. Nutr. 14*:269 (1964) .

16. Benjamin, F., Bassen, F. A., and Meyer, L. M.: *Am. J. Obstet. Gynecol., 96*:310 (1966) .

17. Bhavani, B. and Gopalan, C.: *Indian J. Med. Res., 47*:234 (1959) .

18. Bloch, H., Lipsett, H., Redner, B., and Hirschl, O.: *J. Pediatr., 41*:300 (1952) .

19. Brewer, T. H.: *Metabolic Toxemia of Late Pregnancy. A Disease of Malnutrition.* Springfield, Thomas (1966) .

20. Burke, B. S., Beal, V. A., Kirkwood, S. B., and Stuart, H. C.: *Am. J. Obstet. Gynecol., 46*:38–52 (1943) .

21. Cabak, V. and Najdanvic, R.: *Arch. Dis. Child. 40*:532 (1965) .

22. Capper, A.: *Am. J. Dis. Child, 53*:443 (1928) .

23. Cassady, G.: *Pediatr. Clin. North Am., 17*:79 (1970) .

24. Castellanos, H. and Arroyave, G.: *Am. J. Clin. Nutr., 9*:186 (1961) .

25. Chaudhari, S.: *Br. Med. J., 2*:825 (1951) .

26. Chow, B. F.: In N. S. Scrimshaw and J. E. Gordon (Eds.) : *Malnutrition, Learning and Behavior.* Cambridge, M.I.T. Press (1968) .

27. Chow, B. F., Blackwell, R. Q., Blackwell, B. N., *et al.: Am. J. Public Health, 58*:668–677 (1968) .

28. Clements, F. W.: *Infant Nutrition: Its Physiological Basis.* Baltimore, Williams and Wilkins (1949).

29. Coffey, R. P. and Jessup, R. F.: *Ir. J. Med. Sci., 393*:391 (1958) .

30. Cornblath, M.: *Pediatrics, 33*:388 (1964) .

31. Cowley, J. J. and Griesel, R. D.: *J. Genet. Psychol., 103*:233 (1963) .

32. Cravioto, J.: In N. S. Scrimshaw and J. E. Gordon (Eds.) : *Malnutrition, Learning and Behavior.* Cambridge, M.I.T. Press (1968) .

33. Cravioto, J.: In P. Gyorgy and O. L. Kline (Eds.) : *Malnutrition is a Problem of Ecology.* Basel, S. Karger (1970) .

34. Dalderup, C.: *Vitam. Horm. 17*:223 (1959) .

35. Darby, W. J., Bridgforth, E. B., Martin, M. P., and McGanity, W. J.: *J. Obstet. Gynecol., 5*:528 (1955) .

36. Davies, C. S.: In Chicago Yearbook Medical (1968) .

37. Dawkins, M. J. R., Martin, J. D., and Spector, W. G.: *J. Obstet. Gynaecol. Br. Commonw., 68:*604 (1961).

38. Dawson, A. M.: *J. Obstet. Gynaecol. Br. Commonw., 69:*38 (1962).

39. Deodhar, A. D., Rajalakshmi, R., and Ramakkrishnar, C. V.: *Acta. Paediatr.* (Stockh.), *53:*42 (1964).

40. Dobbing, J.: In N. S. Scrimshaw, and J. E. Gordon (Eds.): *Malnutrition, Learning and Behavior.* Cambridge, M.I.T. Press (1968).

41. Douglas, J. W. B.: *Br. Med. J. 1:*1008 (1960).

42. Drillien, C. M.: *The Growth and Development of the Prematurely-born Infant.* Baltimore, Williams & Wilkins. (1964).

43. Drillien, C. M.: *Pediatr. Clin. North Am., 17:*9 (1970).

44. Eastman, N. J. and Jackson, E.: *Obstet. Gynecol., 23:*1003 (1968).

45. Editorial: *J.A.M.A., 167:*470 (1958).

46. Edwards, C. H., McDonald, S., Mitchell, J. R., *et al.: J. Am. Diet. Assoc., 44:*109 (1964).

47. Flexner, L. B.: In H. Waelsch (Ed.): *Biochemistry of the Developing Nervous System.* New York, Academic Press (1955).

48. Flexner, L. B.: In J. E. Birnen, H. A. Imus, and W. F. Windle (Eds.): *The Process of Aging in The Nervous System.* Springfield, Thomas (1959).

49. Frazer, J. L.: *J. Chronic Dis., 10:*97 (1959).

50. Frazer, J. L. and Watt, H. J.: *Am. J. Obstet. Gynecol., 89:*532 (1966).

51. Giles, C. and Shuttleworth, E. M.: *Lancet, 2:*1341 (1958).

52. Glowinski, *et al.:* Foreign mail. *J.A.M.A., 180:*83 (1962).

53. Gopalan, C.: *Bull. W.H.O., 26:*203–211 (1962).

54. Gopalan, C. and Belanady, M.: *Fed. Proc., 20* (Suppl. 7, pt. 3) :177 (1961).

55. Gruenwald, P.: *Biol. Neonate, 5:*215 (1963).

56. Gruenwald, P.: *Public Health Rep., 83:*867–872 (1968).

57. Gunther, M.: *Proc. Nutr. Soc., 27:*77 (1968).

58. Hale, F.: *Texas Med. J. 33:*228 (1937).

59. Hammond, D. C.: *Proc. Soc. Exp. Biol. Med., 19:*1 (1960).

60. Hansen, H. A., and Rybo, G.: *Nord. Med., 76:*853 (1966).

61. Hauck, G.: *J. Obstet. Gynecol. Br. Commonw., 30:*885 (1963).

62. Hecht, F.: *Obstet. Gynecol., 22:*47 (1963).

63. Hepner, R. and Bowen, M.: *J.A.M.A., 172:*427 (1960).

64. Hepner, R., Gruenwald, P., Dawkins, M., and Hepner, R.: *Sinai Hosp. J.* (Balt.), *11:*51 (1963).

65. Hillman, R. W. and Hall, J. E.: In M. G. Wohl and R. S. Goodhart (Eds.): *Modern Nutrition in Health and Disease,* 4th ed. Philadelphia, Lea & Febiger (1968).

66. Hsueh, A. M.: *Fed. Proc. 29:* (1970).

67. Hytten, F. E.: In C. F. Mills and R. Passmore (Eds.): *Proceedings of*

6th International Congress, Edinburgh, 1963. Edinburgh & London, E. S. Livingstone (1964).

68. Illingworth, R. S. and Kilpatrick, B.: *Lancet, 265:*1175 (1953).
69. International Society for Geographic Pathology: *Pathol. Microbiol., 24* (4) :425 (1961).
70. Jackson, R. L.: In N. S. Scrimshaw and J. E. Gordon (Eds.) : *Malnutrition, Learning and Behavior.* Cambridge, M.I.T. Press (1968).
71. Jayalakshmi, V. T., Ramanathan, M. K., and Gopalan, C.: *Indian J. Med. Res., 45:*4 (1957).
71a. Jelliffe, D. B.: *Infant Nutrition in the Subtropics and Tropics.* Geneva, W.H.O. (1968).
72. Kaelber, C. T. and Pogh, T. F.: *N. Engl. J. Med., 280:*1030–1034 (1969).
73. Kerpel, Fronius E.: *J. Pediatr., 56:*826 (1960).
74. Knobloch, H. and Pasamanick, B.: *N. Engl. J. Med., 266:*1045, 1092, 1155 (1962).
75. Laurence, C. and Klipstein, F. A.: *Ann. Intern. Med., 66:*25 (1967).
76. Layrisse, M., Aguero, O., Blumenfield, H., *et al.*: *Blood, 15:*724 (1960).
77. Leathem, J. H.: In *Reproductive Physiology and Protein Nutrition.* New Brunswick, Rutgers University Press, (1959).
78. Lenz, W.: *Med. Genetics,* Chicago University Press, Chicago (1963).
79. Lin, E. C. C., Rivlin, R. S., and Knox, W. E.: *Am. J. Physiol., 196:*303 (1959).
80. Lubchenco, L. O., Horner, F. A., Hix, I. E., *et al.*: *Am. J. Dis. Child., 102:*752 (1962).
81. Maternal Nutrition and The Course of Pregnancy, National Academy of Sciences, Washington (1970).
82. McBurney, R. D.: *West. J. Surg. Obstet. Gynecol., 55:*363 (1947).
83. McGanity, W. J., Bridgforth, E. B., Martin, M. P., Newbill, J. A., and Darby, W. J.: *J. Am. Diet, Assoc. 31:*582 (1955).
84. McGanity, W. J., Cannon, R. O., Bridgforth, E. B., Martin, A. B. M. P., Densen, P. M., Newbill, J. A., McClellan, G. S., Christie, A., Peterson, J. C., and Darby, W. J.: *Am. J. Obstet. Gynecol., 67:*491, 501, 539 (1954).
85. McKeown, T. and Record, R. G.: *J. Endocrinol., 9:*418 (1953).
86. McKeown, T. and Record, R. G.: *Br. J. Prev. Soc. Med., 11:*102 (1957).
87. McWilliams, M.: *Nutrition for the Growing Years.* New York, London, Sydney, John Wiley & Sons (1967).
88. Mengert, W. F. and Tacchi, D. A.: *Am. J. Obstet. Gynecol. 81:*601 (1961).
89. Millen, J. W.: In *The Nutritional Basis of Reproduction.* Springfield, Thomas (1962).
90. Millen, J. W., and Woollam, J.: *Proc. Nutr. Soc., 19:*1 (1960).
91. Miller, J., Williams, H. B., and MacArthur, J. L.: *Am. J. Obstet.*

Gynecol., 78:303 (1959).

92. Monckeberg, F., Beas, F., and Perretta, M.: *Rev. Chil. Pediatr., 27*:187 (1956).
93. Monckeberg, F. *et al.: Pediatrics, 31*:58 (1963).
94. Naeye, R. L.: *Arch. Pathol., 79*:284–291 (1965).
95. Naeye, R. L.: *Am. J. Obstet. Gynecol., 95*:276 (1966).
96. Nelson, M. M. and Evans, H. M.: *Nutr. Abstr. Rev., 25*:667 (1954).
97. Nelson, M. M., Zuspan, F. P., and Mulligan, L. T.: *Am. J. Obstet. Gynecol., 94*:310 (1966).
98. *Nutr. Rev., 18*:35 (1960).
99. O'Brien, J. R., Usher, R. H., and Maughan, G. B.: *Can. Med. Assoc. J., 94*:1077 (1966).
100. Owen, J. D. and Glienke, C. F.: *Obstet. Gynecol., 20*:531 (1962).
101. Patel, J. C., and Kocher, B. R.: *Br. Med. J., 1*:924 (1950).
102. Payne, P. R. and Wheeler, E. F.: *Nature* (Lond.), *215*:1134–1136 (1967).
103. Perloff, W. H. *et al.: J.A.M.A., 155*:1307 (1954).
104. Platt, B. S., Heard, C. R. C., and Stewart, R. J. C.: In H. N. Munro and J. B. Allison (Eds.): *Mammalian Protein Metabolism*. New York, Academic Press (1964), vol. 2.
105. Platt, B. S. and Stewart, R. J. C.: *Maternal and Child Care, 3*:539–543 (1967).
106. Platt, B. S. and Stewart, R. J. C.: *Dev. Med. Child. Neurol., 11*:174 (1969).
107. Platt, B. S. and Stewart, R. J. C.: *World Rev. Nutr. Diet.*, vol. 13 (1971).
108. Pritchard, J. A.: *Am. J. Obstet. Gynecol., 77*:74 (1959).
109. Pritchard, J. A.: In *Maternal Nutrition and the Course of Pregnancy*. Washington, National Academy of Sciences (1970).
110. Pritchard, J. A., Baldwin, R. M., Dickey, J. C., and Wiggins, K. M.: *Am. J. Obstet. Gynecol., 84*:1271 (1962).
111. Rajalakshmi, R. and Ramakrishnan, C. V.: In G. H. Bourne (Ed.): *World Review Nutrition and Dietetics*, vol. 14. Basel, S. Karger (1971).
112. Reboud, P., Groulade, J., Groslambert, P., and Colomb, M.: *Am. J. Obstet. Gynecol. 86*:820 (1963).
113. Reisman, L. E.: *Pediatr. Clin. North Am., 17*:101 (1970).
114. Reisman, L. E. and Matheny, A. P.: In *Genetics and Counseling in Medical Practice*. St. Louis, Mosby (1969).
115. Robinson, C. H.: *Basic Nutrition and Diet Therapy*. London, Macmillan (1970).
116. Robinson, J. C., London, W. T., and Pierce, J. E.: *Am. J. Obstet. Gynecol., 96*:226 (1966).
117. Rossier, A.: *Dev. Med. Child. Neurol., 4*:483 (1962).

118. Rumbolz, W. L. and McGoogan, L. S.: *Obstet. Gynecol., 1:*294 (1953).
119. Scott, K., Usher, R., and MacLean, F.: *J. Pediatr., 63:*734 (1963).
120. Scrimshaw, N. S.: *Am. J. Obstet. Gynecol., 54:*428 (1947).
121. Scrimshaw, N. S.: *Nutr. Rev., 20:*33 (1962).
122. Scrimshaw, N. S.: *Am. J. Clin. Nutr., 14:*112 (1964).
123. Seitchik, J. and Alper, C.: *Am. J. Obstet. Gynecol., 71:*1165–75 (1956).
124. Shelly, H. J.: *Br. Med. J., 1:*273 (1964).
125. de Silva, C. C. and Baptist, N. G.: In *Tropical Nutritional Disorders of Infants and Children.* Springfield, Thomas (1969).
126. Silverman, W. A. and Sinclair, J. C.: *N. Engl. J. Med., 274:*448 (1966).
127. Simonson, M., Sherwin, R. W., Anilane, J. K., Yw, W. Y., and Chow, B. F.: *J. Nutr., 98:*18 (1969).
128. Smith, E. K., DeAlverex, R. R., and Forsander, J.: *Am. J. Obstet. Gynecol., 77:*326 (1959).
129. Soichet, S.: *Am. J. Obstet. Gynecol., 77:*1065 (1959).
130. Stearns, G.: *J.A.M.A., 168:*1655 (1958).
131. Steinke, J. and Driscoll, S. G.: 5th Congress of International Diabetes Federation. Amsterdam, Netherlands (1964), p. 69.
132. Stephens, J. W., Page, O. C., and Hare, R. L.: *Diabetes, 12:*213 (1963).
133. Stewart, R. J. C.: *Proc. R. Soc. Med., 61:*1292–1295 (1968).
134. Stewart, R. J. C. and Platt, B. S.: *Proc. Nutr. Soc., 27:*95–101 (1968).
135. Stoch, M. B. and Smythe, P. M.: *Arch. Dis. Child., 38:*546 (1963).
136. Sybolski, S. and Tremblay, P. C.: *Am. J. Obstet. Gynecol., 103:*257 (1969).
137. Tarjan, R., Kramer, M., Szoke, K., and Linder, K.: *Nutritio Dieta, 5:* 12 (1963).
138. Thiersch, W.: In *Ciba Foundation Symposium on Congenital Malformations* G. E. W. Wolstenholme and C. M. O. Connor (eds.) London, J. & A. Churchill (1960).
139. Thomson, A. M.: *Br. J. Nutr., 5:*158 (1951).
140. Thomson, A. M.: *Proc. Nutr. Soc., 16:*45 (1957).
141. Thomson, A. M.: *Br. J. Nutr., 12:*410 (1958).
142. Thomson, A. M.: *Br. J. Nutr., 13:*509 (1959).
143. Thomson, A. M. and Billewicz, W. Z.: *Br. Med. J., 1:*243 (1957).
144. Thomson, A. M. and Billewicz, W. Z.: *Proc. Nutr. Soc., 22:*55 (1963).
145. Thomson, A. M. and Hytten, F. E.: *Proc. Nutr. Soc., 19:*5 (1960).
146. Thomson, A. M. and Hytten, F. E.: *Proc. Nutr. Soc., 20:*76 (1961).
147. Tjan, H. L. and Oey, H. K.: *Am. J. Obstet. Gynecol., 84:*1316 (1962).
148. Tompkin, W. T. and Wiehl, D. G.: *Am. J. Obstet. Gynecol., 62:*898 (1951).
149. Tompkin, W. T. and Wiehl, D. G.: In *The Promotion of Maternal and Newborn Health.* New York, Milbank Memorial Fund (1955).
150. Udani, P. M.: *Indian J. Child. Health, 12:*593–611 (1963).

151. Varkki, C., Venkatachalam, P. S., Srikantia, S. G., and Gopalan, C.: *Indian J. Med. Res., 43:*291 (1955).

152. Venkatachalam, P. S.: *Bull. W.H.O., 26:*193–201 (1962).

153. Venkatachalam, P. S., Kalpakam, S., and Gopalan, C.: *Indian J. Med. Res., 48:*511 (1960).

154. Venkatachalam, P. S. and Ramanathan, K. S.: *Indian J. Med. Res., 54:* 402–409 (1966).

155. Warkany, J.: *J.A.M.A., 168:*2020 (1958).

156. Warkany, J. C.: *Bordens Rev. Nutr. Res., 21:*1 (1960).

157. Warkany, J. C., Cravioto, J., and Stephen, J. M. L.: *Adv. Protein Chem., 15:*131–238 (1960).

158. Warkany, J., Monroe, B. B., and Sutherland, B. S.: *Am. J. Dis. Child., 102:*249 (1961).

159. Weber, W. W., Mannunes, P., Day, R., and Miller, P.: *Pediatrics, 34:* 533 (1964).

160. W.H.O. Expert Committee on Human Genetics, 2nd Report. *W.H.O. Tech. Rep. Ser.,* 282, (1964).

161. W.H.O. Expert Committee on Nutrition, 6th Report, p. 143 (1962).

162. *W.H.O. Tech. Rep. Ser.,* 27 (1950).

163. *W.H.O. Tech. Rep. Ser.,* 302 (1965).

164. Wiener, G.: *J. Spec. Educ., 2:*237 ((1968).

165. Wigglesworth, J. S.: *Br. Med. Bull., 22:*13–15 (1966).

166. Winick, M.: *Pediatrics, 71:*390 (1967).

167. Winick, M.: 53rd Annual Meeting FASEB, Atlantic City, New Jersey (1969).

168. Winick, M.: *Pediatr. Clin. North Am., 17* (1):69–78 (1970).

169. Winick, M.: *Am. J. Obstet. Gynecol., 109:*166 (1971).

170. Winick, M. and Noble, A.: *J. Nutr., 89:*300 (1966).

171. Winick, M., Noble, A., and Coscia, A.: *Pediatrics, 39:*248 (1967).

172. Winick, M. and Rosso, P.: *Pediatr. Res., 3:*181 (1969).

173. Woodruff, A. W.: *Br. Med. J., 1:*1297 (1955).

174. Wybregt, S. H. *et al.*: *J. Pediatr., 64:*796 (1964).

175. Zamenhof, S., Van Manthens, E., and Margolis, F. L.: *Science, 160:*322 (1968).

Chapter VI

MALNUTRITION AND FOOD HABITS

INTRODUCTION

General Criteria in the Establishment of Food Habits

THE HUMAN RACE IS distributed all over the globe, living under all kinds of climatic conditions ranging from very cold to very hot, very humid to very dry, and from sea level to a height of 20,000 feet or more. Their food habits are greatly determined by their circumstances and indigenously available food supply. Besides these factors, no clear-cut answer to why different groups of people, living under similar environmental conditions, eat different foods and why they rigidly adhere to their patterns of eating can be given. Basically there are three kinds of diets (animal foods, vegetable foods, and mixed foods) which in their own way pressurize the individuals, living under any one category, to form certain types of food habits. The animal sources of food are habitually eaten by people like hunters and fishermen (Eskimo, Lapp, Samoyed, Fuegian) and pastoral nomads (Khirghiz, Masai, Somali).[5] The plant sources of food are eaten largely by those overpopulated areas of the globe where animal foods are scarcer, e.g. populations of India, Pakistan, Burma, China, parts of Southeast Asia and Africa. Mixed diets, consisting of foods from animals as well as other protein sources, are eaten by comparatively well-off natives of Europe, North America, Australia, New Zealand, and parts of Asia, South America and Africa.[5] Their dietary habits are largely determined by circumstance and indigenously available food supply as mentioned above, but the purpose of this article is to determine what additional factors, such as social structure, cultural patterns, religious sanctions, economics, and above all, the level of education (which largely determines the extent of unscientific superstitions in dietary matters), are responsible for certain food habits which contribute to the perpetuation of underntrition and malnutrition. Flexibility in food habits plays a part in determining the nutritional status of the people all over the world that make them strong, well built and tall, as are the people of Europe and North America, or less strong, less healthy and of smaller stature, as are found elsewhere. It is evident that food habits play a great contributing role in the prevalence of undernutrition or malnutrition in large areas of Asia, Africa, and South America.

Humans also differ from animals because to most of us food is not merely a source of satisfying hunger or even providing nourishment for the body, but in many respects is a representation of an individual culture, religion, social security, and prestige. Food has many meanings for individuals, and it can arouse many emotions—pleasure, confidence, and even violent fanaticism.[14] Food is generally a means to express one's mood and individuality, and in the same manner, food is an integral part of a culture, and many social events are closely interrelated with serving those foods which are demonstrative of an individual's identity with the culture.[18] Food habits must, therefore, be carefully studied by a nutritionist before he ventures into making judgments with respect to its goodness or badness. One must remember that there are no bad foods, only bad diets.[5] One must consider that besides physiological needs, there are always important pleasurable aspects of food, and many people would prefer to starve rather than accept foods which are unfamiliar. After continued refusal to eat, the real physiological need may not always correspond to a conscious psychological need or want.

> In the Hippocratic writings, foods or food theory were linked to human physiology and human physiology to physics, and even to metaphysics. As in all ancient medicine, the idea predominated that certain elements should be properly blended and balanced in the rational world. In the body, also, there should be some kind of balancing of the elements through a proper combination of humors. The diet a man selects should be in agreement with the balance of elements in his body.[2]

While recognizing the sanctity of established food habits and need for least interference, one has to cope with the fact that faulty dietary practices have greatly contributed to initiation and prevalence of protein-calorie malnutrition in certain areas. For example, in Southeast Asia, rice which is devoid of carotene (provitamin A) and also deficient in essential amino acids is considered perfect as a weaning food for the children, yet the cultural pattern will not permit the use of numerous green vegetables so abundant in the tropical area as a source of pro-vitamin A or another food source of high-quality protein, such as poultry. Numerous instances can be cited where the children suffer from deficiency diseases, not because of the inadequate means but because of the traditional and rigidly enforced food habits which fail to support good growth and development in the periods of fast growth of the children. It is in these situations that the nutritionist, the public health worker, and the national government have to initiate a program that does not smack of interference yet is potent enough to modify the diets, so as to safeguard the health and well-being of the people of an area.

Geographic Variations in Food Habits and Their Implications

It is extremely hard to discuss in a small space the various geographic variations in food habits all over the world. The following accounts present brief glimpses of important die-taries or those which are believed to contribute to undernutri-tional states of its people. The reader is referred to important descriptions of the *National Research Council Bulletin*,[23] Cuth-bertson,[5] Burgess and Dean,[2] Pyke,[25] Lowenberg *et al.*,[14] and McKenzie.[18] Orr and Gilks [24] in a summary of the dietary details of Masai, Bantu, and Kikuyu tribes described that Akikuyus among the Bantus and Kikuyus live mainly on cereals (maize, millet, sweet potatoes, plantains). Game, fish, birds, and eggs are ignored. Goats are mainly used as currency rather than as a source of milk or meat, and very little cow's milk is available, particularly to children. Masai tribes, on the other hand, are pastoral and make liberal use of meat, milk, and blood. Zulus also have good diets, but their children suffer because of the cultural custom of serving them at the end after most of the food has been used up by adults.

In Nyasaland children are not allowed eggs for fear of bladder disease, and pregnant women are not given eggs for fear of having bald-headed children. Similarly, tomatoes are believed to cause blisters on a child's skin. The children suffer varying degrees of undernutrition because of these beliefs, and consequently, the food habits revolve around using lots of cereals.

Cereals are also the mainstay of most people in Asia, and an average Asian derives 70 to 80 percent of his energy requirements from the cereals of one kind or another. In most places, green leafy vegetables are used by the population, but fruits are comparatively scarce. The food habits in India are largely determined by the heavy pressure of population and traditional methods of agriculture and livestock raising. A large section of the population is vegetarian, depending only on plant sources of protein, due as much to religious influence as to the scarcity of the animal source of protein. Milk has a respectable place in the food habits of the people but is not regularly taken because of its scarcity. The fish resources have not been developed, but if fish, meat, and poultry are made available at prices within the reach of the consumer, most of the population will make use of them. Heavy pressure of population and scarcity largely determine the kind of protein-rich foods incorporated in their pattern of traditional food habits. The importance of population pressure can be estimated from the fact that India is about one third the size of the U.S.A. and has to support approximately three times the population of the United States. The food habits of the Chinese people, although showing a great deal of cultural individuality, are also greatly determined by the scarcity of animal protein as required by a population as big as 750 million. The production of beef, mutton, milk, pig, poultry, and eggs is quite low. Russel [27] and Wiltfogel [30] estimated that rural population of China derives 91.8 percent of their calories from cereals, 5.2 percent from vegetables, 2.3 percent from animal products, 0.5 percent from sugar, and 0.2 percent from fruits.

Most Indonesians like to eat rice, vegetables, fried meat, salted fish, egg with raw green vegetables and fruits with a meal.

Such foods would provide a very well-balanced diet for adequate growth and maintenance; but Indonesia also has the same problem as the rest of Asia, i.e. population pressure and consequently lower economic level of existence. Most of the poor families cannot afford more than rice and a bowl of vegetables with very little animal proteins, with the result that protein malnutrition, particularly among children, is a serious problem. Malaya has also a similar diet pattern consisting of rice, raw vegetable leaves, and pulses. Milk is available in very small quantities, and meat and eggs can be afforded only occasionally.

In Latin America, in general, maize and beans dominate the food habits, although in Panama rice is a more integral part of the dietary pattern compared to maize and milk, and meat products are not as available as much as the population would like to have. Fruits, such as bananas, oranges and apples, are used in fair quantity. The Caribbeans use boiled fish and maize. Milk consumption is low, but an adequate quantity of proteins is provided by fish. Rice, yams, and coconut are an integral part of food habits. The dietary pattern of the Caribbean people is comparatively sound from the nutritional point of view.

Food habits of most of Western Europe consists of eating wheat, potatoes, accompanied by a fairly large consumption of dairy products, poultry, meat, fish, green vegetables, and fruits and are nutritionally well balanced to maintain adequate growth in the younger population. The people in general are tall and heavy compared to those from countries of Asia and Africa. The percent of protein-calories derived from animal sources in Europe is 41, compared to approximately 34 percent in Latin America, approximately 19 percent in Africa, and approximately 17 percent in the Far East.[5] In North America, 71 percent of the protein calories in the diet are derived from animal sources and are very much representative of the food habits of the people in this area. There is a heavy reliance on the consumption of meats and milk with every meal. The food habits of the people in North America are greatly influenced by the growth of science and technology and their liberal use in agriculture in order to produce farm and meat surpluses. Murry and

Blake [22] in the U.S. Department [196] *Yearbook of Agriculture* pointed out that

> The distribution of the food dollar in the United States was 35 cents for meat, poultry, fish or eggs; about 24 cents for beef, pork, veal, and lamb; 5 cents for poultry; 4 cents for eggs; and 2 cents for fish. Vegetables and fruit took 18 cents of the dollar. More than half of this was spent for fresh varieties. Milk and milk products, excluding butter, took 14 cents. On flour, cereals, bread and other baked foods 11 cents were spent; 12 cents were divided fairly evenly among fats and oils, sugar and sweets and other miscllaneous items. Beverages took nearly 10 cents. [5]

This pattern of consumption gives a fairly good idea of the food habits of the North Americans as a whole with small variations in the farm families and city families, such as the former used more eggs than the latter, and the urban population consumed more beef and poultry than the country people. The problem of undernutrition is not present in North America because most people are aware of their nutritional needs. A classic example is provided in a survey by the European Productivity Agency of the Organization for European Economic Cooperation, that many people eat fish more by habit and because they think they need it, rather than because they have a special desire for this particular food. As a matter of fact, the main problem in North America is of overnutrition. A study of Iowa school children revealed that 17 percent of the girls and 11 percent of the boys were obese. [19]

In Europe, one may differentiate between an English meal, a French meal, a Spanish meal, or a Polish meal, and the food habits of the people are somewhat rigid; the situation in North America is more or less flexible. There are seemingly no rigid food habits, and Italian pizzas, Chinese or Mexican preparations are becoming as popular as steaks, hot dogs, and hamburgers. The American food habits based on the culture of science is proving a potent force in changing food habits even in rigid traditional societies. The powdered milk of the United States is readily accepted even by those tribes who will never drink milk from any other cow except their own and where boiling milk is as much a heinous crime as a murder. Eskimos no longer have as much fascination for their foods if they can turn to western groceries.[25] According to Pyke, "The social forces which impel Europeans and Americans to embrace the products of large-scale food technology, that render the worldwide catering of the Hilton hotels irresistible from Istanbul to Amsterdam, exert the same effect over the emerging nations of Africa, Asia and South America." The conclusion that could be drawn from the geographical variations in food habits is that in the countries which are industrially not well developed, social, cultural and religious influences are as strong in determining the food habits as is the availability of nutritionally desirable foods, whereas in the highly technological West, economic and agricultural capability plays a major role in determining what people eat.

Food Habits and Their Contribution to Malnutrition

The dietary habits of a people are generally based upon the foods locally grown, but sometimes food priorities are outrightly misplaced because of ignorance. For example, cash crops, such as coffee, tobacco, cotton, may replace the food crops, or the food imported from other areas may be heavily starchy. The locally produced poultry or milk may be sold to cities to earn some cash, thereby the health of the family is bartered for money. Such consequences follow as a result of poverty and ignorance. But in those areas where poverty and ignorance are mixed with misplaced social or cultural traditions, the situation is compounded, and the faulty food habits result in gross deficiencies of the nutritional state. An illustrative example may be found in India, where the northern regions would prefer to grow food crops, and the southern part of India devotes its energies to raising cash crops. The resulting difference is an obvious contrast in the health and growth patterns in the two regions. McCarrison [16,17] carried out some controlled studies on rats to depict the dietary differences between northern and southern parts of India. Pyke [25] has described that

> Groups of young rats, twenty in each, were fed on certain diets of India, care being taken to simulate in every detail the culinary practices of the races concerned. The experiment was so conducted that factors such as climate, atmospheric temperature, rainfall, age, body weight, sex distribution, caging, housing and hygiene were the same

in all groups. And then he went on to detail the results of the experiment—how the average weight of the animals fed on the Sikh diet of freshly ground whole wheat made into cakes of unleavened bread, milk, butter, ghee, curds, legumes, fresh carrots, cabbage and other vegetables and meat once a week, was 235 grams at the end of the trial while, on the other hand, the groups of rats fed on the Madrasi diet weighed only 155 grams. Their diet was composed of washed polished rice, legumes, condiments, vegetable oil, coffee with sugar and a little milk, ghee used sparingly, and cocoanut.

Similar differences are observed among the agriculturally oriented Kikuyu tribe, who raise cash crops and consume largely cereals, tubers, plantains with small quantities of legumes and green vegetables. This tribe, when compared to Masai who are a pastoral people, use their cattle products (blood, meat and milk) in addition to cereals, bananas, and beans. The Kikuyu are generally lethargic, lacking in stamina, and subject to disease. The Masai are taller, heavier, and endowed with 50% greater muscular strength.[25]

In most cases where food habits are deeply entrenched under the influence of local culture, the blame for malnutrition is laid at the door of the inappropriateness of a particular food, hot or cold nature of the food, or some disease associated with a certain kind of food, or simply to some supernatural force. In these circumstances, malnutrition is due not to lack of availability of the right type of food in that particular area but to ignorance, e.g. fish, a major source of protein, is prohibited to young children in Malaya because it is believed to produce worms. The young toddler, after the new pregnancy, is weaned primarily on cereals and, being deprived of body-building proteinaceous foods, is very much susceptible to infections and infestations. The latter are treated, or so to say, mistreated with semistarvation diets of rice water, barley water, and weak tea.[25]

IMPORTANCE OF FOOD HABITS

It cannot be denied that faulty food habits in vast areas of the world have played a major role in the contribution of protein-calorie malnutrition, particularly the protein malnutrition. Protein malnutrition is generally prevalent where foods are habitually poor in protein but provide calories through starchy foods ranging from inadequate to excess. Unfortunately, in some countries where malnutrition is common, and understandably so, among the lower strata of the society due to low intake of protein-rich foods, it is not uncommon to see protein malnutrition among the children as well as adults of the somewhat economically well-off and wealthier classes as well. This gross neglect of body needs is not always due to lack of purchasing power or availability of protein-rich foods but is a simple matter of well-established food habits which are oriented towards a heavy reliance on starchy foods. It is, therefore, of utmost importance that any effort to alleviate the problem of protein malnutrition must accompany a thorough understanding of the importance of food habits of a particular group of people with respect to their religious, cultural, or social existence.

Hunger and Appetite

The food habits in an individual are formed early in life when a child is fed lovingly, and a certain food develops the image of a source of great pleasure and delight. That food becomes so deeply ingrained in the psychology of an individual that in later life he would need the same food to derive the pleasure of eating.

The foods to which a particular set of people are used to for a long time are, therefore, the only kinds of food or foods which satisfy their appetite and which are somewhat more satisfying than eating a nutritious food in order to satisfy their hunger. Robinson [26] recently defined these terms that,

> Hunger is the urge to eat and is accompanied by a number of unpleasant sensations. It follows a period when one has been deprived of food and is generally associated with contraction of the stomach. The individual begins to feel irritable, uneasy and tired. If a blood sample is taken at this time, the blood-sugar level is somewhat low. When food is taken, the individual begins to feel better almost immediately.

The appetite on the other hand is, "the anticipation of and desire to eat palatable food." The habitual foods satisfy the appetite as well as hunger, whereas strange foods, irrespective of their high nutritive value, may kill the hunger for food and do not satisfy the appetite. Hunger and appetite must, therefore, be considered separately, and as Burgess and Dean [2] pointed out, "Hunger is perhaps more familiar to the physiologist and appetite to those concerned with the psychological aspects of related but not identical phenomenon." Existing food habits are, therefore, based on cultural, social, and economic factors, and a concerted effort must be made to understand them in those contexts and very cautiously interfered with, if necessary, keeping in mind all the above aspects. It is well known that people choose to starve rather than accept unfamilar foods. In controlled conditions, it has been observed that after a period of 14 to 21 days, the hunger striker loses hunger as well as appetite. It appears then that real physiological needs may not always correspond to a conscious psychological needs or want.[2] The case of immigrants into distant countries is well illustrative of the above point. Immigrants to the United States generally change their language and dress quickly, but the food habits remain distinctly on the old pattern for a long time. Even religious affiliations change easier than the food habits. Under certain circumstances when the stress of employment conditions force them to eat unattractive foods during the working hours, it results in somewhat rigid attitudes towards familiar foods. In this case, an unattractive lunch may be more nutritious and satisfy the hunger and the physiological requirements but not the appetite for food, which they try to satisfy in the evenings at home by gorging on the traditional foods.

Food Habits, Should They Be Interfered With?

Man is a creature of food habits that have been acquired during the course of raising. In those societies where a wide variety of food is eaten and the children are exposed to foods with varying tastes and textures, change in food habits is relatively not difficult even if the dietary habits have been practiced long enough to be a part of a culture. The wide acceptance of foreign foods, e.g. pizza and Mexican preparations in the U. S., is an example. In such societies, most men are not ordinarily conscious of their diet as constituting a set of habits. In old traditional societies, however, where a particular diet is the staple food, it has been established that the food habits, whether they are adequate in providing the required nutrients to the body or contribute to malnutrition, are firmly fixed in the mode of living of an individual. These food habits must be viewed not only in terms of nutrition or economics but along with the social, cultural, and religious setup of which a particular group is an intricate part. The main justification often given in favor of interfering with food habits is that the world food supply of traditional foods is inadequate for the good nutrition of the present generation, and if a concentrated effort is not made to change to nontraditional food sources and add to the quality of protein-rich foods, serious catastrophic shortages of food might exist in the coming decades that could make protein-calorie malnutrition a global problem, threatening the whole future of human civilization. A conservative estimate shows that for the expected world population in 1980, the supply of cereals would have to be augmented by 50 percent and that of protective foods [2] by 70 to 90 percent.

It can never be sufficiently emphasized to those concerned with improvement of the nutrition standards of the malnourished populations that interfering with food habits, unless they are on a voluntary basis, may defeat its very purpose because adding something unfamiliar to the diet may break an individual apart from his social cohesiveness and do more harm than good. Most nutritionists, having been either trained in the West or involved with Western ideas, must also not make the mistake of introducing some of the common foods to which they themselves are accustomed but are quite foreign to the populations they are dealing with. A classical case has been given by Anderson and Calvo [1] that the food of the Otami Indians did not include meat, dairy produce, fruits or vegetables of conventional kind considered necessary in the Western world for a nutritious diet. Instead they made their meals from tortillas and from local plants, such as malva, bediondilla, tuna, nopales, magney, garambullo, yucca, purslone, pigwood, sorrel, wild mustard flowers, lengua de vaca, sow thistle, and cactus fruit. They drank pulque, an intoxicating beverage, made from the juice of the century plants. The diet was analyzed at MIT, and it was found that it provided a better nutritional balance than was present in the diet in the U. S. at that time. A remark made by an old woman, as it was recorded by a dietitian in a Central African village, has been quoted by Le Gros Clark [4] which may not be inappropriate here. "You Europeans think you have everything to teach us. You tell us we eat the wrong food, treat our babies the wrong way, give our people the wrong medicine. You are always telling us we are wrong. Yet if we had always done the wrong thing, we should be dead. And you see, we are not." This, according to Clark, not only sums up the paradox that at times is implicit in any encounter between modern science and the traditional cultures of mankind but also emphasizes the cultural blocks that a nutritionist may have to face in order to change things for the better.

Food habits should be interfered with only when it is certain that they are contributing heavily to the malnutrition of the population, and even then, efforts should be made to supplement their traditional foods to overcome the deficiency so as to give it the semblance of least interference in their culture pattern. Methods of combating malnutrition, such as genetically manipulating their staple food to make it protein richer, should be evolved, and food habits should be touched as a last resort.

METHODS OF STUDYING FOOD HABITS

Most of our present knowledge about the food habits is derived from the research and experimental studies carried out during World War II. It was during that period that, for the first time, nutritionists and social scientists worked together on the problems of studying food habits and improving nutritional standards. A number of methods are employed to study the food habits of the people and will be dealt with in a very brief manner. The reader is referred to two important monographs, National Research Council Bulletin No. 108 on the problem of changing food habits, and *Malnutrition and Food Habits* by Burgess and Dean [2] and Clark [4] for detailed studies. It is of extreme importance to know about food habits, how they are established, and how a child learns to eat and like or avoid a certain kind of food. Unfortunately, in most of the countries where the protein malnutrition is a serious health problem, it is extremely difficult to collect accurate information because the purpose of inquiry is likely to be misunderstood. The methods commonly employed to study food habits are the following: (1) *Market Research:* It relates to studying various aspects of food habits. It starts with the productivity of a country and studies the consumption patterns as related to the purchasing power of the people in question. An analysis of the by-products of market research has occasionally provided information useful to the public health nutritionist. (2) *Fact Finding Surveys:* They include an inquiry into various aspects of food habits, how infants are fed, and what is the level of nutrition education of the mother. It is often found that mothers who are most in need of advice with respect to infant raising practices are the ones who seek it least frequently. This method of investigation includes a study of daily menus, variations in food consumption during the week, month, or year. (3) *Attitude Surveys:* They include an investigation into the attitude of the people towards beverages, preference for nonalcoholic or alcoholic drinks, cost and local influences on their attitudes. In one investigation, it was found that attitude towards beverages was largely determined by (a) preference for nonalcoholic or alcoholic drinks; (b) cost, cheapness, or expensiveness; and (c) certain local or provincial influences. (4) *Field Observations:* Data on general food habits can also be collected by general field observation, such as questioning the educated people, although they may prove to be limited in their knowledge of their fellowman.

All these methods of studying food habits have grave pitfalls, and unless all of them are employed with adequate controls on a particular community, a highly inaccurate picture about their food habits may emerge.

FOOD HABITS AND SOCIETY

Food Habits and Social Values

Food is a symbol of close relationships, friendliness, and social acceptance, and food fancies and food habits are part of a social setup that helps to identify the individual as a part of the whole and makes him feel secure. Community habits or the food habits of a social group may benefit the health and physiological well-being of the members or hurt them, leaving them undernourished. These are, nevertheless, potent factors which cannot be ignored by an individual. An enlightened and educated member, knowledgeable of the role of nutrients in body building, may modify the social regimen but cannot ignore the social customs completely. A food habit is not a passing whim or fancy but is a feature of the society completely integrated into its structure and social values and hence may or may not be wholesome with respect to their nutritive value,[4] and according to Burgess and Dean,[2] food habits are so deeply significant that they rank alongside language or reading habits in importance. "What people are willing to eat is determined by a complex system of attitudes, ideas and assumptions that form the local cultural patterns. These include religious restrictions, taboos, ideas pertaining to the merits and demerits of a food, and other attitudes which are as yet little understood." [14]

It will be interesting to discuss a few important factors which lead to the formation of food habits that are difficult to repudiate with a conscious effort. The safest generalization that can be made about the social psychology and food habits is that they are formed at a very young age and are a direct link with the individual's sense of security, emotional stability, and physiological well-being. The food fancies built in the child's early experiences in a particular way become deeply ingrained. They are related not only to the smell of the food, taste of the food, texture of the food but also to emotional security that a mother's pleasant smile provides along with the food. The family environment also influences the formation of food habits. Its members accept certain foods better when the entire family is together for meals in a happy relaxed atmosphere. The undernutrition or malnutrition of the children, therefore, is directly linked with the food habits of the adults.

If the family or the social group to which it belongs has enough food of the right quality and prepares food wisely, then every member including children will be better fed. In most cases it is the certain manner of preparation of the same food items that determines the food habits of a group; for example, beans prepared by Mexicans or Indians are not the same as prepared by Americans, although these are the same beans. Rice to a Puerto Rican is rice only if it is short grain rice and has a little lard added to it.[2] A person eats a certain food because he not only likes its taste, but also because it includes familiar qualities such as the smell, the roughness, smoothness, temperature, color, dryness, softness or hardness, many of which are very important to an individual because he has preserved them through his growing years.[2] Most individuals have certain well-formed tastes that are with them from infancy and stay until death. The individual all along this period always seeks and enjoys those kinds of foods that give him pleasure as well as social identity.

Besides social values, social customs also play an important role in determining not only the food habits but also the physiological well-being of its members. This can be categorized into two areas. At an individual level, the food habits of the mother governed by social customs are an important influence on the eating habits of the children and their health status. Occasionally, she may pass on her dislikes for certain foods important for the satisfactory growth of the child or may force on them her likes of foods that may or may not be satisfactory. At the social level, social customs can also stretch certain concepts of privacy in food habits a little too far. For example, in northern Arabia, even the husband and wife would not like to eat in front of each other and may or may not eat the same preparation. In most parts of Arabia, no woman will eat before men, and there is a widespread notion that one should not be seen eating by anybody. In Sudan, there used to be a common practice, not common these days, to cover the mouth when eating and drinking. In order to preserve the social custom of maintaining privacy in food habits, school children in some countries are given long noon hours so they can go home and eat with their families.

Food Habits and Social Prestige

The compulsion of custom as related to social prestige plays an important role in forming certain food habits; even if these habits are not rigid, they take a chunk off an individual's budget. This money could well be spent on food items that could go a long way in supplying the food needs of the growing children as well as adult members of the family. Let us take, for example, the drinking habits of an individual as related to his social life. These habits may be extremely harmful for his own health and that of his immediate family, but they become important in terms of happiness and well-being of a community of which he is an integral part. Drinking liquor or beer is an essential form of fulfilling certain social obligations. For example, it is the most effective form of pleasing a boss, a reward for help by a friend, and for cementing loose friendships. In Africa in certain countries, tribal councils cannot be held or marriages consummated without adequate amounts of beer, irrespective of whether the person's budget affords it or not. Huntingford [8] gave an apt description of the Nandi tribe's preoccupation with beer, in spite of lack of food at home for the infants.

> The European who sees a Nandi continually getting drunk, although he is at the same time short of food, does not realize that beer is a social necessity and not merely an enjoyment. If a Nandi cannot from time to time give a beer party, even a small party, he will lose social standing; he will be considered mean and will not be asked by his neighbors to partake of beer. He will be, unofficially but none the less effectively, pushed out of his rightful place in the Koret (i.e., parish).

The nutritive value of this drink (beer) for adults may not be ignored because, having been produced from germinated grains (contributing vitamin C as well as several B vitamins), this beer may be a source of calories as well as energy, but the point of discussion here is how important social customs are to an individual as to sacrifice his family's health to discharge those social obligations. An FAO study in Dakar indicates, and according to the author's observations it is true of most parts of India as well, that social customs or social obligations determine the proportion of family income that is allotted to food purchase. Increased incomes from better crops do not go to improve food levels but to satisfy a desire for social prestige through bigger and more elaborate weddings, birth ceremonies, and funerals. In a sophisticated society, like that of North America, high prestige and expensive foods, such as roasts or steaks, are served when guests are invited, and hamburgers or beer are not served,[29] even if that is all that the family can afford. Lowenberg *et al.*[14] showed by a diagram the relationship between social and physiological needs and the rightly placed or misplaced priorities.

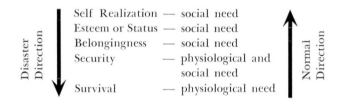

This scheme of priorities is applicable not only to the African tribal way of life but also to highly advanced and sophisticated societies of the West. All over the world, men have been discharging social obligations at the cost of the family's health. For example, in many communities in India such obligations, such as providing new dresses to the visiting relatives at the time of birth of a child, take priority over investing money on the proper recovery and health of the mother. Similarly, the family's health is sacrificed in order to set aside money to provide dowry for a daughter's marriage, and under the direct impact of these social obligations, it is not uncommon to see undernourished or malnourished children in homes, which are seemingly well off. As Huntingford[8] described for African communities, the social obligations in Indian society are also as compelling and without fulfilling them, an individual may find himself quite effectively pushed out of his rightful place in the society.

Foods for Relieving Tensions

Eating familiar and satifying foods are always associated with a feeling that everything is well with the world around him. Such feeling originates in the crib, with the baby foods given by a smiling mother, assuring the child his personal well-being as well as the stability of his surroundings. In tense moments, food seems to give solace as well as satisfaction that no other source apparently provides. Adults learn to eat whenever they are under tension. A survey of Lowenberg *et al.*[14] showed that 75 percent of his group ate more when under tension. In most circumstances foods prove a great tension-relieving factor. Since tension is a part and parcel of the modern life, a habit of resorting to food under the slightest tension could have grave consequences. If the food is available, most adults would consume calories well beyond their physiologic needs and tend to become obese and as a result become prey to a number of metabolic disorders. Under tension most men and women have learned to resort to foods that are of doubtful nutritional value. In this category come the habits of drinking tea or coffee, alcoholic beverages, smoking and chewing tobacco, chewing beetle leaves or even smoking pot (drugs that affect the nervous system). It should not be surprising if the total sales of these commodities with doubtful nutritional value but certainly harmful to human physiology are more than that of the nutritious foods, such as meat, dairy products, vegetables, fruits. In the United States alone, more than 22 billion dollars worth of alcoholic beverages are sold. Excessive consumption of these beverages leads to penury, cirrhosis of the liver, obesity, and increased mortality due to traffic accidents, but men and women used to them cannot limit their consumption because it helps in relieving their tensions.

The harmfulness of tobacco, as a source of nicotine and its contribution to respiratory complications, is well established. Nevertheless, the social habit of smoking or chewing tobacco is so well established all over the world that a poor laborer in India sacrifices the health of his infants to provide himself the delight of smoke. In that country, despite shortage of money for food, 6 to 8 percent of the income is spent on smoking. Its uselessness is well established in highly advanced countries of the West, but its hold on these societies is probably as well entrenched. During the last war, Britain, desperately short of food, chose to limit food imports rather than restrict supplies of tobacco. It is quite interesting as well as shocking that vast areas of good quality lands are devoted in almost all the countries of the world to the production of nutritionally useless crops. This land, put to producing food, will eliminate shortages of food that these countries are experiencing. United States may well be able to afford to put aside land to grow 1,400 millions lb of tobacco a year, but can India (producing 1,100 million lb) and China (producing 1,000 million lb) afford this wastage of their good land? Economically they can afford it because it is a cash crop and brings in money, but if the purpose of the land is to grow food for the people, then it is a bad strategy. Poor countries like Algeria, Bulgaria, Puerto Rico, and Yugoslavia devote a great deal of their good land to the production of tobacco.[25]

Tea and coffee are other widely-used tension-relieving foods, whose nutritive value is not only doubtful, but they are also implicated in raising blood cholesterol,[31] and countless individuals in many societies are addicted to their consumption many times a day. These individuals deliberately deprive themselves of proteins, minerals, and vitamins (lacking in these beverages) and add calories due to accompanying sugar intake, with the resulting obesity, but they cannot break the habit. Pyke[25] described that tea and coffee imbibing, "May become a dietary habit so compulsive that to break it without understanding its strength can disrupt a whole society. Industries can be brought to a standstill if a tea-break is carelessly displaced."

The disruptive effect of the use of various drugs in the communities, resulting in malnutrition or metabolic and mental disorders at the individual level and loosening social cohesiveness and dignity at the social level, is quite clear and need not be discussed in detail. These drugs are introduced in order to relieve some mundane tensions and end up in individual and social tragedies.

FOOD HABITS AND CULTURE
Cultural Aspects of Food Habits

A culture, such as Western culture, Indian culture, Chinese culture, African culture, has a very important influence in shaping

the food habits of a community, irrespective of whether it contributes to good nutrition or bad nutrition. Such cultural patterns
do reflect the economic poverty or prosperity of a particular region, but even if economic situations change for the better or
worse, the cultural patterns of food are invariably adhered to.
United States is somewhat an exception, probably because it
has been the "boiling pot" of many cultures and has drawn its
citizens from different cultures all over the world. Prosperity
and opulence has also played a role in growing American adven-
tures in unfamiliar foods. An average American wants to eat a
great variety of foods and will not mind trying Mexican, Italian,
Chinese, and other foods. Beyond trying foods occasionally, an
American also has a cultural pattern of food habits of his own.
He can live on hamburgers and hot dogs but not on pizza alone.

Numerous examples can be cited where irrational dietary
habits under the influence of local culture successfully prevent
the use of available food in human health and welfare. The classical example of this cultural impact is the prevalence of protein
malnutrition among children in certain areas where the protein-
rich foods are available but are not given because of cultural prejudices and ignorance and the resulting faulty weaning practices.
Nutritious foods are labelled too hot or too cold, light or heavy,
and are withheld from the child until he is, by the criteria of the
culture, better able to resist their ill effects.[28]

Many cultures also accept a high mortality rate for pre-school
children as normal and natural and determined by the will of
God.

A cultural heritage has always proven stronger than economic
and social circumstances and has influenced human destiny in
many ways, including food habits. Our choices of foods are expressions of ourselves as individuals and as members of a certain
cultural group. For example, a man tends to get married to a
girl who has a similar cultural background because it tends to preserve his food habits, and the marriage proves harmonious in a
number of ways, particularly with respect to the meaning of a
particular food and its method of consumption. For example, oats
are well accepted as food in Scotland, but some countries in the

vicinity believe it to be fit enough only for the horses. Corn, also a staple diet in a number of regions, may be detested as food by the Irish or the Germans, who may consider it chicken feed.[14] Most Mexicans prefer tortillas of white maize to that of yellow. Under these conditions of dietary rigidity, some unhappiness in an intercultural marriage may be understandable with respect to cultural meanings of certain foods.

When a particular food is a part of a certain cultural setting, a nutrition worker or health educator is bound to be faced with failure if he tries to persuade its substitution by a more nutritious food. His attitude should be that the traditional food and the manner in which it is prepared is great, but it should be supplemented with legumes or other protein-rich sources.[13] Plantain is a classical example; it contains only 1% protein and is poor nutritionally except as a source of calories, yet it is an integral part of some African cultures as a staple food: this fact must not be ignored by nutrition workers, and its significance in African culture must be well understood.

> There is a legend that Kintu, the founder of Buganda, first introduced the plantain. Today native beer is fermented plantain. The placenta is buried under a plantain tree. Food is steamed in plantain leaves. The baby is born on a fresh leaf, and a shroud can be made of old leaves. The significance of the plantain, both as a symbol of the Buganda people and of the general 'goodness' is emphasized by the fact that the badge of the women's club has a plantain tree on it. When the traditional ruler, the Kabaka, attends a special function, the road along which he will pass, is lined with freshly planted plantain shoots.[5]

Cooking reveals the culture of a country, and a country's soul is reflected in its food. "The creative skill of an intricate dish well cooked and served and enjoyed by the family provides immense material satisfaction. A dinner for two in soft candlelight provides immense individual pleasure and background for romance." [14] Foods prepared in a certain manner, dictated by cultural history of the region, have the properties of emotional satisfaction and give the individual a social and cultural dignity. All of us have a certain image of food to which we are linked culturally. A forcible change of circumstances which leads to consumption of unfamiliar foods can be very frustrating. Even the same food having an unfamiliar look and feel could be disappointing. This is especially true of small children. They are particularly sensitive to texture of the foods as much as taste. In the United States, people react favorably to velvety ice cream, crisp rolls, fluffy mashed potatoes, but the same people may not like to eat greasy meat and lumpy mashed potatoes. There is nothing more frustrating than to see your favorite food presented in an unattractive manner. The worst punishment that can be given, which has been tried in jails, is to get the favorite foods of the people to be fed and mash them in their presence into an unattractive lump of food and serve them. The nutritive value is there, but the culture is killed.

As another example, wheat imported from the United States was rejected in India because of different color and glutin properties and its difference from their own brand. It is strange but true that people rate the same brand of coffee as weaker when served in thin china cups than when served in heavy pottery mugs.[14]

That food habits are greatly determined by past history is exemplified by the Indian and Chinese cultures. The people belonging to different regions of these vast countries seem to have little in common with each other, but an analysis of food habits clearly reveals a cultural unity between all the Indian people or the Chinese. In India, the people in different regions (north, south, east, west, and central) have different languages and from their physical appearances seem to be different people, but surprisingly the manner of preparation of foods, the meaning of foods in religious rites and eating habits show a great similarity. The food habits unite the Indian people culturally, and it makes their political and economic unity easier and more meaningful.

It may not, therefore, be right to assume that the human is a biochemical engine and will consume anything that nurtures its body. Biologically, human beings are truly omnivorous, and their "engine" will take any kind of organic stuff offered to it, but culturally, there is much more than that to human nutrition. Human beings suffer the worst kinds of malnutrition and nutritional deprivation, but will not eat the most abundant foodstuff around them if it does not agree with their culture. A food for one man in one part of the globe may prove an article of repugnance on another's part, and certain foods accepted as delicious and nourishing in one culture may be viewed with disgust and actually cause sickness to a person of another culture. Men eat or abstain from eating particular foods for no apparently good reason and when asked cannot explain why they reject certain foods. Eating of insects, rich as they are in nutritive value, is an example of food that is not only liked but considered a delicacy among certain people and rejected with detest by other human populations. An average American or European will hate to eat insects as a part of his menu, but in Japan all kinds of insects form part of the diet and are highly prized. Dragon flies, locusts, crickets, and beetles are a delicious food among Ifugao tribesmen in the Philippines. In India a vegetarian who is culturally bound to eating only the plant food will refuse to eat any animal foods offered to him. Among the nonvegetarians, one who will eat one kind of animal flesh may refuse to eat another kind of meat because it does not agree with his cultural background. For example, a man from one class or community may relish the chicken legs but may stubbornly refuse to eat frog legs, or a person may eat beef but will reject pork and vice versa.

Also in the area of nutrition of the infant there are certain cultural influences which determine the kind of foods the child is going to eat. In most eastern countries, where joint family systems still prevail and the grandparents live with their children, the grandmother will have absolute authority on how to feed the baby. She takes this role upon herself because of her early experience in child raising, and to all practical purposes, she dictates what the child should be given and what must not be given. In most instances, this feeding program reflects the cultural influences without regard to the nutritional needs of the child. For example, if the grandmother believes that purging the child relieves him of gastrointestinal problems, the child will be purged, irrespectivie of what the family doctor says or believes. The priority of food service in a household is another cultural pattern that occasionally becomes the main reason for malnutrition among children. For example, it is the Zulu custom that men should eat first followed by women, and if there is any food left, it should be given to children.[5] The custom is based on lack of appreciation for the needs of the children and is governed by the local necessity that the warriors get the best food to maintain their strength. Fortunately, in India, which is another area of widespread under-nutrition, the priorities of serving food in the family are rightly placed, and the children get their share first before the elders are served.

Customs and Superstitions as Related to a Particular Culture

The compulsion of custom is not merely characteristic of an individual but is true of a social group, a community, or even a whole nation. It expresses itself in a number of ways. For example, there are cultural taboos on a food irrespective of its nutritive value and cultural interpretation of certain foods which may or may not be rational. These biases in favor of or against a particular food are a result of certain experiences which are passed on from generation to generation and become a part of a cultural setup.

As with foods, illness and states of well-being are understood differently in different cultures and may be the result of a mixture of ancient and modern ideas.[2] Diseases are associated with the use of certain articles of food and are believed to be avoided if that particular food is not consumed. For example, milk is very much valued in numerous countries as a nourishing food, but in some cultures, it is rejected with revulsion as an animal mucous discharge. Due to certain cultural reasons, milk is generally avoided in Thailand. One can make a sizeable list of food superstitions all over the world that could be linked to cultural or religious influence. In Indonesia, virgins are encouraged to eat bananas, cucumbers, or pineapple in order to ensure physical perfection according to a belief. In certain parts of India, mangoes are believed to produce jaundice. Children are branded on the abdomen to improve the gastrointestinal system. Children are deprived of supplementary foods up to one year with the cultural belief that they cannot digest them, and certain ceremonies are established in order to ensure the continuance of such customs.

If a child develops any kind of upset at a time when a supplementary food is being given, the illness is blamed on the food and is henceforth discontinued.[2] Cultural influences often prove to be potent obstacles in any effort to relieve the suffering population (infants, children as well as adults) of protein-calorie malnutrition or other deficiency diseases. It is, therefore, important to learn of the cultural or historical origin of certain prevalent ideas about foods and diseases because in those countries where protein-calorie malnutrition is prevalent, and the situation needs to be remedied, a full understanding of the cultural influences in attitudes towards health and disease, education, economic and agricultural conditions, and last, but not the least, cultural prejudices towards different kinds of foods is essential. Numerous examples can be cited in which communities suffer from undernutrition and malnutrition, not because of lack of food but because of the cultural patterns which encourage a starchy food and discourage another kind of food which may be protein-rich and needed by the members of the community.

There are certain cultural practices which are not only a result of superstitions but appear to be quite mystic in their origin. The African continent is full of such examples, and the reader is referred to an excellent monograph, *Folk lore in the Old Testament* written by J. G. Frazer.[6] A few examples may be quoted here. Among certain tribes exists a superstition against boiling the milk because of the belief that such a process will not only dry up the milk in the cow, but the animal may also die of the injury. This practice may be classified in the category of sympathetic magic. Among the Masai of East Africa boiling milk "was a heinous offense, and would be accounted a sufficient reason for massacring a caravan." The tribes firmly believe that robbery and murder may harm individuals, but something like boiling milk may hurt the sustenance of the whole tribe. Cuthbertson[5] explained that because of this strange belief, in the first edition of the Hebrew decalogue there are no such commandments as, "Thou shalt not steal," or "Thou shalt do no murder," and instead there is a commandment, "Thou shalt not boil milk." Also, only the close family could use the milk produced by one's cows, and under no circumstances will the family supplement its food supply from outside the kin group. Women are also believed to exert an evil influence on the cattle during their menstruation period, and it is customary in a number of tribes to exclude milk from the diet of girls when they reach the age of puberty.

A somewhat similar belief, based on sympathetic transmission of disease, is present in some parts of West Bengal, India, that during the process of boiling milk, if it overflows from the utensil, it may burst the nipples of the cow that supplied it. This practice may have its origin from the precious nature of the milk that it may not be wasted during the process of boiling. Similarly, a cultural belief that cow's milk results in diarrhea in young infants is fairly strong in the minds of some people, and the children are kept away from it. Probably such a belief arose from the adulteration or contamination of the milk available in the market.

Some African tribes also take great pains to make sure that the milk is not contaminated by vegetables in the stomach and must not be eaten together in the same meal. A belief that a mixture of the two articles of food in their stomachs hurts the health of the cows is very strong in their minds. Another superstition relates to eating game meat by Zulu women in the belief that, "If they do, they will bear wild and immoral children. It is believed that if women or girls eat horsemeat, their children will have big ears, and pregnant women do not eat pumpkin porridge for fear that the child will have birth marks." [5] A number of cultural taboos on food, otherwise nutritious, exist in India as well,[5] and relief from them would contribute to removing the undernutrition to some extent. For example, in West Bengal young mothers or boys are discouraged to eat eggs because they are believed to cause debility. Milk and fish meat must not be consumed in the same meal for fear of getting leprosy or leukoderma. Brain must be avoided because it is likely to cause premature graying and baldness. The eating of goat tongue by children and young women may make them talkative. Goat legs eaten by children may lead to underdevelopment of the knee and ankle joints, and pig's stomach eaten by young women will darken their complexion.

In Bangladesh, a pregnant or lactating mother is put on a dry diet and not allowed to have fluids, which makes it difficult for her to produce and maintain a supply of milk. In Indonesia even nursing mothers are advised to take less food than required, and in Malaya, fish is not given to children because it is believed to produce worms.

An excellent study by Carstairs[3] in *Health, Culture, and Community* shows that for rural Indians a sickness may not only be a physical impairment but also a moral crisis caused by certain acts considered immoral. Instead of a clinical diagnosis and treatment, a sick person may be prescribed moral atonement in addition to or even instead of medicine.

FOOD HABITS AND RELIGION

In some societies, religion has played an important role in determining the food habits of the people and has to some extent influenced the general health of its followers for the better or worse. Among the major religions of mankind, Buddhism preached effectively against the custom of eating animal food. More than 2,500 years ago, when a predominantly Hindu India was liberally practicing animal sacrifices for religious rites and animal foods were an accepted part of the daily menu of the people, Buddha preached the sanctity of animal life, interpreting the old Hindu belief of transmigration of soul in a new way, by telling people that the flesh and blood of the animals is no different from their own, and furthermore, any of these animals could have the soul of any of their ancestors. Buddha's influence successfully prohibited the taking of life for pleasure or eating, and one of the most powerful kings of the ancient times, King Ashoka, led a crusade against harming animals by humans. Under the influence of Buddhist thought, a large number of people all over Asia are traditionally vegetarians and will refuse to take any animal food except milk under any circumstances and are happy living on heavily starchy food. A strict Hindu or Buddhist completely abstains from meat, but liberal Hindus will eat meat of a sheep or a goat but not that of a cow, which is considered sacred. Mahatma Gandhi, the father of the Indian nation, in his youth intellectually agreed that if sheep or goat could be eaten, why not cow and also agreed to eat a little bit of beef preparation. But his Hindu culture and rejection of beef were so strong in him that the food made him violently ill.[29] Under the circumstances, when a nutritionist, trained in the West's oriented science, sees malnutrition amongst millions of Indians (a country believed to have one fifth of the total cattle population of the world) his immediate reaction would be to ask the people to forget about the irrelevant religious ideas and eat the protein-rich cattle. Of course, the question remains: Is he justified to give such advice?

In contrast to Hindu and Buddhist belief in the sanctity of animal life and an evident prevalence of malnutrition in these societies, the Christian religion is anthropocentric (taking man as the pivot of the universe) which believes that all creatures in the universe are for the use of man to the best of advantage. This philosophy is in contrast to Hindu and Buddhist ideology that animal life is as sacred as human and has as good a soul as human. Christianity believes in full use of nature and natural objects including animals for the good of human species. This philosophy is probably the major factor in the development of science and technology in the Christian West. Taking over the role of master of nature, the Christian West eliminated poverty, hunger, and malnutrition by most systematic and scientific use of nature and natural objects. With the blessings of religion the western explorers created abundance in this world, plenty of food for everyone, with scientifically managed cattle farms and mechanized agriculture. "The dominant western religion, teaching the supremacy of man and his absolute right to exploit his environment has enabled food to be produced with matchless efficiency." [25] This is not the right place to pass judgments or to comment on the different philosophies. The fact remains, however, that a Hindu and a Buddhist who reveres cattle are somewhat undernourished, and his Christian brother, who grows cattle to eat, is adequately nourished.

Religion has played a significant role not only in the food habits of the communities but also to some extent in determining the priorities of its use because among those communities religion is not merely a ritual but a drive, such as a drive of hunger.

"Religion is a philosophy or code with which a fabric of a community is permeated and by which its values are influenced." [25] For example, alluding to some Chinese and probably Hindu beliefs, food must be set apart for the dead ancestors before it is distributed to the living family. Certain communities use a great proportion of their food supplies for religious purposes, making turmeric or other noneconomic religious activities, in spite of the fact that they live on subsistence levels and could use their energies in producing more food.[25]

Besides religion, foods have also played some role in politics of certain countries. In India, the fasts of Mahatma Gandhi had great political repercussions and were used successfully to arouse the masses to unify for their demand for independence, and most political observers will say that these fasts were effective as political campaigns. The Boston Tea Party could also be similarly interpreted as being interrelated to food and economics, and tea, being a part of the daily food in the American way of living, greatly stimulated the politics of the American Independence.[29]

CHANGING FOOD HABITS CONTRIBUTING TO MALNUTRITION

Resistance to Changes

The experience of many health workers in most countries shows that food habits of the people are considered an extremely personal matter and are as much an indication of self-expression as are the clothing, reading habits, or political attitudes. Food habits are an 'integral part of the whole fabric of life and cannot be changed in isolation." [14] It took at least 200 years for the potato to be accepted in Europe and 100 years for the tomato. In order to understand why people resist any change in their food pattern, one must understand that food is not merely a vehicle of satisfying hunger, but familiar foods represent an emotional clutch, a source of psychological and physiological satisfaction and, above all, a source of security that everything is well in the world as far as they are concerned. Burgess and Dean [2] aptly remarked that, "Unfortunately there appear to be psychological, sociological and cultural factors which create barriers against rapid changes in food habits and which are less well understood than the impersonal aspects of nutrition and malnutrition." Food habits are particularly hard to change in those societies where they have been built into a child's early experiences. Various kinds of foods also develop different expressions and meanings, such as certain foods, irrespective of their nutrition value, are associated with a particular status—social, economic, or religious. For example, in a multicultural society like India, Hindus wouldn't eat a particular food because it is considered the food for the Muslims or vice versa. A change to anything similar to the forbidden food will, therefore, be greatly resisted. Taste and texture are other important factors about which people show a lot of resistance if asked to change. Occasionally, it may not be the food itself that is resented, but the way it is cooked or presented to them, because this kind of change reflects some change in circumstances and gives them a feeling of insecurity. Mexicans eat beans and so do the Indians, but since they are prepared in a different manner, they are not the same food. Bread used in the United States is made from the same wheat as bread (chapatis) made in India, but an average Indian will refuse to eat American bread if it is substituted for his chapatis.

This brings us to the problem of whether we should leave the people to themselves and let them follow their food habits, even if from the nutrition point of view they are faulty and contribute to undernutrition and malnutrition. This is not a positive approach and shows a lack of understanding of the human behavior. Most men and women will change their food habits if they are convinced that such a change does not reflect lack of security, is not a change for the change sake, improves their health, and above all does not affect their social status or image. Margaret Mead,[20] having studied food habits in rural communities, believed that it is not difficult to change the food habits if the substitute foods are cheaper and delicious to eat.

Ignorance and illiteracy play an important role in showing a stubborn resistance to any change in food patterns. In these circumstances, improving the educational level and exposing them to the practical benefits of better nutrition reduces this resistance towards accepting a new and unfamiliar food. Education and changes in economy bring about an atmosphere in which social changes are possible, and food habits, being a part of social life, also change or are modified for the better in a manner such that the participants are sometimes not aware of it.

Voluntary Changes in Food Habits

Under certain changed circumstances, certain individuals or communities change their pattern of food habits and adopt the new foods almost spontaneously. This sudden change in food habits for the better or the worse may be an adaptive mechanism to the changed circumstances, for example, change of place of occupation from a village economy to an urban economy. Firstly, the foods of their home village may not be available or the family may not have enough money left to buy those foods after paying rent, clothing, and other necessities of urban life. Most societies these days are undergoing a period of rapid changes, which disturbs the old patterns and results in a new way of life. With social changes, however, an average person's demands increase more rapidly in the area of material goods, such as house, furniture, and means of transportation, rather than in the area of improving food. He may still eat more of the same thing. But when the social conditions change, it is only a matter of time that new foods and new packages in which new foods come are also accepted. Eskimos and Australian aborigines, having come into contact with Western way of life, turn to Western groceries eagerly. A member of a Bantu tribe, when he leaves his village to work in a mine, easily adapts to the foods offered to him.

The experience of gaining social prestige is another instance where spontaneous changes in food habits take place. It is based on the desire to eat foods that are associated with social prestige. If the so-called prestige foods are nutritious, the change is for the better, but this is not always the case and may result in poorer foods than the traditional diets. For example, taking to white bread (not enriched) instead of tortillas, tea instead of buttermilk, coffee instead of atole. When circumstances are favorable or when members of a community become knowledgeable about the nutritional value of another easily available food, it is surprising to see a large number of people taking the change so willingly, as if previous food habits did not mean much to them. The rice-eating Bengali and a South Indian in 1944 would prefer to starve rather than eat wheat flour,[21] but as wheat becomes abundant and cheaper, and convinced of its nutritional superiority, millions have taken to it cheerfully.

Voluntary changes in food habits also take place among individuals or communities emigrating to countries where the available foods are different from those of the immigrant group— Orientals, Italians, Poles, Hungarians, Czechs who immigrated into United States were so much attracted to the higher wage pattern that they did not mind eating the foods available to them during the working hours, and once initiated, they developed a liking for American foods. It is not surprising to find in the United States a person who has not eaten the food of his home country for years and is not at all unhappy about not getting it.

It may be interesting that once a group accepts new foods and makes it their own, they develop somewhat rigid food habits for acquired foods and find it hard to change them. An interesting example is the plantation workers among the Puerto Ricans whose so-called traditional food of dried fish, rice, and lard was determined by the commercial interests of the New England companies. Attempts to modify them by advising them to introduce fresh fish and vegetables met with extraordinary resistance. Lack of resistance or voluntary acceptance of new foods in the first place was due to its association with better economic opportunities, whereas an attempt to modify their diet only to provide them better nutrition was misconstrued as interference in their personal likes or dislikes of foods. In a somewhat similar experiment during the World War II, McCance and Widdowson [15] remarked that, "If people can once be induced to accept a change of diet, they are likely to become so used to it that they may never wish to revert."

The most difficult problem in food habits arises where people are malnourished and have learned to blame their state of health to factors other then nutrition. In such precarious situations, the health worker's responsibility is indeed very heavy. Not only a change in food habits is needed, which is not a change for change's sake, but is meaningful, but at the same time, the subjects concerned are convinced that they are accepting them voluntarily. Then only a lasting change has been brought about.

Methods of Changing Food Habits

Man is a product of his circumstances and so are his food habits. In the present day, human beings in vast areas and in large numbers are eating foods that contribute heavily to undernutritional and malnutritional status of their health. The national governments in these countries are increasingly aware of the growing calamity. A fight against prevalent undernutrition and malnutrition cannot be waged successfully by improving only medical and health facilities. It is essential at the same time to improve the quality of food ingested by the people, which essentially means changing their patterns of eating, or in other words, interfering with their eating habits. A nutritionist or a health worker, unless well equipped with the knowledge of how to effectively change the people's food habits, is likely to be completely frustrated. In traditional societies, familiar foods, irrespective of their nutrition value, are so much a part of their daily existence and so clearly interwoven into their social, cultural, and religious life that it requires a deeper understanding to facilitate a change for the better and thereby improve their health.

Enforced Change

This is the last method that should be tried to change the food habits of the people. You may have the best intentions in the world, but if you try to force upon a certain people a change that they don't understand, they will resist the change with all their energy, and in this way, instead of helping them, you are hurting them. For example, if a particular traditional food is withdrawn from the market and instead people are asked to consume another nutritionally better product, people will not accept the change and may even pay a higher price to get their familiar or traditional items of food. Burgess and Dean [2] in their treatise on food habits have explained that, "Every time we fail to tell the people the reasons for our actions, we are reducing the status of the people and their state of responsibility. Too often in the past, we have not accorded to the people whom we are attempting to change, full dignity and full rights to change in every respect." Any enforced change may be partially or wholly successful only under certain conditions, such as (1) majority of the people understand, appreciate, and accept the necessity for a profound change; (2) the people are convinced about the goodwill of the government towards them, but any political propaganda by an opposition party could nullify this condition; and (3) the skill on the part of the government agents (nutritionists, health workers, and officials) in their attempt to demonstrate the superiority of the new product compared to the old one.

Education

Education and enlightenment are the best vehicles of a desired change. A change in people's attitude toward health and disease is most important if any lasting changes for the better have to be brought about in their food habits. A child at school is the best teacher at home. A school lunch program and the accompanying education could go a long way in diffusing those ideas to the child's home. Children at school could take to small-scale farming in vegetables and fruits and be explained their importance in the menu. Schools can also make children part of the shopping group for the dairy products or other products from the grocers and have the teacher explain their significance on the spot. Children then can be persuaded to use those principles of nutrition at home with their evening meals or over the weekend. Most parents modify their meals and go along with children's tastes and likes. In this manner, the school could effectively modify the food habits or popularize a new product for its nutritional value. Education in fundamentals of nutrition can also help to educate the parents. A mother, somewhat informed about nutrition, will not use money to buy a soft drink for her baby and will instead invest it in milk. Education is important for the people to have good aims. Educational process may include things like providing practical suggestions for preparing foods in attractive ways, but while doing so, one must respect the likes and dislikes of a person or a community. It is very unwise to teach attractive beef preparations to a member of a Hindu community and pork preparations to a Muslim.

Image of Food

Beans prepared in a Mexican style are not the same food as beans prepared in an Indian style because their flavor is going to be different, because of the different manner of preparation and use of different varieties of spices. Flavor arouses the receptors of taste and smell, and an unfamiliar or unfavorable response to them could lead to rejection of the food. The image of the food is a part of social living and cannot be divorced from people's food habits. In Britain, a nourishing soup was not accepted until its color was changed from white to brown.[2] It is a well-known fact that color of a food can greatly increase or decrease one's appetite or desire for a particular food.[5] Besides the manner of preparation and the color, a social image of the food is equally important. Nuts may be rich in proteins, but if their social image is low, they will not be accepted. Polished rice versus unpolished rice may be another example. A new food product rich in nutrients may be produced by a subsidy from the government to keep its price low, so that people of the lower socioeconomic group may buy, but it may not be sold because of its poor social image and the belief that this food is meant for the poor people. The same food, if it is somewhat higher priced and is accepted by the well-off classes, will be easily taken by the poorer classes as well. Sometimes new foods with very low nutritive value become popular among the poorer classes only because they are consumed by the well-off classes and add to their already-deficient diets. The popularity of sodas (soft drinks) and white highly milled wheat flour instead of whole wheat flours are some of the examples. It is, therefore, extremely important to create a social image of a new food product if it is released in the market.

Persuasion

This is by far the best approach to try to change or modify the food habits. This involves a long process of explanations about the deficiencies in their traditional foods, advantages of modifying their traditional foods, and taking new food products. The experience of numerous field workers indicates that when persuasion is the only method used, a desire for certain kind of change is widespread because they are aware that something is wrong with their health which cannot be explained in terms of effects of supernatural powers, as their witch doctor or self-centered politician will like them to believe. It is always better to persuade people to modify than to change the food altogether, i.e. increasing the use of nutritious foods along with the traditional foods. If a nutrition worker tells a Puerto Rican that his beans and rice are the main reason for his undernutrition and he should instead use tomato and milk, he is not likely to be successful. But if he understands the psychology of the people and highly approves of their beans and rice and asks them to add something, like milk to their diet, things would improve. The task of changing food habits is a problem of culture building. One need not destroy the old one to introduce the new.

In the process of persuasion, a number of approaches, such as group-decision method and request method, can be followed and have been discussed in detail in a monograph on the problems of changing food habits, published by the National Academy of Sciences, Washington, D. C.[23]

Dr. Jelliffe has life-long experience working in Uganda and other developing countries. He has suggested that food habits should not be interfered with unless they have to be and, at best, effort should be made to modify them in a manner that helps to uproot the superstitions that led to their formation in the society in the first place.[9-12] The following approach may be tried:

1. Beneficial practices among communities, such as prolonged periods of breast feeding, should be approved and encouraged, and they may be complimented for such a custom.

2. Harmful practices, such as not giving fish to infants when available or not giving milk or other supplementary foods or purging the babies with castor oil because of some beliefs or super-

stition, should be discouraged or an attempt be made to correct them by friendly persuasion and convincing demonstration.

3. Neutral practices, such as massaging the body with oil or some tribal custom of handling the baby, which have no harmful effect, should be left alone and should not be interfered with.

4. Unclassifiable habits, such as mother's pre-chewing foods for the babies, needs further observation and research and may not be interfered with till more is known about them.

IMPACT OF TECHNOLOGY ON FOOD HABITS

High levels of industrialization and sophisticated technology in food storage, transport, and marketing not only help to make the best use of a country's supply in foodstuffs but can also create agricultural surpluses with the result that the consumers have a wide choice of foods to choose from for their dining table. Technological application to the preservation of food by canning, refrigeration, and freezing help make a particular food available all the year round, and when accompanied by mass transit system and cheap transportation, the availability of a great variety of food materials to the buyers becomes assured. This improved technology, therefore, has a direct bearing on the standard of living and food habits of the people. A high standard of food consumption is found in those countries where the farmer enjoys the benefits of technological advances in agriculture, preservation, and marketing.[2] The food habits in these countries are largely determined not by old traditions but by energy demands of the industrialized society and the wide variety of foods available in the supermarkets. In the United States, more than 100 kinds of cereals are available for breakfast; about the same number of variety for lunch meats and cheeses are available for lunches and the available variety for supper can be imagined by the fact that an average-sized supermarket carries 15,000 different items.

In traditional societies, where certain cultural factors prohibit the introduction of mass-scale food technology, the food habits are bound to traditional patterns mainly because of a subsistence earning. Lack of education and ignorance also play their part in making the food habits rigid; for example, in a country like India, where religion has a strong hold on the minds of people about taking animals' lives, large-scale meat processing plants based on modern technology cannot be established. In such countries expansion of technology must be accompanied by a campaign on the social level, as well as an enlightened education system. With the expanding populations, the pressure of which is more likely to be felt in extremely overcrowded Asia, the food technology based on use of scientific methods of agriculture and modern storage, transport and marketing facilities is the only ray of hope in providing adequate nutrition based on culturally based food habits and, at the same time, adding to the variety of foods to be eaten.

REFERENCES

1. Anderson, R. K. and Calvo, J.: *Am. J. Public Health, 36:*883 (1946).
2. Burgess, A. and Dean, R. F. A.: In *Malnutrition and Food Habits.* London, Travistock (1962).
3. Carstairs, G. M.: In B. D. Paul (Ed.): *Health, Culture, and Community.* New York, Russell Sage Foundation (1955), p. 107.
4. Clark, F. le G.: In G. H. Bourne (Ed.): *World Review of Nutrition and Dietetics.* Basel and New York, Karger (1968), vol. 9, pp. 56–84.
5. Cuthbertson, D. P.: In H. H. Beaton and E. W. McHenry (Eds.): *Nutrition.* New York, Academic Press (1964), vol. 2.
6. Frazer, J. G.: In *Folk Lore in the Old Testament.* London, Macmillan (1923).
7. Gravioto, B. R. *et al.*: *J. Nutr., 23:*317 (1945).
8. Huntingford, G. W. B.: *Colonial Research Studies No. 4,* HMSO (1950).
9. Jelliffe, D. B.: In *Infant Nutrition in the Subtropics and Tropics.* WHO Monograph No. 29 (1955).
10. Jelliffe, D. B.: In P. Gyorgy and A. Burgess (Eds.): *Protecting the Pre-school Child.* London, Travistock (1965).
11. Jelliffe, D. B.: In "Proceedings of the American Medical Association Western Hemisphere Nutrition Conference," Chicago (Nov. 1965).
12. Jelliffe, D. B.: In *Infant Nutrition in the Subtropics and Tropics,* WHO, Geneva (1968).
13. Jelliffe, D. B. and Bennett, F. J.: *Fed. Proc., 20* (pt. 3, suppl. 7):185 (1961).
14. Lowenberg, M. E., Todhunter, E. N., Wilson, E. D., Feeney, N. C., and Savage, J. R.: In *Food and Man.* New York, John Wiley & Sons (1968).

15. McCance, R. A. and Widdowson, E. M.: *Med. Res. Council Spec. Report. Ser., 254* (1946).
16. McCarrison, R.: *Br. Med. J., 2:730* (1926).
17. McCarrison, R.: *Indian J. Med. Res., 19:61* (1931).
18. McKenzie, J. C.: *Proc. Nutr. Soc., 28:103–109* (1969).
19. McWilliam, M.: In *Nutrition for the Growing Years.* New York and London, John Wiley & Sons (1967).
20. Mead, Margaret: *Nat. Acad. Sci., Nat. Res. Coun. Bull. 108,* Washington, D. C. (1943).
21. Mottram, V. H. and Graham, G.: In *Hutchinson's Food and the Principles of Dietetics,* 10th ed. London, Arnold (1948).
22. Murray, J. and Blake, E.: *Yearbook Agr.,* U. S. Dept. Agriculture (1959), p. 609.
23. *National Research Council Bulletin,* vol. 108, Washington, D. C. (1943).
24. Orr, J. B. and Gilks, J. L.: *Med. Res. Counc. Spec. Report Ser., 155* (1931).
25. Pyke, M.: In *Food and Society.* London, John Murray (1968).
26. Robinson, C. H.: In *Basic Nutrition and Diet Therapy.* London, Macmillan (1970).
27. Russell, E. J.: In *World Population and World Food Supplies.* London, Allen and Unwin (1954).
28. Scrimshaw, N. S. and Behar, M.: In B. H. Beaton and E .W. McHenry (Eds.): *Nutrition; Vitamins, Nutrients Requirements and Food Selection.* New York and London, Academic Press (1964), vol. 2.
29. Williams, S. R.: In *Nutrition and Diet Therapy.* St. Louis, C. V. Mosby (1969).
30. Wittfogel, C.: In I. Galdston (Ed.): *Human Nutrition, Historic and Scientific,* Monograph III. New York, New York Academy of Medicine International Univ. Press (1960), p. 61.
31. Yudkin, J.: *Lancet, 2:155* (1957).

Chapter VII

FIGHT AGAINST PREVALENT MALNUTRITION

Protein AND PROTEIN-calorie [malnutrition are the most serious nutritional problems that lead to deaths as well as retarded mental development amongst numerous infants and preschool children.] In the developing countries of the world its prevalence in the severe form varies from 1 to 9 percent, whereas in moderate form, it is as common as 50 percent among children of the preschool age. These figures become very serious when we become aware of the fact that more than three quarters of the human population is crowded in the overpopulated developing countries. It is also intriguing that 70 percent of the total animal protein is eaten by less than one third of the human population.[12] In addition to protein malnutrition, other deficiencies, particularly that of vitamins, are as prevalent among people who are nutritionally poor in protein and/or calories.] The rapid increase in human population and a corresponding reduction in per capita food-producing land has added to the difficulties in improving the nutritional status of the people involved. Gigantic efforts are required even to maintain a status quo in the nutritional level when increases in population are taken into account. Children in the developing countries are the hardest hit because of (1) cultural influences, under which the adult population does not appreciate the nutritional needs of the growing children; (2) demands of a large family and arrival of additional babies (because of unrestricted population growth, the number of children approximates half of the population of some of the developing countries) ; and (3) insanitary conditions of living, in which the undernourished children become prey to all kinds of diseases and infections that abound in their environment. The parents in these countries are generally unable to avoid the stress and strains that the above-mentioned factors put on a growing child, with the result that some die, some manage to reach adulthood with average functioning ability, whereas others are permanently impaired with respect to their mental development, thus adding to the steadily deteriorating quality of the human species. Dr. Parpia, Director of the Central Food and Technological Research Institute, Mysore, India, pointed out that

By the time a child reaches 18 months of age, 80% of his central nervous system has already developed. Ninety percent of his brain structure has been built by the time he is four years old. If he is without sufficient protein of the right kind during this period, the damage to his brain can never be repaired.[88]

Dr. Scrimshaw, head of the Department of Nutrition and Food Sciences at Massachusetts Institute of Technology, summarized the results of the recent research efforts that "not only are malnourished children smaller in size and more susceptible to infections, but they may be prevented from attaining their full mental capacity and also their full social development." [88]

Fortunately, human society has produced men and women who are not only compassionate towards other fellow beings but who as the leaders of their communities find persistent hunger and malnutrition totally unacceptable from moral and social point of view, and also because it impedes the progress of a nation in every sphere.[27] The leaders of most of the developing countries appreciate the problem and have set aside part of their resources to fight the prevalent malnutrition in their midst. They are also assisted by a number of international agencies in their task. The task of preventing the prevalent protein-calorie malnutrition involves the dedicated efforts of differently trained people, for example, politicians, economists, teachers, plant pathologists, geneticists, agricultural veterinarians, physicians and nurses, and the absence of any one of them from the team will leave a gap in the struggle.[62]

There are certain differences in various countries in the strategy of how the fight is to be undertaken, but the basic goals everywhere are the same and may be stated as the following: better nutrition must be provided to people of all ages, especially to growing infants, preschool, and school children, and all impediments towards attaining this goal should be removed. Most of the nutrition workers agree, however, that the main focus of efforts should be educational in a broad sense because without a long-term desirable change in the people's knowledge, attitudes and behavior about factors causing dietary deficiencies, we may only touch the periphery of the problem or solve it on a short-term basis. For long-term solutions in planning program in nutrition, it may be worth quoting the guidelines suggested by Food and Nutrition Board of the National Academy of Sciences.[47] They have real merit for wide adoption.

> 1. Establish departments of nutrition in universities with specialists in clinical nutrition, biochemistry, physiology, dietetics, and food management.
> 2. Organize and support curricula for training medical students, nurses, dietitians, have demonstration agents, and public health educators in nutrition sciences.
> 3. Assist and support dietary surveys, nutrition clinics, and research programs on problems of greatest local and national importance, including special emphasis on preschool children.
> 4. Establish food technology laboratories in one or more agricultural colleges, with specialists in bacteriology, food analysis, food engineering, and food management.
> 5. Organize and support training programs in food sanitation, quality control, research and demonstrations, emphasizing the production and processing of high-quality protein foods and prevention of protein-calorie malnutrition in early childhood.
> 6. Organize councils on food and nutrition to coordinate programs and advise the secretaries or ministers of agriculture, health, education, commerce, and economic development.

These guidelines will prove ideal for a long-term prevention of nutritional deficiencies among the population and will create a highly organized team of leaders in every field or indirectly concerned with it who will not only build a strong society but will regulate its growth in proportion to its resources.

In the fight for prevalent malnutrition, however, one has to think of the measures which do provide a long-term relief but whose effects are also visible in the present. This program would include treatment of the moderate and severe cases of malnutrition, rehabilitation of the vulnerable groups progressing towards malnutrition, increasing the level of food production and instituting family planning methods to slow down the rate at which the new babies arrive, so that better attention could be paid to the development of nutritional standards of the existing population. The combat strategy may be outlined as follows:

1. Treatment of moderate and severe cases of kwashiorkor should be prompt and all-out efforts be made to rehabilitate the children before any impairment in their functional capacity becomes a permanent part of their life. Details will be discussed in the following chapter on clinical approaches to fight malnutrition.

2. Diagnosis and admission of children, having mild to moderate degrees of malnutrition, to nutritional rehabilitation centers, where they are given nutritionally rich supplementary foods. Day-care centers, elementary schools, or other child-care institutions should also be involved in providing nutritious foods to children of vulnerable condition so as to prevent their regression into more severe form.

3. Elaborate public health measures to control infectious diseases are as important as improving food resources. There is an established synergism between malnutrition and infections, and most children who die of gastroenteritis or respiratory problems are basically malnourished individuals.

4. Increasing the level of food production is the most important strategy in the struggle against prevalent malnutrition, but equally important is a thorough study of the dietary habits of the people, because unfortunately in the traditional societies people prefer to starve rather than eat unfamiliar foods. The details of dietary habits contributing to malnutrition and people's resistance towards change have been discussed in an earlier chapter. The field observations on the rigidity with which the people hold on to their food habits indicate that those who advocate the use of mass-scale technology to produce unfamiliar food products rich in all the nutrients to feed the undernourished masses do not have a good grasp of the behavior of the human species. A human body is not merely a biochemical engine, and people do not eat nutrients but eat and relish meals that may not give them adequate health but provide them social and emotional security and preserve their identity. This is not to

undermine the advantages of mass-scale production of new food products but to emphasize that such a product may not be accepted by the masses of undernourished people who are ignorant, illiterate, and whose lives are guided mostly by religious, cultural, and social traditions. The main advantages of mass-scale production of a single new food product may be that

Expert knowledge can be put to use to design the formulation in such a way that the introduction of a single food item can bring the diet of a particular group up to adequacy in every respect; by judicious choice of materials the most economic use can be made of available materials and, most important, of the nutrients already available in the normal diet—an example of this is the possibility of utilizing the supplementary effect of proteins; technological expertise can be applied to utilize protein materials which, as such, would be unacceptable as food, by presenting them in an attractive, palatable form; the product can be formulated so as to contain the necessary nutrients in high concentration. This has the advantage of minimal disturbance of the food pattern, as only one new item, in fairly small quantity, need be introduced; and in the design of the product, cognizance can be taken of the good preferences and eating habits of the particular population group concerned, while the product can be made and presented in such a manner as to fit in with normal eating habits.[27]

Such a product, however, should be acceptable to children and their parents—cheap, processed from local ingredients, easily stored, and mixed easily with staple foods. The food should be bland in taste capable of use as a drink and rich in high-quality protein, vitamins, and minerals.[55] In the writer's opinion, the new food products can make a significant contribution to improving the health standards only when it is presented to the people after adequate demonstration; for example, in the nutritional rehabilitation centers, hospitals, school lunches, day-care centers, and mass-scale free supplementary feeding programs. In introducing the masses to an entirely new or unfamiliar food, one has to recognize that to change the food habits of a population is a formidable undertaking, and keeping this fact in mind the most effective strategy of improving the health may be to concentrate on the production of larger quantities of traditional crops whose seeds are genetically manipulated to overcome certain amino acid deficiencies, supplementing staple foodstuffs during central processing with additives which improve its quality without changing its taste or appearance.[35] At the same time, efforts should be made to improve dairy animals and their care to augment the milk and other dairy products. Adequate attention is also needed in the development of fresh water or marine fisheries accompanied by an efficient transport system of reaching the consumers in the fresh form. India catches more than 2 million tons of fish in the coastal waters but does not have adequate transportation facilities to take it to the consumers in the inland areas.

5. An elaborate system of mass education about infant feeding practices, advantages of breast feeding, nutritional requirements of the growing children and nutritional needs at all ages and conditions, such as during pregnancy, lactation, and old age, is needed, and the success of this program be thoroughly evaluated periodically. Details have been discussed in the chapter on nutrition education.

The following discussion of combatting prevalent malnutrition is based on the writer's awareness of the fact that human beings cannot be coerced into changing their life patterns and recognizing that the dignity of the individual, their dietary habits should not be interfered with beyond a certain point, even with the best of intentions.

NUTRITIONAL REHABILITATION CENTERS

Among the children showing signs and symptoms of nutritional deprivation, a majority of them show moderate degrees of malnutrition which do not require their admission to the hospitals. At the same time, they are considered ill enough to be allowed to stay at home, eating the same diets which precipitated their physical condition. It is essential, therefore, to establish nutritional rehabilitation centers (NRC) as separate institutions or attached to outpatient clinics of children's hospitals. Jelliffe [41] outlined two purposes for the NRCs: First, to expose the mothers of malnourished children to nutrition education for a fairly prolonged period, and secondly to rehabilitate the child recovering from kwashiorkor or suffering from moderate protein-calorie malnutrition. The biggest advantage of these centers is that they could be a clinical facility that can be manned mostly by paramedical personnel and can relieve the professional physician to attend to more serious cases.

The idea of NRCs was developed by Bengoa [8] in 1955 and has been supported ever since by a number of workers.[9,10,11,41,71,76,80] Algeria, Colombia, Costa Rica, Guatemala, Haiti, Uganda, Venezuela, and Tanzania have established such centers, the largest number of them being in Colombia.[24] Bengoa [10] and Jelliffe [41] outlined the objectives of nutritional rehabilitation centers as follows:

a. To reduce mortality due directly or indirectly to malnutrition in young children;

b. To reduce the incidence of malnutrition;

c. To improve the nutritional status of vulnerable groups such as pregnant and lactating women, infants, young children and school children;

d. To improve the family diet in general;

e. To create in the community an interest in better nutrition;

f. To promote and encourage other local agencies and to cooperate with them in implementing measures, such as those designed to assume availability of foods in the light of the pressing nutritional needs and the nutritional requirements, in general, of the population.

The children suffering from mild to moderate degrees of kwashiorkor or marasmus can be classified into two categories: (1) those who are diagnosed at a clinic to be nutritionally deficient but have no clinical complications and do not require any medical therapy; and (2) those children who not only show symptoms of nutritional deficiency but also have certain infections or other clinical complications. The first category of children may be put into an institution where they could be regularly provided with well-balanced diets, whereas the latter ought to be admitted to the type of rehabilitation center where, in addition to good diet, the children are adequately treated for their clinical symptoms. The day nutritional rehabilitation centers operating in a number of countries will be sufficient for the needs of the first category of children. For the second category, however, residential type of rehabilitation centers are important.

The day NRCs are organized similar to day nurseries or kindergartens. The children as well as malnourished pregnant or lactating women spend six to eight hours a day at the center six days a week and take their three meals there. The mothers of the children are encouraged to be with the child and help in cleaning the center as well as in preparing meals for the children and get practical instructions in child-care practices from the supervising nurse. Bengoa, who originated the concept of NRC, stressed that mothers' education should be the main aim of the rehabilitation centers, and the center's nutritionist, dietitian, nurse must take pains to give detailed practical demonstrations to the mothers. A mother well educated in principles of nutrition will take better care of the health of older children and her husband. This supplementary feeding program in the day NRCs may be supported by new food products manufactured from inexpensive local resources (see New Food Products). In addition to feeding children at the center, the possibility of selling the nutritionally rich new food products at low prices, probably subsidized by the government, must be thoroughly investigated. This could serve to popularize these products and serve as an intermediate procedure between the commercial system and free distribution.[41]

The residential rehabilitation centers require large resources with regard to staff and equipment, and whereas the day centers can pull along without the presence of professional physicians all the time, the residential NRC must have in addition to nutritionists, dietitians, and nurses the services of trained doctors, particularly pediatricians. In general, mothers are encouraged to accompany the child to the center and are treated as a junior staff, participating fully in the care of the child involved. The residential NRCs operate in close association with a hospital to take care of any change in clinical complications in a child. Bengoa[11] has described that residential-type centers are generally located in the urban areas and serve mostly as convalescent centers for children who had been successfully treated for severe types of malnutrition but not yet fully recovered to be discharged for fear of relapse or as a center for those children who had been treated for diarrhea at a rehydration center. The NRCs play an extremely important role in helping the hospitals serve larger number of patients and ensure the complete recovery of the treated patients, particularly those who have come from the remote rural areas and have no access to other medical care. The NRCs also provide a great opportunity for the research worker to collect data about the clinical and biochemical problems involved in nutritional rehabilitation of a malnourished child.[11] This data could be usefully employed elsewhere to improve the activities of NRCs.

As stressed earlier, the education of the mothers is an important objective of the NRCs, and the fulfillment of this objective can serve a very useful purpose, i.e. once the staff of those centers is convinced about the learning ability and proficiency of the mother in nutritional requirements and cooking and serving processes, the patients, who are clinically relieved of their symptoms but not adequately recovered from a nutritional point of view, can be sent home. A follow-up study could be continued with the patient's family through periodic contacts. This method would make available the facilities of the center for a larger number of needy patients. In the NRC, every attempt is made to use locally available foods as well as cooking utensils, so that the educational impact on the mother will not be wasted.

The NRCs have their own handicaps, particularly in the area of the number of people they can serve. In the developing countries where protein-calorie malnutrition is quite prevalent among the population, a few NRCs here and there may not even touch the periphery of the problem, but it may be argued that the one NRC in an area might have an overall beneficial influence in the community, and one mother educated in the center may spread her acquired knowledge among a large number of women in her neighborhood. The nutritional rehabilitation center, if incorporated in the community development program and if it maintains an active dialogue with the people of all socioeconomic levels, can serve as a useful model for preventive measures in the area's fight against prevalent malnutrition in the community.

PUBLIC HEALTH ACTIVITIES

Most often in places where malnutrition is widespread in communities and not restricted to certain individuals, its presence is not due to deficient diets alone but to prevalent infections, insanitary conditions, and lack of personal hygiene. In those areas, the combat strategy against malnutrition should not merely be a correction of dietary deficiencies but should include all-out public health measures. Malnutrition may be a primary factor in debilitating these children, but their constant exposure to a variety of infections seems as important. These infections are greatly responsible in stunting the growth of the child. In a study of a Guatemalan village nearly one fifth of the children had eight or more episodes of diarrhea during their first two years of age,[83] and similar fate is shared by millions of children in the other developing countries where sanitary conditions are less than satisfactory, and many of them die of either malnutrition or infection in the second year of life. The psychomotor development of children such as these has been found retarded by more than seven months at one year of age.[83]

The reasons for the poor sanitary environment, particularly in the rural areas, are many. In most tropical countries, the number of trained physicians are grossly inadequate. Also, most of the physicians are concentrated in the urban areas due to better amenities of life as well as a better income, and the rural areas tend to be ignored. Low incomes, predominantly starchy foods, insanitary conditions, religious and cultural superstitions, ignorance, and illiteracy all play their role in compounding the picture with the result that the most vulnerable group of the community—the children—suffer from protein-calorie malnutrition and infections, among which diarrheal diseases and respiratory infections are most common. Also present are schistosomiasis, trypanosomiasis, guinea worm, and hookworm infections.

Bengoa listed 12 principles on which the public health activities of a community (for the control of malnutrition in young children) should be based.[10,41]

	1. Treatment in hospitals and outpatient clinics;
	2. Supplementary feeding programs for malnourished children;
	3. Development of weaning foods based on inexpensive local resources;
Treatment,	
Nutritional,	4. Education of mothers on child-feeding practices;
Rehabilitation,	5. Immunizations;
and	6. Periodic surveillance of the population at risk (early diagnosis and treatment);
Prevention	
	7. Nutritional rehabilitation through special units in day nurseries, kindergartens, and so on;
	8. Control of diarrhea;
	9. General nutrition and health education;
Promotion of	10. School feeding and educational programs;
Better	11. Combined programs of education and food production (school, family, and community gardens);
Food Habits	
	12. Planning family diet.

The importance of these activities has been discussed in detail by Jelliffe.[41] In the writer's opinion, top priority should be given to preventive measures, such as immunizations of children and periodic surveillance of the population at risk. A comprehensive immunization program, particularly in rural areas of all developing countries, is a prerequisite to any public health measure. This program should include immunization against smallpox, tetanus, diphtheria, pertussis, polio, measles, and tuberculosis. In areas with high incidence of malaria, semisuppressive chemoprophylaxis or chloroquine should be made available to all the susceptible populations. Besides immunizations, a well-organized team of health workers and paramedical people should be employed in order to survey periodically and collect data on any clinical condition appearing in individuals in different age groups. Mobile teams can go from village to village and the population at risk be examined right at their homes, so that on-the-spot instructions in sanitary conditions and public health measures can be given, depending on the condition. The influence of on-the-spot education is likely to be more lasting. Diarrhea is probably the most devastating illness that always seems to go hand in hand with poor diets, poverty, and unhygenic homes. Public health measures should include the training of the mothers in recognizing the early signs of dehydration and oral administration of sugar solution with salt in it. This should lead to a sufficient understanding on the part of the mother that she takes the child in its early stages of diarrhea to the hospital or the rehydration center, where intragastric, intraperitoneal or intravenous fluids may be administered.[40,58,72] In any fight against malnutrition, the most vulnerable group, i.e. the child population, must take priority in public health measures, supplementary feeding programs, or even the allotment of available space in the hospitals or outpatient clinics. Bengoa [11] outlined a program for combating malnutrition among the young children, which is explained in Figure 17.

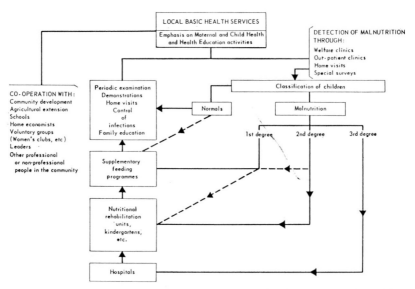

Figure 17. Program for the protection of young children from malnutrition (Reproduced from Bengoa).

PREVENTION OF NUTRITIONAL ANEMIA

Nutritional anemia was defined in a WHO technical report as a condition in which hemoglobin values are lower than the normal due to a deficiency of one or more essential nutrients, regardless of the cause of such a deficiency,[102] and the following fields of study were recommended: " (a) Absorption of iron from tropical diets; (b) Dermal losses of iron in tropical regions; (c) The part played by blood losses due to hookworm in the etiology of anemia; (d) Tissue iron stores; (e) The role of protein deficiency in anemia; and (f) The incidence of iron deficiency anemia in infants and children in the tropics." Detailed accounts of nutritional anemias are available in excellent reviews by Woodruff [103] and Vitale *et al.*[99] Nutritional anemias are an acute problem affecting large populations in most developing countries. In the children suffering from protein deficiency, biochemical indications of iron, folic acid, and ascorbic acid deficiencies are always present, and hypochronic iron deficiency anemia (suckling anemia) occurs during infancy all over the world, particularly in the tropical and subtropical countries. In these countries, it is estimated that the daily iron intake is not only inadequate, but a significant part of available iron is not absorbed because of bulk cereal foods with a high content of phosphates and phytates.[86] In the tropical climates, the loss of iron in the sweat and in urinary excretion is also more than in other places. Other nonnutritional factors, such as infections, may lead to hepatic losses. Under such physical conditions, even a small burden of hookworms can produce anemia because of smaller amount of blood in a child accompanied by higher needs of iron and protein.[41] The main strategy in fighting nutritional anemia includes the improvement of foods, fighting the infections, and prophylactic use of iron.[85]

The improvement of food and the dietary habits are the most important steps in the prevention of anemia. Faulty food habits, which do not provide adequate protein, aggravate the situation and lead to anemic condition. Platt *et al.*[70] observed that infant pigs, when given low-protein diets show some anemia, but when a low-protein diet was given with extra carbohydrates, the anemia was more pronounced. In most developing countries where anemia is prevalent, the traditional foods provide bulk carbohydrates which may provide nearly sufficient calories but not enough protein. The macrocytic anemias are, therefore, due to protein deficiency and are an "expression of the generally abnormal metabolism in a malnourished organism." [3] Ironically, it has often been seen that in anemic patients, the response of protein diet foods is often very slow. This led to the belief that protein deficiency and anemia are not causally related. Allen and Dean [1] observed, however, that during protein deficiency the hemo concentration masked the anemic condition which became evident only after serum albumin increased and plasma volume expanded under the influence of protein-rich diets, and an apparent increase in anemia resulting from treatment of kwashiorkor may give the impression that protein supplements are not having any beneficial effect in the treatment of anemia.

After a detailed investigation, particularly in Israel, Poland, India, Mexico, and Venezuela, a WHO scientific group on nutritional anemias recommended certain preventive measures. These may be usefully summarized here:

General Sanitary and Dietary Measures

In areas where hookworm infection leads to iron deficiency the eradication of the parasite must be pursued rigorously. Sanitary measures, particularly in rural areas, should be strengthened. In some areas, iron deficiency has also been caused by use of refined products, e.g. the refined sugar with little iron content has become more popular compared to the unrefined sugars which contain a significant amount of iron. Educational programs in sanitary methods and richer diets, such as encouraging the consumption of vegetables, pulses, and iron-rich foods, are essential.

Food Enrichment

Fortification of food, particularly wheat flour and baby foods with iron, is urgently needed in a number of countries. Other foodstuffs should be carefully selected for iron enrichment depending on their use and physiological absorption, according to the climatic conditions. It is, however, very important to implement programs designed to provide protein- and iron-enriched foods for infants and children for an effective prevention of protein malnutrition.

Iron Supplementation in Pregnancy

Iron needs of pregnant mothers are usually not met with the diets available in most developing countries, and iron deficiency is widespread in pregnant women. Detailed investigation of the optimum iron needs are urgently needed, but 60 mg daily of supplemental iron must be given during the second and third trimesters. The best long-term approach to the prevention of anemia in pregnancy is the fortification of the iron content of food.

Mass Treatment of Iron Deficiency in School Children

The WHO study group recommended that in this vulnerable group, the children must be screened by periodic surveys for parasitic infections and hemoglobin levels and treated with iron supplements, where needed. In most developing countries, a national screening program is worth undertaking.

Research

A coordinated research effort in nutritional anemia should be undertaken with a view to have a long-term control. The problems that need special attention are (1) prevalence of iron, folate, and vitamin B_{12} deficiency in infants and pre-school children; (2) absorption of food iron and the enrichment of iron content in food; (3) effects of cooking, processing, and storage on folates and vitamin B_{12} and their malabsorption in tropical climates; and (4) immunological diagnosis and prevention of parasitic diseases.

In the United States, where protein-calorie malnutrition is negligible compared to developing countries, iron deficiency is not very uncommon, particularly in the infants beyond six months of age, adolescent girls, and among women in their reproductive period.[51] The iron losses during menstruation among adult women are twice as much as in the adult male. These women have to eat more foods which not only contain significant amounts of iron but also from which the iron can be absorbed by the body. For example, iron in wheat can be poorly absorbed compared to iron in meat. Egg yolks, commonly considered as foods of high biological value, also impair the absorption of iron.[94] Inorganic iron is better utilized by the body, and fortification of commonly known foods, such as bread, will be ideal for prevention of iron deficiency or iron deficiency anemia. In the United States, however, the situation is somewhat complicated because of decreasing intake of total food, particularly bread, with increasing age, because of the fear of obesity.

> When the total caloric intake is low and approximately 40% of the calories are supplied as fat and 20–25% as sugar, there is little room in the diet for iron containing foods. Improved manufacturing methods, use of stainless and aluminum utensils and emphasis on cleanliness have lowered the total iron intake.[51]

BREAST FEEDING AND DEVELOPMENT OF WEANING FOODS

Breast Feeding

The incidence of kwashiorkor and to a great extent marasmus as well is most common between the ages of one and three. Kwashiorkor is also referred to as a disease of the weaning child because before the age of weaning, the child gets most of its nutritional requirements fulfilled from the mother's milk. Unfortunately there has been a steady decline in the practice of breast feeding the infant all over the world, and if this trend continues, the battle against the prevalent malnutrition will be much harder to win. There is increasing evidence that the trend of bottle feeding with cow's milk is increasing not only among the educated elite but also among the general populations in many tropical countries.[39]

As Jelliffe [39] put it

> The modern tendency to regard the female breast almost exclusively as a symbol of sex may also make her less inclined to 'risk losing her figure.' Also it must be admitted that many of the doctors and nurses in the United States of America and Europe appear to have little knowledge of the advantages of breast feeding and almost routinely start on artificial bottle feeds.

The first year of the infant is very critical from the point of view of mental development as well as physical growth. The importance of the latter can be imagined from the fact that a baby trebles its birth weight at the termination of the first year. In view of the great importance of satisfactory nutrition during the first year, it is quite disturbing that this ancient practice of breast feeding the baby is being discontinued in a number of areas where economic and industrial development of the region and public health facilities are inadequate to cope with problems that are associated with artificial feeding. In the United States, less than 20 percent of the infants are breast fed, but the artificial nursing facilities are so superb that no malnutrition among infants has been observed that could be directly attributed to lack of breast feeding, but this is not true of areas like Asia, Africa, and South America.

In these areas a rejection of breast feeding practice will lead to a disaster of unimaginable magnitude, and the battle against malnutrition will be lost.

Davies [23] believes that a steady decline in breast feeding practices and increasing sophistication of artificial feeding is due to emancipation of women. This may be the case in advanced countries of the West where methods of artificial feeding are quite adequate, but in developing countries, the main reason for the discontinuation of this practice is mainly the unthoughtful imitation of Western ways as well as a fashion and to some extent due to hard economic realities that women have to go to work in order to join the husband in earning a living wage for their families. In the developing countries, where the mothers are giving up the beneficial practice of breast feeding, the problems of artificial feeding are so immense that the child suffers unnecessarily, and there is an increasing incidence of nutritional marasmus and infective diarrheas due to the overdiluted and contaminated milk usually given to such unfortunate children who are deprived of the readily available and sterile milk in the mother's breasts. There are numerous problems associated with bottle feeding, particularly in the developing countries, and it is extremely difficult for an average mother to carry out bottle feeding successfully because of [39]

1. *Expense.* Milk is very expensive and not available in quantities needed to feed the babies alone, leaving aside children,

adults, and old people. In Uganda, for example, it will cost one third of daily wages of a laborer to feed one baby on milk bought from the market. Also it is extremely difficult to obtain milk that is uncontaminated.

2. *Hygiene.* In the developing countries, the dwelling places of most of the lower sections of the society are far from clean, and it is almost impossible in those places to prepare a sterile formula for feeding and storing it for the next use. Feeds are liable to be contaminated with dust or insects.

3. *Education.* Finally, the mothers in these areas are not educated enough even to understand and follow the instructions to mix different types of feeds necessary for artificial feeding. The results of this discontinuation of breast-feeding practice are most dissatisfactory and lead to a startling increase in number of semistarved, marasmic babies suffering from infective diarrhea.

The writer fully shares the views of Jelliffe and other prominent nutritionists that a vigorous campaign be made to restore the original status of breast feeding as a means of rearing the child during the first year of its life. The advantages of breast feeding are so many, and some of them may be mentioned here.

1. *Composition of human colostrum and milk.* Small amounts of colostrum are secreted in the first two or three days. It is yellowish and thicker than regular milk but is endowed with more protein, more fat, and definitely larger quantities of essential vitamins and minerals. Within a few days, it changes to bluish-white regular breast milk whose nutritional composition has been adapted for the growth of the human infant for thousands of years. The average amount of protein is 1 percent, carbohydrate 7 percent, and fat 4 percent, and it contains approximately 20 calories to the ounce.[26] The amount of vitamins in mother's milk varies with the mother's diet, but such deficiencies in the breast-fed infant have been rarely observed. The composition of human's and cow's milk are quite different, and although the latter can be humanized to a great extent and children thrive on it, the precise constituents of the breast milk cannot even be grossly mimicked biochemically.[39]

Breast milk is easily digested and in large part leaves the stomach in 1½ to three hours, depending on the quantity.[26] The mineral composition of breast milk is perfectly suited to the newborn kidney and has an important homeostatic effect during the first four weeks of life.[23]

2. *Sterility, easy availability, and economy.* The greatest advantage of breast feeding lies in its sterility and easy availability. The breast milk is not contaminated, and this is not only a great safety factor, but the child enjoys a greatly reduced risk of illnesses and infections. The breast milk contains antibodies against certain enteroviruses [39] and immunoglobulins present in human milk and inhibit viral and bacterial multiplication when they reach the gastrointestinal tract.[46] Evidence indicates that the incidence of colic diarrheas and constipation is less in breast-fed babies than in those fed on cow's milk.[26] Besides these advantages, the free availability and economy in the family's budget should be important considerations in not switching to artificial feeding.

3. *Emotional stability.* Not only is breast feeding adequate nutritionally, but closer physical contacts between the mother and the infant assist the development of certain emotional links. In India, breast suckling is not considered merely an ingestion of food but is an important link or continuity between the mother and the child. This may be particularly true of prematurely born babies, and if breast feeding is substituted by bottle, an inadequate and improper use of it may even result in interruption in brain growth during its most critical period of development.

Levin *et al.*[53] compared the babies fed on breast milk and cow's milk and found similar weight gains, serum protein levels, and incidences of infection. But when the advantages of breast feeding are considered in terms of less trouble in keeping the milk sterile, easy availability, and immunological properties, the breast feeding is the wisest thing to do. Ebbs [26] pointed out that in spite of similar growth patterns with human's and cow's milk, the differences in properties of essential amino acids and source of the vitamins must be considered while selecting the method of infant feeding. "Perhaps steady growth with continuous nutritional stability in the breast-fed infant may contribute more to the succeeding years of the life of the individual." [26] Osborn [67] reported larger numbers of coronary artery lesions in young adults who were bottle fed compared to those who were breast fed during the first months of their life, and Mellander *et al.*[57] showed lesser number of dental caries in the breast-fed babies. Sudden deaths referred to as "crib deaths" or "cot deaths" are more frequent among the bottle-fed compared to the breast-fed babies.

> Cow's milk protein may be absorbed from the gut during its increased permeability in the first days of life, and regurgitation and aspiration into the lungs of even a small amount of milk at a later date might cause a severe anaphylactic reaction leading to pulmonary oedema, and death in a sensitized infant.[23]

Weaning Foods

The duration of breast feeding varies from three months to two to three years, depending on the lactating ability of the mother and the economics of the family in affording supplementary foods. In some developing countries, where the practice of breast feeding is a tradition, it may be continued over a long period of time because it assures some supply of good quality milk. The quantity of breast milk gradually decreases after four to five months, and the nutritional demands of the infants gradually increase with the result that the child cannot be kept on breast milk alone and must be provided with weaning foods to satisfy his demands for proteins, calories, as well as vitamins and minerals. In the technologically developed countries of the West, a large variety of baby foods in ready-to-serve jars are available, and the average mother can gradually wean the child to bottle milk and these weaning foods. In the Eastern countries, where no organized industry for baby food that can supply the needs of the population exists, the children are weaned on homemade cereals. These starchy foods do not supply the child with adequate proteins as well as vitamins and minerals. This kind of food regimen, at a time when his nutritional demands are increasing due to the demands of growth, proves disastrous for the child, and he starts going down the hill. If breast feeding is completely abandoned due to either lactation failure or second pregnancy, the problem becomes all the more difficult. It is always hard to get sterile milk in a ready-to-serve form in some of those countries, and contaminated formulas lead to infective diarrheas. Ironically in most cases, the mothers in the traditional societies stop solid foods under the belief that the child may not be able to ingest them and gives a diluted gruel made from flour and water. This not only does not supply enough proteins but also not enough calories. The child's energy needs are not met, and he starts metabolizing the tissue proteins to provide for the basic energy levels. Kwashiorkor and marasmus, the basic nutritional states, are most often observed at the weaning age. This is further complicated by lack of essential vitamins, and a complicated etiology results.

Toddlers and preschool children are the most affected populations that suffer from undernutrition and malnutrition. Numerous studies indicate that kwashiorkor and marasmus are most common between the ages of one and three years. For an effective fight against malnutrition prevalent in this age group, a satisfactory supply of weaning foods is essential. In the planning of and production of such foods, the WHO protein malnutrition committee suggested that the final product must take into consideration the following factors: (1) the amino acid content of the individual ingredient and biological quality of protein in the final product; (2) possible presence of toxic factors; (3) desirability of using foods of local origin; and (4) its suitability for feeding the weaned infants in terms of promoting growth and general well-being. It is logical to encourage the use of animal proteins in the preparation of weaning foods but in view of the fact that there is a general scarcity of animal protein, particularly in overpopulated countries of the East, the desirability of using vegetable proteins has been generally advocated. In general, oil seeds and nuts, oil seed meals, and isolates, and legume seeds have been used in the preparation of weaning foods, and wherever possible, skim milk powder and fish flours have been used. Legumes and nuts are important sources of proteins and can be usefully utilized. Some of the important weaning foods produced in Asia, Africa, and South America may be mentioned.

TABLE V

SOME WEANING FOODS MANUFACTURED IN ASIA, AFRICA, AND SOUTH AMERICA

Name of Food	Ingredients	References
Bal Amul	Soybean and powdered milk	Subrahmanyan et al.[92]
	Vitamins and some amino acids	
Balanced	Cereal malt (37%)	Chandrasekhara et al.[19]
malt food	Low fat peanut flour (40%)	
	Roasted pulse (Bengal gram) flour (10%)	Subrahmanyan et al.[92]
	Skim milk powder (10%)	
	Added to it–essential vitamins and minerals	
Enriched	Low fat peanut flour (25%)	Subrahmanyan et al.[91]
macaroni	Wheat semolina (22.5%)	
(ringlets)	Casein (2.5%)	Subrahmanyan et al.[92]
	Tapioca flour (50%)	
	With appropriate amounts of thiamine, riboflavin, calcium pentothenate, vitamins A and D, and calcium carbonate	
Nutro	Wheat semolina (80%)	Subrahmanyan et al.[90]
macaroni	Low fat peanut flour (20%)	Subrahmanyan et al.[92]
	Fortified with vitamins and calcium	
Nutro	Peanut flour (25%-30%)	Subrahmanyan et al.[90]
biscuits	Wheat flour (35%-40%)	Subrahmanyan et al.[92]
	Sugar (18%)	
	Shortening (15%)	
	Salt (0.75%)	
	Calcium carbonate (0.5%)	
	Glucose (0.5%)	
	Thiamine, riboflavin, niacin, and vitamins A and D	
Indian	Peanut flour, ground	Subrahmanyan et al.[89]
multipurpose	Bengal gram flour	Altman and Ditmer [2]
food	Vitamin and mineral premix	
	Calcium phosphate, thiamine, riboflavin, vitamins A and D	
Bal Ahar,	Wheat flour, whole-grain	Scrimshaw and Parman [81]
formula 2A	Cottonseed flour	Altman and Ditmer [2]
	Bengal or red gram flour	
	Vitamins and minerals, calcium phosphate, iron, salt, thiamine, riboflavin, nicotinic acid, vitamin A palmitate	

TABLE V—Continued

Name of Food	Ingredients	References
Biscuit meal (Uganda)	Peanuts, whole, ground	Dean [25]
	Cornmeal	Altman and Ditmer [2]
	Milk, skim, dried	
	Cottonseed oil	
	Sucrose	
Pro Nutro	Cornmeal, whole-grain, white and yellow	Altman and Ditmer [2]
	Soybeans, dehulled	
	Peanuts, dehulled, shredded	
	Milk, skim, dried	
	Whey powder	
	Sugar	
	Malt-extract solids	
	Wheat germ	
	Fish protein concentrate	
	Torula yeast	
	Salt	
	Bone phosphate	
Incaparima, Formula 9	Corn whole, ground, cooked	Bressani and Elias [14]
	Sorghum flour, cooked	Behar and Bressani [7]
	Cottonseed flour	Altman and Ditmer [2]
	Torula yeast	
	l-Lysine hydrochloride	
	Calcium carbonate	
	Vitamin A	
Incaparina, Formula 14	Corn, whole, ground, cooked	Bressani and Elias [15]
	Soybean flour	Altman and Ditmer [2]
	Tortula yeast	
	DL-Methionine	
	Calcium phosphate and vitamin A	
Incaparina, Formula 15	Corn, whole, ground, cooked	Behar and Bressani [7]
	Cottonseed flour	Bressani *et al.*[16]
	Soybean flour	Altman and Ditmer [2]
	Torula yeast	
	l-Lysine hydrochloride	
	DL-Methionine	
	Calcium carbonate	
	Vitamin A	
Peanut milk	Peanut milk fortified calcium and vitamins	Subrahmanyan *et al.*[92]
Dried milk substitute	Soybeans (2 parts)	Autret and van Veen [6]
	Peanuts (1 part)	Shurpalekar *et al.*[84]
		Subrahmanyan *et al.*[92]

These foods have proven excellent substitutes for milk and animal proteins and promote comparable growths in children, but the problem of malnutrition among toddlers and preschool children is so big in magnitude that the development of these foods is only a beginning of the fight against malnutrition, affecting more than 300 million children in the world. Technology based on large-scale production, distribution, and marketing is essential to make these wonderful foods available in the remote rural areas of the developing countries, where the need for them is the greatest. A beginning in the long struggle against child malnutrition has been made. Let us hope we bring some light to the lives of those for whom a state of undernutrition and malnutrition has been a way of life for generations. Speaking of the situation in India, where 80 percent of the young children suffer from varying degrees of protein malnutrition, Dr. H. A. B. Parpia, Director of the Central Food Technological Research Institute, Mysore, declared that

> The protein malnutrition of India could be conquered if oil seed proteins were used more efficiently and were supplemented by grain legumes and amino acids to make up their deficiencies. Weaning food biscuits, ice cream, beverages and sweets can all be made cheaply from vegetable protein. If we were to avoid the possibilities of even greater famines than India has experienced in the past, these new and unconventional food products will have to be exploited, and as soon as possible.[88]

IMPROVED PRODUCTION OF LOCAL FOODS

Increasing the Production of Traditional Foods

As discussed in the preceding chapter on food habits, it is evident that people do not change their dietetic patterns easily even though they contribute heavily towards their undernutritional status. The most practical strategy under these circumstances is to increase the production of habitual foods. In view of the unchecked steadily growing human population, it is estimated that, "The supply of cereals and proteinous foods would have to be increased by 50 and 80% respectively by 1980, allowing only for a marginal improvement in nutritional standards."[18] Every effort should be made to increase the production and consumption of pulses and nuts which are richer in proteins as compared to cereals. Particular attention has to be paid to the use of oil seed proteins for humans, most of which at present are used for cattle feeding after extracting the oil. The irony of the situation is that most of the food increases must be made in countries where the per capita incomes and per acre yields are among the lowest in the world, and agricultural practices are more or less primitive. In the advanced developed countries, the food production has been at a much higher rate than the growth in population, and the reverse has been true of the poorer countries of the world with the result that the gap between the rich and poor nations has become wider, and never before has the emergency to improve upon the food situation in overpopulated poor countries been greater than it is today. There is enough scientific knowledge available if it is applied in the fields to produce more foods and applied in the homes to curtail the population growth. The main strategy in providing additional food consists of increased production of traditional cereals (e.g. rice, wheat, maize, sorghum, millet) with supplementation of common foods and development of new food products richer in required nutrients. This strategy may not work, however, if some of the fundamental problems that lead to chronic food shortages are not fully solved.[34] Some of them are

1. *Land reforms.* In most of the developing countries, lack of ownership of the land is a big hindrance in boosting farm production. The custom goes back to the medieval ages. The rich people used to buy lands and lease it to the peasants on either a contract basis or sharing half the produce. The farmer, after giving away half of the produce to the landlord, was never left with enough grain to feed his family. The rich landlords lived in the cities remote from their farms and never cared to improve the lands, and the farmer, being a tenant, had no incentive to put in any capital investment because he could be evicted any time and thereby lose all the investment. The developing countries are paying attention to land reforms and to the fact that the land should belong to the person who tills it. The rich landlords, residing in urban areas, have sufficient political influence, however, to hinder the implementation of any government-sponsored re-

forms. In those circumstances where the farmer finds himself helplessly exploited, he either suffers in silence or rises in revolt, and many revolutionary movements have arisen strengthening the hands of the communists who take up their cause. The Nexalite movement in India is a recent example of restlessness on the part of the farmers. In the writer's opinion, for any meaningful effort to increase the production of food, the land reforms must receive top priority. Also, land holding in most developing countries has been decreasing due to repeated fragmentation generation after generation among the many children of a farmer, and cooperative farming needs to be introduced where modern agriculture could be carried out on a scientific basis and to the advantage of all parties.

2. *Soil fertility and lack of irrigation water.* Land has been constantly used for centuries without any significant input except probably cow dung and is no longer as fertile. The dependence on rains and the lack of dependable amounts of irrigation water further complicate the situation. Heavy doses of fertilizers, nitrogen, and phosphates, and an assured supply of irrigation water are needed to enrich the soil to get better yields.

3. *Desert formation.* The pressure of population evident particularly in Asia where half the human population lives has resulted in excessive use of the land without adequate input. Overgrazing by cattle has also contributed to the destruction of water-retaining vegetation and has resulted in the formation of semi-arid and arid zones out of very fertile areas. Preventive measures need to be rigorously imposed by assuring a constant water supply and planting grasses and vegetation.

4. *Mechanized agriculture.* In lands where soil fertility has been depleted by constant use with an erratic supply of water, the traditional methods of agriculture, using ploughs by animals, will not improve the yields. The governments in the developing areas have to take the initiative and provide the necessary resources to the farmers to change this sad state of affairs. An industrial base for the production of agricultural machinery, fertilizers, insecticides, and pesticides is needed and, above all,

what is needed is an easy operating credit system for the farmer to make use of this technology on the farms.

5. *Research in plant breeding, elimination of pests and disease control.* Highly skilled breeding of plants in order to select the desired qualities of protein contents, yield, and resistance to diseases needs highly developed systems of agricultural research and the trained personnel to produce an army of second-generation scientists. Some developing countries have paid adequate attention to the formation of agricultural universities, stimulating team research activities and intensive breeding programs. Mexico and India have done very useful research in the last decade with the help of advanced countries, and these countries are helping others by spreading their knowledge in plant genetics, breeding, and disease control.

Crops with Better Protein Quality and Higher Yields

Increasing protein quality of cereal crops, which form 60 to 80 percent of the total food intake in many countries is an important feature of the campaign to eradicate human malnutrition. New varieties of cereal crops are coming up with emphasis on higher yields and better protein quality. Putting enough nitrogen in the soil is the quickest and easiest way of improving the protein content; for example, in India, the protein content of wheat has been raised from 9 to 10 percent to 16 to 17 percent. The other method of improving the nutritional value of the cereals is the use of gene mutations and selective breeding. The reader is referred to a nutritional symposium of the *Federation Proceedings of the American Society for Experimental Biology*, volume 25, 1966, for valuable contributions in this area. It has been shown conclusively that the protein composition of the endosperm of maize seeds can be changed considerably by one gene mutation (opaque 2), and additional mutation of another gene (floury 2) could enhance the protein composition still further.[59,61,64,65] Experimental feeding of animals showed that the mutant variety of maize promoted growth three times faster than the controls. The mutant hybrid varieties have been developed in almost all the cereal crops. Special mention, however, may be made of a hybrid between durum wheat (triticum) and rye (secalis) generally referred to as triticale. It is a new man-made cereal produced after lots of research work and contains 18% to 20% protein compared to 10% to 16% protein in wheat and also contains more of the limiting amino acid of wheat, i.e. lysine, an essential amino acid for good nutrition and growth. As a commercial crop, triticale has certain additional advantages over wheat because it resists dry weather and could prove an ideal high-protein crop in the semiarid areas of the world. Further research in triticale is going on, particularly in India, at a very urgent pace because of its potentialities.

During the last decade, crossbreeding and using heavy doses of fertilizers with adequate irrigation facilities have increased the yield of major cereal crops in a fantastic manner, so much so that the resulting increase in productivity has been referred to as "green revolution" in developing countries.

> As of mid–1968, both the food situation and food production prospects in Asia have changed almost beyond belief. The Philippines is self-sufficient in its staple food—rice—for the first time since 1903. Iran, with a substantial expansion in wheat acreage, is actually a net wheat exporter this year. Ceylon's rice harvest climbed 13% above the previous record, as it both expanded the area under cultivation and raised yields. Pakistan's wheat crop was estimated to be 30% above the previous record; India's total food grain crop was 32% above the previous year's drought-depressed crop, and 12% above the previous record.[17,66]

Streeter [88] submitted a report of the activities of the Rocke-feller Foundation in India during 1969 and discussed the numerous new varieties of major cereal crops developed in India and all over the world, which show yields 100 to 700 percent more than the conventional varieties, and the reader is referred to this monograph. To summarize, a few varieties may be mentioned here. In the production of new wheat varieties the genetic material was collected from all over the world. Some material contributed towards dwarfness in order to avoid falling down because of winds; other genetic material contributed towards high-yielding ability; some other traits gave the desirable color of the kernel, and some others provided rust resistance, good milling and baking qualities, or higher quantity of protein, and now a wheat variety called "Kalyan Sona" in India, "Mexipak" in Mexico and Pakistan occupies more cultivated area in Asia than any other. "Sonalika" is another important wheat variety of India whose yields are almost as much as Kalyan Sona but has a larger kernel and matures earlier and is considered important from the point of view of a farmer trying to raise more than one crop a year. "Chotti Larma," another variety, ripens its heads earlier than the stalks and can be raised regardless of the late season weather. In the evolvement of these different species, special attention is paid to their rust resistance. Rust kills millions of acres of wheat every year. With different varieties endowed with genetically different kinds of resistance the nation is helped as a whole, so that if one variety is under attack, the entire wheat crop does not suffer. A number of other varieties of wheat have proved highly effective in raising the yields per acre and percent content of protein (e.g. Sonora 63, Sonora 64, Mayo 64, Lerma Rojo 64A), raising the per-acre yield four times India's national average.

Rice is the staple food of about 1½ billion people and is probably the most important and most widely used cereal in the world. So far the success story of rice has not been so spectacular as that of wheat, but a number of new rice varieties have come up which have greatly raised the hopes of winning the battle against food shortages and prevalent malnutritional conditions existing in the developing countries of the world. A new variety "T (N)-1" is a short-stemmed sturdy dwarf, utilizing heavy doses of fertilizer and much higher yields. "Jaya" and "IR8" are two other varieties that have proved top-yielding crops in India. In both of them, however, the kernels are coarse and crack badly in hulling and milling and are not as fancy as "Padma" or "Basmati," which are somewhat low yielding but are very fancy.

Maize has undergone a revolutionary change, and breeders have produced many new varieties, ten in India alone, that yield 50 to 100 percent more than the conventional crops. Corn is somewhat deficient in lysine and tryptophan and efforts are being made to increase the lysine content and at the same time develop a variety that accepts larger amounts of fertilizer and resists falling over.

Brilliant experimental work has been done in a number of laboratories, particularly at Purdue University by Mertz, Nelson, and collaborators.[59,60,61,65] Nelson [64] showed that in terms of protein quality, the mutant maize proteins may be equivalent to the milk protein, and in the areas where maize is the staple diet, this could make a significant contribution in improving the diets of millions of people who are fighting desperately to eliminate the prevalent malnutrition in their midst. Sorghum and millet are other crops of great nutritional value for humans and farm animals on which sustained research efforts are needed to improve their nutritive value. Nelson believed that

> Since genes exist that change the amino acid pattern of maize in a desirable fashion, there is ample reason to believe that genes changing the amino acid pattern of other cereals exists and could be isolated, and if this strategy proves successful in all the vegetable crops, there may not be much room for despair.[64]

This kind of over-optimism about the future of the "green revolution" discussed here may prove extremely costly in terms of human sufferings if new problems arising from new technology are not taken care of at the right time. Wharton [66,101] struck a pessimistic note and believed that further spread of new varieties of cereal crops may not be as fast as earlier successes might suggest because of the following obstacles:

1. Most of the new varieties require irrigation and careful water control systems which require huge capital investments. The developing countries may not be able to afford this spending without substantial external assistance, which may or may not be available. For example, the Mekong River development requires approximately 2 billion dollars investment over the next two years in order to improve the agricultural economy of Southeast Asia.

2. A very efficient system of storage, transportation, and marketing the affluent quantity of new grains is required.

3. Large quantities for agricultural inputs, such as farm supplies, equipment, fertilizers, insecticides, and pesticides, are needed to be available at the right time, in the right quantities, and at the right places.

4. The new varieties require new skills on the part of the

farmers with respect to planting dates, depth of planting, fertilizer rates timings, and pesticides, which may be difficult to learn for the tradition-bound illiterate farmers of most developing countries.

5. Market fluctuations of prices in the time of surplus may prove a great disincentive for the farmer to produce more and put in larger capital investments in the land. For example, the International Rice Institute estimates that the average Filipino rice farmer requires about 20 dollars per hectare when traditional methods are used, but must invest approximately 220 dollars when the high-yield IR8 rice variety is grown. The new yield is three times greater, and the net return four times greater, but the farmer must have credit to finance the operation and an assurance of return. A means must be found to tap the money markets in the urban sector.

If the difficulties mentioned above are solved in time, the "green revolution" in the making may reach a "take-off" stage and become a potent force in eradicating prevalent malnutrition and undernutrition. But if it fails, the world may once again be faced with a desperate situation as was brought to light at the time of drought and near-famine conditions in India during the years 1965–66, but on a much larger scale.

Supplementation of Cereals and Common Foods

The cereals most widely consumed all over the world are deficient in only one or two amino acids which make their proteins biologically inferior to animal protein containing well-balanced amino acid ratio. The widespread and predominant use of cereals in the diets have resulted in varying degrees of undernutrition and malnutrition, and according to one estimate, more than 50 percent of the world population is undernourished.[36] In view of this and the rapidly increasing world population, one has to look hard to find sources to improve the nutritional standards of the human population which are not only practical but are also within the economic reach of most people or their governments. One logical answer is to supplement the habitually used cereals deficient in certain amino acids with synthetically produced ones.[36,52] During the recent times, the industrial production of certain amino acids at relatively low cost has made their utilization for supplementing vegetable sources of proteins a practical feasibility. By fermentation methods, amino acids can be prepared from low-grade materials which are not suitable for human consumption. Such a measure could be extremely useful not only in the prevention of kwashiorkor but also to improve the diets of the undernourished populations.[82] A South African group of nutritionists have made an important contribution by showing a definite improvement in kwashiorkor symptoms by the use of vitamin-free casein or a mixture of synthetic amino acids. In most cases not only a distinct improvement in anorexia, apathy, cutaneous lesions, and edema is observed, but the amino acid mixture provides a satisfactory "initiation of cure."

Laboratory investigations have shown that wheat proteins are improved by supplementation with lysine,[38] maize production by lysine, tryptophan, and threonine,[79] rice, ragi, sorghum and millet proteins by lysine and threonine.[52] Supplementation with these amino acids leads to a marked increase in nitrogen retention in children fed these cereals supplemented by appropriate amino acids.[34,74,97] Lysine, tryptophan, and isoleucine supplementation of maize diets, supplying children and adults with 0.5 to 1.0 gm protein/kg/day results in significant increase in retention of nitrogen in all the subjects.[97]

Supplementing oil seed proteins (with much higher protein content than the cereals) with the deficient amino acid is another method of providing additional high-quality protein to the human population. Supplementation of soybean protein with methionine raises its protein efficiency ratio (PER) to a level almost equal to that of milk proteins.[42] Howe *et al.*[36] showed that supplementation of lysine, threonine, and methionine, singly or in combination, raised the PER of oil seed proteins to the level of animal protein, casein. Similarly, supplementation of sesame with lysine,[44] peanut with lysine, methionine, tryptophan, and threonine,[96] cotton seed with lysine and methionine,[15] and of chick-pea proteins with methionine [78] will have the same effect.

It is, therefore, technically possible as well as desirable to

TABLE VI

EFFECT OF FORTIFICATION OF VEGETABLE PROTEIN FOODS WITH
DEFICIENT AMINO ACIDS ON THEIR NUTRITIVE VALUE

(Reproduced from Narayana Rao and Swaminathan, 1969)

Protein Food	Protein Efficiency Ratio [1]	Reference
Soya bean	2.4	Parthasarathy *et al.*[68]
Soya bean + DL-methionine (0.6%)	3.2	
Soya bean + MHA (0.6%)	3.2	
Sesame	1.7	Joseph *et al.*[44]
Sesame + L-lysine (2.4%)	2.9	
Peanut	1.6	Tasker *et al.*[96]
Peanut + L-lysine (2.2%) + DL-methionine (0.6%) + L-threonine (0.8%) + DL-tryptophan (0.2%)	3.2	
Wheat	1.2	Hutchinson *et al.*[38]
Wheat + L-lysine (0.4%)	2.4	
Rice	1.0	Pecora and Hundley [69]
Rice + DL-lysine (2%) + DL-threonine (1.2%)	2.0	
Maize	0.6	Sauberlich *et al.*[79]
Maize + DL-methionine (0.1%) + L-lysine (0.5%) + DL-tryptophan (0.1%)	2.2	

[1] Level of protein 10%.

supplement the cereals and oil seed protein with synthetically produced amino acids. Such a procedure will also cost much less than other foods which have the same quality protein content. It is, however, not possible to produce the oil seeds in such large quantities as compared to cereals, and more emphasis has to be put to improve the quality of cereal proteins.

> It must be recognized, in view of the rapidly expanding populations, that hundreds of millions must continue to subsist entirely on cereal grains. These people are almost certain to benefit from the judicious supplementation of these foods with lysine, lysine and tryptophan, or lysine and threonine. In addition, there is no other method at present by which the protein quality of the food of many of these undernourished people can be improved without a concurrent sacrifice of available energy-yielding food which hungry people can ill afford.[36]

Mixing fish flour in the traditional foods is another important procedure of supplementary fortification for traditional foods. In Mexico, a simple and practical method of incorporating fish flour into basic foods without changing traditional dietary habits has been very successful (for example, adding fish flour into breads, cookies, biscuits, or adding 10% fish flour in noodles used commonly in soups). In all these foods neither the flavor, the odor, nor the texture has been modified by the addition of fish flour.[18] If a resistance toward adding nutritious supplements arises from a small group with vested political interests, it may not be impractical to legally enforce enrichment of common foods.

NEW FOOD PRODUCTS

Need for New Foods

The human populations on this planet are not equitably distributed. The largest state in terms of area is Soviet Russia, which has a population of about 200 million people. Next door China is much smaller in size but has a population of approximately 800 million people. Next door India is about one third the area of the United States and has a population load of about 560 million people. Southeast Asia is all the more crowded. In these areas, a choice between augmenting the production of animal or vegetable sources of protein has to be tipped in favor of the latter simply because these overpopulated areas can't afford to concentrate on the large-scale production of animal protein, in spite of the fact that there is a general recognition of high biological value of proteins of milk, eggs, and poultry and meats. It is estimated that production of animal proteins needs three to six times more land compared to equivalent amount of vegetable proteins.[74] For example, grass can yield protein up to 600 lb/acre/annum, but these figures are reduced to 370, 269, 90, and 54 lb for the production of beans, wheat, milk, and meat, respectively.[87] The available acreage in the overpopulated developing countries can, therefore, be better utilized if the land is put to use for the production of vegetable sources of protein compared to animal protein. The situation in India is especially critical from this point of view. Unused land hardly exists, and arable land cannot be used to produce milk and animal protein to feed its ever-increasing population. Calculated in terms of world supplies, the animal proteins are grossly inadequate, and it is becoming evident day after day that feeding infants with conventional foods (animal milk and other dairy products) will become more difficult in the near future despite efforts to increase dairying and stock raising. It is important, therefore, to look for foods which are protein rich, palatable, digestible, and of good biological value.[41]

It is a recognized fact that undernutrition and malnutrition states are most prevalent in those areas of the world which predominantly use cereal foods deficient in one or two of the essential amino acids. It is also a well-recognized fact that nutritional deficiency states are caused not because of imbalance in protein quantity but because of protein quality.

Even with a diet of rice, the cereal with the lowest protein content, the protein intake approaches the recommended daily allowance of the FAO (1 gm/kg/day) which is higher than would be required if all the proteins in the food were of high biological value and much higher than the requirement suggested by the Food and Drug Administration.

Research efforts during the last 15 years in the development of new food products, based on different vegetable proteins, have revealed that new foods produced by a scientifically based combination of different amino acid patterns could be as efficient in promoting growth as the animal proteins, and their development has raised a new hope in our struggle in overcoming the prevalent malnutrition and undernutrition. A large number of scientists engaged in research in the development and evaluation of processed foods firmly believe that the scarcity of animal protein can only be overcome by substituting its need by new food products based on vegetable sources. For details, the reader is referred to a monograph *Processed Plants Protein Foodstuffs* [4] and some other articles by prominent workers.[15,22,74,75,92,93] At present these foods have been produced commercially on a small scale and have been found to be well accepted. In the writer's opinion, for a successful fight against malnutrition, a large-scale quality-controlled production of these foods is important, accompanied by a highly efficient storage, distribution, and marketing system so as to reach the people in remote rural areas where they are needed the most. Besides their availability, a vigorous educational campaign is needed which is based on visual proof of their ability to improve the health standard of the people. A successful battle against prevalent malnutrition can be waged only if these high-quality protein foods, supplemented with additional vitamins and minerals, are so widely accepted as to become a part of their daily diet.

Principles of Production and Composition of Important New Food Products

The most important sources of vegetable proteins produced in large quantities in the developing countries are the specially processed oil seeds, such as peanuts, soybeans, cotton seeds, sesame, and sunflower, legumes including beans of different varieties, and cereals, such as maize, wheat, millet, sorghum, and rice.[73] A chemical chromatographic or microbiological analysis of amino acids reveals that cereal proteins are deficient in lysine, whereas legume proteins contain adequate quantities of lysine but contain lesser amounts of methionine and tryptophan. The oil seed proteins are somewhat deficient in lysine, methionine, and threonine. None of these foods could become a complete food by itself, and the absence or deficiency of one essential nutrient in human food may jeopardize the biological utilization of others. If the cereals, beans, or oil seed proteins are mixed in quantities in proportion to their amino acid pattern, they compensate for each other's deficiency in amino acids, and the new food product will have as good a balanced ratio of essential amino acid as milk and will be as potent as milk in promoting growth or maintaining good health. With this basic principle and after thorough researches on the biological value of proteins from new food mixtures, a number of them have been formulated and trial studies on animals and humans completed. Some of the important food products and their ingredients have been given in Table VII.

The FAO/WHO expert committee on nutrition suggested

TABLE VII

LIST OF IMPORTANT NEW FOOD PRODUCTS [41,45]

Product	Country	Composition	Protein Content (%)
1. Inca-Parina 1.1	Guatemala	Maize, cotton seed flour, vitamin A, lysine, $CaCO_3$	27.5
1.2	Colombia	Same plus defatted soya flour	27.5
2. Fortifex	Brazil	Maize, defatter soya flour, vitamins A, B_1 and B_2, DL-methionine, $CaCO_3$	30.0
3. Pro-Nutro	South Africa	Maize, skim milk powder, peanut, soya, FPC, yeast, wheat germ, vitamins A, B_1 and B_2, niacin, sugar, iodized salt	22.0
4. Saridele	Indonesia	Extract of dry soya, sugar, $CaCO_3$, vitamins B_1, B_{12} and C	26.0–30.0
5. Protone	UK, Congo	Maize, skim milk powder, yeast, vitamins, minerals	24.40
6. Arlac	Nigeria	Peanut flour, skim milk salts, vitamins B_1, B_2, B_{12} and D	42.0
7. Indian MPF	India	Peanut flour, chick-pea flour, vitamins A, B_1 and B_2	40.0
8. Prolo	UK	Soya flour, DL-methionine, minerals, vitamins A, B_1, B_2 and PP	49.0
9. Alpine MPC	USA	Marine protein concentrate	80.0
10. FAP	Morocco	Fish protein concentrate (FPC)	80.0
11. Superamine	Algeria	Wheat, chick-peas, lentils, skim milk powder, sugar, vitamin D	20.0
12. SM	Ethiopia	Teff, peas, chick-peas, lentils, and skim milk powder	15.0
13. Bal Ahar	India	Mixed wheat flour, vegetables and defatted oil seed flour, vitamins, Ca	22.0–26.0
14. Lactone	India	Vegetable protein-toned milk, ground nut protein isolate, glucose, syrup, minerals, vitamins, water blended with buffalo milk	0.12
15. Aliment DE Sevrage	Senegal	Millet flour, peanut flour, skim milk powder, sugar, vitamins A and D; Ca	20.0
16. CSM	USA	Maize (precooked), defatted soya flour, skim milk powder, $CaCO_3$, vitamins	20.0
17. Supro	East Africa	Maize or barley flour, torula yeast, skim milk powder, salt, condiments	24.0

that in the planning of new food mixtures, the following criteria must be taken into consideration:

(1) the amino acid content of the individual ingredients and the final product; (2) the possible presence of toxic or interfering factors; (3) the need for obtaining exact specifications for each of the components; (4) the necessity of avoiding processes that may damage protein quality; (5) the desirability of using products of local origin; (6) the low cost and good-keeping quality of the products; (7) suitability of the product for feeding weaned infants; and (8) the acceptability of the product to the consumers. At the same time, the processed protein foods should possess high nutritive value and should have a significant supplementary value to the diets normally consumed by the people in the region. Although the primary objective should be to provide a supplementary source of protein of good quality, it is desirable that a vegetable protein food should also contain or be fortified with adequate quantities of vitamins and minerals that are likely to be lacking in the diets.[30,92]

The manufacturing processes should satisfy most of these criteria; for example, optimal heat processing eliminates partially or wholly the nonnutritional or toxic factors present in the vegetable proteins and improves its nutritional value.[54] Their suitability in weaning infants has been proven by numerous feeding experiments, and if made available in larger quantities at moderate prices, the consumers have shown a definite preference for them.

Special mention may be made here of the unique position of peanuts in an overpopulated country, like India, where prevalent undernutrition is of a great magnitude. India produces 40 percent of the world production of peanuts and properly utilized could provide significant quantities of good quality protein when it is incorporated at 20% level in the average poor vegetarian diets of India. Feeding trials on school children, given one oz of peanut flour besides their regular diets, have shown significant increases in height, weight, and hemoglobin content over control groups not receiving additional supplements.[50,63] In India, the common cereals, particularly wheat and maize and barley, are eaten in the form of flat-pan cakes, "chapatis" (unleavened bread). It is most convenient to mix peanut flour in the cereal flours. A number of mixed flours are available in India but not in quantities needed by the population. For example, mysore flour is a blend of 75:25 of tapioca flour and peanut flour. Paushtik flour is a blend of wheat flour, peanut flour, and tapioca flour in the ratio of 75:8:17. The essence of the problem is to provide 40 to 50 gm of protein from these protein mixtures which will adequately supplement the 10 to 15 gm of protein derived from the traditional foods.

Nutritive Value of New Food Products

The isolated protein from the vegetable sources are devoid of fibers and other interfering materials, such as odoriferous and bitter taste, trypsin inhibitor, phylates and are almost completely digested.[5] Having solved the problem of digestibility, attention is given to their growth-promoting patterns compared to egg proteins and milk proteins. A number of studies on the nutritive value of these products have been carried out and have shown that vegetable proteins of moderately high nutritive value can promote adequate growth when fed at somewhat higher levels.[74] As the world supply of animal protein gets scarce in view of the exploding human population, the economic significance of these foods becomes self-evident as well as logical. Studies on the regeneration of plasma proteins, as compared to milk proteins, indicate that the rate of regeneration is somewhat slower with vegetable protein mixtures in the early stages, but given sufficient time, return to normal values with vegetable proteins alone,[95] but when small quantities of skim milk powder are added to predominantly vegetable protein mixtures, the rate of regeneration of plasma albumin is distinctly improved. A 2:1 blend of peanut protein isolate and skim milk, in which the latter provides only 15 percent of the total protein, is as effective as skim milk powder itself in the regeneration of serum albumin in kwashiorkor children.[13] In feeding experiments with children, the Indian multipurpose food (a mixture of peanut flour and chick-pea flour with added vitamins and minerals) produces highly significant improvement in height, weight, RBC counts, hemoglobin, and nutritional status compared to the control group receiving regular vegetarian foods.[43] When this formula is supplemented with 20% skim milk powder, it results in a marked improvement in kwashiorkor patients within eight to ten days.[92]

Vegetable protein isolates have shown the property of homogeneous mixing with other traditional food products and, being bland in taste, they are not easily observed. As substitutues of milk and animal proteins, they have proven excellent in improving the general nutritional standards of the undernourished population, but when they are used along with milk or animal protein with a view to economizing or making the best of the available quantities, their nutritional value is all the more enhanced. A blend (1:1) of solubilized proteins and skim milk contains 60% to 61% protein and can be readily fortified with essential vitamins and minerals and prove effective as a medium of diet therapy for malnourished children and as a supplementary weaning food for the infants. The success of the new food products, however, depends on whether or not the people involved understand the necessity and significance of these foods and the marketing efficiency of their distribution. A United Nations' report [33] in 1968 adequately describes the conditions of the success of these new foods.

> The greatest obstacle to the commercial use of new protein foods is not so much in their production in a safe, nutritious palatable and sufficiently inexpensive form, but the requirements for effective marketing and promotion. Excellent products have remained laboratory curiosities because they were not presented to the public in a culturally acceptable manner or were not properly distributed in association with a well-designed educational and promotional campaign.[1]

Galliver [3] suggested that for food products to become successful, as a diet or a supplementary food among the masses, a manufacturer has to

> (1) develop products which are acceptable to the local population and which will fit into their existing or already changing eating habits; (2) ensure raw materials supply; (3) establish sound production methods and quality control; (4) establish a sensible price structure which results in a selling price which the consumer can afford and which offers a fair profit to the producer; and (5) bring the virtues of the product to the attention of the consumer, i.e., promote and advertise.

ROLE OF INTERNATIONAL AGENCIES IN THE FIGHT
AGAINST MALNUTRITION

Some international agencies recognize malnutrition as a public health problem of international importance and have devoted their energies and money to fight the menace in the best possible way. However, in those areas of the world where this battle has to be fought most devotedly, the geometrically growing populations without concomitant increases in food production are making things difficult. Any progress made in improving the nutritional status of the people is eaten away by the growing populations, and it is feared that unless the population growth is slowed down, the battle against prevalent malnutrition may be so long drawn out that it may be as good as lost. One of the greatest achievements of the international agencies in this area is that they have made the world aware of the magnitude of the problem and have aroused the active interest of the governments and social organizations of many developing countries to control their population and at the same time combat the menace of prevalent malnutrition. Great attention has been given during the recent years by most of the developing countries in health planning and nutritional programs as part of their overall plans for social and economic development. The work of the following international agencies has greatly contributed to improving the nutritional standards of millions of people all over the world and may be briefly mentioned here. The foremost among them is the World Health Organization (WHO) of the United Nations.

World Health Organization

The nutrition activities of the WHO have been detailed by Dr. Bengoa,[12] the chief of the nutrition unit of the World Health Organization. The WHO is principally involved in the evaluation of protein-calorie malnutrition (PCM) in young children, relationship between PCM and infection, development and testing of new protein-rich foods, nutritional anemias, vitamin A deficiency, endemic goiter, rickets, assessment of nutritional status, nutritional requirements, nutrition activities in health services, coordinated applied nutrition programs and training of personnel. Out of all of these, protein-calorie malnutrition has always been the most serious problem and has been given the rightful place in its programs by WHO. In its severe form the prevalence of PCM varies from 1 to 9 percent, whereas the moderate form may be as common as 10 to 50 percent in the children of the one-to-five-year-age group all over the world.

The WHO has tried to attack the problem from four angles:

1. Early treatment of protein-calorie malnutrition (PCM) by public health measures and by encouraging the establishment of nutritional rehabilitation centers with the help of local governments and agencies or with the support of private foundations.

2. Prevention of PCM in the vulnerable groups of the population by tackling the problem of periodic surveillance of the population at risk and providing adequate dietary protein to this group, identification of socio, cultural, and economic factors influencing the diets of vulnerable groups, by promoting breast feeding practices and by discouraging early weaning. During the last few years WHO has employed more than 150 nutrition experts to advise the various governments in their control and prevention programs.

3. Fight against malnutrition is led by WHO in cooperation with other agencies of the United Nations, such as FAO, UNICEF and ILO, by giving technical assistance to the governments in the elaboration of their national food policies; improved utilization of the available food by improved handling, storage, processing, and marketing methods; increased production of conventional protein foods and improvement of its protein quality by genetic selection; and encouraging the development of vegetable protein mixtures based on locally produced cereals and legumes. WHO has the responsibility of testing these foods for safety and suitability for human consumption. WHO also plays a major role in supplementary feeding programs.

4. Nutrition education programs by encouraging not only the teaching of nutrition in the medical schools but creating a paramedical team of people who are especially trained in nutrition at different ages, climatic conditions and nutrition pat-

terns around the world; nutrition education through demonstration of child-feeding practices to the mothers. The most important function of WHO in the area of education lies in the training of local personnel in collaboration with FAO and UNICEF. Great emphasis has been given to the training of dietitians and public health nutritionists, and on numerous occasions WHO has provided experts to countries to train the technical staff and has also provided equipment and fellowships for training abroad. The Institute of Central America and Panama is a noteworthy example of WHO collaboration with the member states. This institute has not only served the six member states but has made extremely valuable contribution in the area of nutrition research that have proved useful in other parts of the world as well. WHO also sponsored seminars in different parts of the world, e.g. one on weaning foods was held in Addis Ababa, Ethiopia, in 1969.

Besides protein-calorie malnutrition, WHO is actively engaged in other areas of health which are a direct or indirect sequela of faulty diets, such as control of infections that precipitate malnutrition, avitaminosis A, nutritional anemias, endemic goiter, and so on.

Food and Agriculture Organization

The motto of the FAO is providing enough bread for everybody. As mentioned earlier, the FAO and WHO have cooperated in many areas in the fight against prevalent malnutrition. A cooperative world food program in 1962 between FAO and WHO was meant to relieve malnutrition in the developing countries by the use of the surplus foods and encouraging at the same time their social and economic progress. FAO has a joint committee on nutrition with WHO, UNICEF, and UNESCO. This joint approach is aimed at helping all the needy countries of the world in providing more and better food. FAO in 1960 launched a vigorous campaign in its fight against the prevalent malnutrition and hunger and is popularly referred to as the Freedom from Hunger Campaign (FFHC). Most of the countries have their committees of FFHC and function with great dynamism with the help of government and nongovernment agencies, industrial and business concerns, religious and private foundations, in order to free mankind from hunger, undernutrition, and malnutrition. The main purposes of the FFHC are similar to those of the FAO but are orientated towards practical implications of certain techniques that help add to the quantity and quality of the existing food resources. The FAO is also concerned with gathering technical and economic information about food and agriculture and advises governments all over the world in the improvement of their plans in these areas. Under those general guidelines the FAO and the FFHC try to develop local roots among the people who provide food; these organizations also seek to train men in new methods of modern agriculture and women in the appropriate use of available foods and ways and means of feeding their families better food. The FFHC seeks cooperation and participation of the people in its efforts to demonstrate higher productivity of agricultural crops by sagacious use of fertilizers, better quality seeds, improved methods of soil conservation, and irrigation. FFHC also teaches the farmers about the better breeds of farm animals, raising poultry, fishing, and other profitable occupations by providing them with trained people as well as materials and tools. Through the FFHC the FAO tries to reach the farmer who ultimately has to fulfill the goals of the FAO by providing enough food for everybody. Providing teachers and trained personnel is considered the most important function of the FAO. In 1964 the Director General of the FAO, Dr. Sen, extended its scope by organizing a movement involving the young people of the world in the economic and social development of their respective regions. The idea is to provide a trained generation of young people who will not only supply adequate food for everybody, but who will also provide a liberal broad basic leadership in the future. This movement, generally referred to as the Young World Appeal (YWA), has since its inception attracted large numbers of young people and has proved a dynamic organization, where the young generation feels involved in the affairs of not only their own countries but in other less fortunate ones as well. The YWA brings out the idealism in the young generation. It has assisted in a number of very useful projects in a number of developing countries and has contributed with skill, time, and money. To quote a few examples: the YWA has assisted in projects like modernization of fishing boats in Madagascar, development of dairy farms in Kerala, India, and poultry projects in South India. One of the greatest handicaps of any movement to end poverty and hunger from the world is an acute shortage of trained and motivated workers and technicians. From this point the enrollment of the young people can prove a great asset. A special project, as a part of the Young World Appeal, is a project that goes under the name of Young World Food and Development (YWFD). It is aimed at aiding certain economic, agricultural, and educational programs in the developing countries with a view to fire the young people with a missionary zeal to participate in programs designed to develop leadership skills, literacy, interest in science, and education as well as develop in them a spirit of self-help.

United Nations International Children Emergency Fund

The UNICEF is a major international agency that recognizes the needs of children all over the world and is completely devoted to alleviating their sufferings. About a billion children in the world today are ill-fed, ill-clothed, suffer sickness, infections, and privation compared to a few hundred million in the prosperous West who get the nutrition they require, the protection they require, and above all, the emotional stability they require. In 1963 the combined income of about 120 developing countries, which comprise about three quarters of the world population, was one fifth of the more developed nations. In such economic circumstances, the most vulnerable groups are the children, and their needs are generally neglected due to a lack of proper appreciation of them. The protein requirements of children are higher than they will be in any subsequent period in their life, and yet in a number of regions, the adults have a precedence over the available food of the family and the children get the left-over food. UNICEF has played an important role in focussing the attention of the world to the needs of children. UNICEF's activities cover the many direct and indirect needs of children.

In meeting the direct needs, UNICEF aids the local agencies (government and private) in developing networks of health services for the mothers and children. The aid may be in the form of specialists, equipment, or medicines. Eradication of certain diseases like malaria, tuberculosis, and trachomas is the major goal of the health service, besides taking care of common infections. General social life of the children and the mothers is an extension of health services of UNICEF because the healthy environments are important for healthy growth of a child. UNICEF has helped in a number of countries, opening social clubs, child welfare clinics and children's institutions. In meeting the needs of the children indirectly, UNICEF has been committed to educational and vocational training of personnel, such as scientists, teachers, doctors, nurses, midwives, and social workers. The success of the whole program depends on the training and motivation of these people. The scientists have been aided by UNICEF in developing high-protein mixtures from locally available foods, such as children's foods developed from cereals or legumes (see Weaning Foods). The UNICEF-aided teachers stimulate education and scientific ideas in areas where superstitions dominate in matters of health, food habits, and food needs and the feeding practice of children and bring to proper focus the needs of growing children. UNICEF also aids the training of local people in the field of nutrition education by providing experts from the outside. The nutritionists and social workers encourage the local efforts to mobilize the local resources in order to provide for their children supplementary feeding programs comprising of milk or other protein-rich foods.

Besides these efforts at improving the lot of children all over the world, UNICEF has done excellent work in the area of providing emergency relief to victims of natural disasters, such as floods and earthquakes. Mention must be made of the dedicated efforts of Maurice Pate, the Executive Director of UNICEF since its founding in 1946 until his death on January 19, 1965. Mr. Pate's persistent efforts and programs of practical action in improving the lot of children made UNICEF a unique organization, serving the needs of children in 118 countries. The 1965 Nobel Prize for Peace to UNICEF was a posthumous tribute to Pate, and as Secretary General of the United Nations, U Thant said, "The credit for UNICEF's unique achievements belong to Maurice Pate as he was truly a great humanitarian."

The United Nations' international agencies, operating with the aid of governments all over the world, private organizations, and help from individuals, have created great hope for the future of mankind. Today, more than ever before, hunger is not a threat to the existence of the human species, in spite of exploding human population. A feeling of despair has already been transformed into one of hope. Some private and semigovernment organizations have also played an important part in dispelling hunger, undernutrition, and malnutrition. Notable among these are the Ford and Rockefeller Foundations, Peace Corps, AID, and Food for Peace Programs and Pan American Health Organization.

Private Foundations

The private foundations concerned with waging a war against undernutrition and malnutrition are many, but the Ford Foundation and Rockefeller Foundation are preeminent among them. Ford Foundation has provided millions of dollars worth of help every year in improving the standards of public health, rural development, and agricultural industries, the lack of which contribute to ill health and poor nutrition. A single most spectacular achievement is the establishment of the International Rice Research Institute in the Philippines. The Ford Foundation has contributed towards lands, buildings, and equipment, and the Rockefeller Foundation has picked up the operational costs. This institute has made significant contributions to the development of new varieties of rice which have more than doubled its production in South and Southeast Asia. IR8 is the miracle rice developed by this center, and work is continuing on the evolvement of other varieties of rice that respond to heavy doses of fertilizer, giving more than two crops a year with a high yield. This research effort, when applied in the fields, will go a long way in creating an abundance of food in those areas which, during the last few decades, have always faced chronic deficits.

The work of the Rockefeller Foundation in helping Mexico, India, Pakistan, and some other countries in the development of high-yielding wheat varieties needs to be recognized as a big leap forward in the main struggle against food shortages and hunger. India, with a population of more than 560 million people today, is self-sufficient in food because of the evolvement of these tough high-yielding varieties, and the generous help provided by these private foundations has to be appreciated. The main aim of these foundations is to help train the local scientists and local field workers and help them take over the local food and agricultural programs because the creation of well-trained indigenous teams is the sure means of ensuring long-term changes.

Other Agencies

Pan American Health Organization (PAHO) is in a sense the regional office of WHO, and established in 1948, this is one of the oldest international health centers. The PAHO has its headquarters in Washington, D. C., and provides advisory services to a number of South American countries in planning and execution of local health programs as well as assisting the training of scientists and field workers in carrying out the details of those programs. The PAHO has created zone offices in all the areas and coordinates their efforts in promoting the production of more food and better nutrition in those areas. The PAHO has done excellent work, and slowly and steadily these areas are moving towards more and better food for everybody.

The establishment of the Institute of Nutrition for Central America and Panama in 1949 is a great achievement in the area of nutrition to carry out the research, training, field work, and advisory details to the six member governments in the area. Highly enlarged in its mission since its inception, this institute has become the Mecca of highly sophisticated nutrition research and has provided a great stimulus in other countries as well by training the visiting scientists from all over the world. The production of high-protein vegetable mixture, incaprina, and its acceptance by the masses is indeed a great landmark in this area's fight against prevalent undernutrition and malnutrition.

Agency for International Development (AID) as an agency of the U. S. Department of State and the Peace Corps, initiated by John F. Kennedy in 1961, and CARE, an agency for person-to-person international aid, are three other agencies which have put up a remarkable effort in solving the food, agricultural, health, and nutrition problems of the developing countries. Whereas AID is a U. S. Government-regulated agency to provide help to the developing countries in the formulation and execution of their agricultural programs, thereby ensuring maximum output of agricultural commodities, the Peace Corp Program has a unique distinction in that Americans go out to share their expertise on a voluntary basis, thereby ensuring better human relations in the process of rendering help. Not only do the Peace Corps volunteers render valuable help to the developing countries in their struggle to raise their standard of living, but by living among them, they develop understanding and friendship that may prove vital in promoting world peace in the future. In the past ten years, more than 25,000 volunteers have served abroad, 50 percent engaged in teaching, 27 percent in rural and urban community development, health, agriculture, and public works. It is the writer's hope that all developed countries will send their best talent on a voluntary basis to the developing areas of the world and not only give them the help they badly need but also gain an understanding of their problems and their struggle to live decently with assured minimum basic needs. Such interchange of international personnel would promote friendships between countries that politicians often successfully mess up and assure a future world that has less hostility and less tension, and there are no hungry people going to sleep.

FIGHT AGAINST MALNUTRITION IN THE UNITED STATES

The United States is the richest country in the world with the highest per capita agricultural production. It is hard for anybody outside this country, much less in the developing countries, which are the recipients of American farm surpluses, to imagine that there are some people in the United States who are undernourished or malnourished. A recent estimate puts at 29 million the number of poor people in the United States who cannot afford to buy adequate quantities of food for their families.[56] For a detailed description of hunger in the United States and what the government is doing to eradicate the problem, the reader is referred to an excellent presentation by Nick Kotz, *Let Them Eat Promises, the Politics of Hunger in America.*[49] A very sketchy outline of this problem is being presented here. The well-fed people in this country seem to have the common misunderstanding: how can anybody be undernourished or malnourished in this affluent society? The so-called poor must be wasting their money on coke, potato chips, and beer. Their undernutrition or malnutrition must, therefore, be because of ignorance, and there is nothing anybody could do about it. In the congressional hearings in 1969, the liberal politicians blamed hunger on lack of money, while the conservatives dismissed malnutrition as a problem exclusively of ignorance. Most nutritionists called as witnesses agreed, however, that both money and education contribute to the problem of the hungry poor.[49] It is clear that few people who live outside the environment of the poor can grasp the full meaning or the ramifications of a life of poverty and ignorance, and a survey of the hospitals can easily show that respiratory and gastrointestinal illnesses are the habitual illness of the poor because there is a synergism between malnutrition and infection.[77] Some of the measures of the U. S. Government to fight prevalent malnutrition and undernutrition may be briefly mentioned here.

1. *Commodity Distribution Program.* Initiated 30 years back to provide food assistance to poor families, the grocery articles (dairy, meats, and cereals) were donated to the poor under the assumption that such a help would save some of their money and help them to purchase other items of food that they liked.

2. *National School Lunch Act.* Enacted by Congress in 1946, nutritionally balanced foods have been given to the school children

in their lunch program. Such programs were designed to give, during the lunch, a diet that would enable the child to grow adequately, even if his home diet were poor, and included articles like half a pint of milk, meat, vegetables or fruits and enriched bread with butter or margarine.[31] The lunches were provided free or at reduced prices to those children who could not pay. In 1968, the Act was revised to include the nonprofit institutions which provide nursery or day care for the children of families in low-income groups.[48]

3. *Food Stamp Program.* It was designed to provide bonus food stamps to low-income families in order to help them buy larger quantities of foods on a limited income. It was started in 1961 by President Kennedy in order to help the needy and make more effective use of this country's productivity [32] and was enacted as a Food Stamp Act in 1964 by the Congress. As an example of how the Food Stamp Program has worked, a four-member family in 1969 in any of the Southern states received $56.00 worth of bonus food stamps if the monthly income of that family ranged from zero to $29.99. The amount of bonus stamps was reduced to less than half (i.e. $26.00) if the family income ranged from $110.00 to $129.99 per month and to $18.00 for a family earning $340.00 to $369.99 per month.[49]

Mayer [50] has greatly criticized the food program of the U. S. Government on the grounds that it has failed to meet the requirements of the needy and, therefore, does not fulfill the aim it was intended to achieve. There are approximately 300 very poor counties that do not have any program because the local authorities did not care to ask the U. S. Department of Agriculture, and in some counties where some programs to help the needy exist, they are discontinued at the harvest time in order to ensure abundant labor at subsistence wages. In some other counties, the commodities do not reach the majority of the poor because of numerous local problems. According to Mayer, only 5.4 million out of 29 million participate in government-sponsored food programs, and not more than one third of the poor children attend the public schools participating in the lunch programs. In numerous places, despite the provision of the law to serve lunch free to poor children, they have to pay the full price for the school lunch or go without it. Even with the best of intentions, participation in the food assistance is dropping with the result that malnutrition among the poor in this country has risen sharply during the last ten years.[56] In 1967, 8.8 million families containing about 30 million persons were listed among the very poor, and only 18 percent of them were covered by the food programs, and out of 6 million school-age children of these families only 2 million received free lunches.

The recent changes made by the U. S. Secretary of Agriculture are expected to improve the situation significantly.

> The first reform is a uniform requirement that every county with a Food Stamp Program in effect must provide every participating family with enough food stamps to enable the family to pay for what the Agriculture Department considers to be a minimum-economy diet for that size family. For a family of four this amount is $106 a month, with corresponding amounts for larger or smaller families. The second change sharply reduced the amount of cash a family must put up to purchase the stamps. For example, previously a family with an income of $150 to $170 a month had to put up $60 to get $88 worth of stamps. But under the revision it now must put up only $42 for the new amount of $106.[37,77]

This revision of the food assistance program is well intentioned and is likely to help the poor to a great extent, but there are still 293 counties and cities which do not run any federal food program, and there are still 3 to 10 million hungry people who are not covered by these programs.[77] President Nixon aptly said in 1969 about hunger and its management that, "Something very like the honor of American democracy is at issue." Kotz [49] has quoted Albert Camus as saying that, "Perhaps we cannot prevent this from being a world in which children are tortured, but we can reduce the number of tortured children. If we do not do this, who will do this?"

UNITED NATIONS' RECOMMENDATIONS FOR CLOSING THE WORLD PROTEIN GAP

(Reproduced from Jelliffe, 1968) [41]

In a report to the United Nations Economic and Social Council, the Advisory Committee on the Application of Science and Technology to Development recommended in 1968 that the following general policy objectives be adopted for closing the world gap:

Protein from Conventional Sources

1. Promotion of increased quantity and quality of conventional plant and animal protein sources suitable for direct human consumption.

2. Improvement in the efficiency and scope of both marine and freshwater fisheries operations.

3. Prevention of unnecessary loses of proteinaceous foods in field, storage, transport, and home.

New Sources of Protein

1. Increase in the direct use of oil-seeds and oilseed protein concentrates by human populations.

2. Promotion of the production and use of fish-protein concentrates.

3. Increase in the production and use of synthetic amino acids to improve the quality of protein in cereals and other vegetable sources, and the development of the use of other synthetic nutrients.

4. Promotion of the development of single-cell protein for both animal feeding and direct utilization by man.

To achieve these objectives, the Committee recommended implementation of the following specific proposals:

1. Increase protein production from conventional plant and livestock sources.

2. Increase protein production from marine and freshwater fisheries sources.

3. Reduce waste of foods contributing to protein supplies.

4. Accelerate the development and growing of genetically improved plants of high protein value and improved agronomic characteristics.

5. Expand the use of oil-seed meals as direct sources of protein in human diets.

6. Support the production and marketing of acceptable fish-

protein concentrates (FPC) for human consumption in developing countries with substantial marine resources.

7. Greatly intensify research on single-cell protein sources.

8. Support the use of synthetic amino acids or protein concentrates to improve the nutritive value of cereal and other plant proteins.

9. Support the promotion and distribution of suitable protein foods in developing countries.

10. Develop and support regional and national centers for research and training in agricultural technology, food science, food technology, and nutrition.

11. Assist centers for the animal and clinical testing of new protein foods for developing countries.

12. Support training of personnel in the fields of marketing (including distribution and promotion), market research (including socio-cultural surveys of consumers), and systems analysis to assist in the marketing and promotion of new protein foods.

13. Expand the number of fellowships for training in nutrition, food science and food technology, and other fields important to the production and consumption of protein foods.

Governments should review and improve their policies and their legislation and regulations regarding all aspects of food and protein production, processing and marketing so as to remove unnecessary obstacles and encourage appropriate activities.

CONCLUSIONS

The future of man's fight against prevalent malnutrition depends mainly on our determination to fight with all the resources at our command and consists mostly of (1) removing ignorance; (2) augmenting food supplies of both energy-yielding and high-quality proteinaceous foods, with special emphasis on the latter; and (3) controlling the exploding human population. An unchecked growth in population will not only increase our task and responsibility but also could weaken our determination. Overawed by the magnitude of the problems in taking care of the existing population, we could tend to get demoralized and be tempted to give up if the rate at which new babies arrive is not diminished. As discussed earlier in a number of places, increasing evidence from research accumulates that malnutrition has a retarding effect on mental development, and these children show lower I.Q. scores as compared to controls belonging to the same chronological age and ethnic group not affected by malnutrition. After adequate rehabilitation of the malnourished, the difference in the development of the adaptive motor and language and personal social behavior tends to decrease.[20,21,28] In view of such findings, we have to watch any lag in our determination to fight the menace of malnutrition because it could have disastrous consequences for the human species on this planet.

Although poverty plays a significant role in faulty dietary patterns, the ignorance about foods and body needs appears to be among the more important causes for the prevailing undernutrition and malnutrition. This is particularly true in cases like Ceylon, an island surrounded by oceans with valuable quantities of fish, where infants and young children are not given fish under the belief that it causes malutrition. Much benefit could result from the existing food resources if people develop an intelligent understanding of the role of foods and modify their cultural or social beliefs and attitudes. Proper education could not only improve the dietary intakes but also can reveal the importance of proper hygiene, wrong notions about diseases, and the necessity to deal with them in the right manner. Without education, the people are not likely to respond to programs necessary for promoting better food intake or healthy food habits.

Augmenting food supplies in the already-overpopulated areas of the world is not a simple matter. One may summarize some of the steps in this struggle which will certainly shed some light on the complexity of the problem.

Mass Psychology

A mass psychology, which could convince individuals of the advantages of better health, has to be created by demonstrating its practical advantages. In a number of cultures a small-sized family with low total food intake and moderate amount of energy expenditure is so much an accepted fact of life that they consider it sufficient and don't feel the need for improvement. A practical demonstration of the direct relationship between diet and productivity or higher earnings is essential. For example, an improvement in caloric intake has been shown to improve the work output in road building, industry or agriculture, thereby increasing the earnings of the individual concerned. The reader is referred to a FAO monograph on nutrition and working efficiency.[29]

Increasing the Production of Habitual Foods

This will involve a whole set of changes in economy, agriculture, and industry. An industrial infrastructure is needed to develop the insecticides and pesticides to save 20 to 30 percent of all the food grains which, at present, are destroyed. The industry also must supply the fertilizers, phosphates, and nitrogen as well as farm machinery, and at the same time it must undertake the manufacture of certain amino acids that are deficient in traditional cereal crops to enrich these foods and balance their amino acid content. Traditional methods of agriculture have to be changed. This will involve improving irrigation facilities, supplying good-quality seeds through an organized seed industry and, above all, educating the farmers in new agriculture in addition to presenting them with the right incentive to adopt the changes with enthusiasm.

Development of Food Industry

A highly developed and sophisticated food industry should manufacture new food products (weaning foods and supplementary foods) from locally produced traditional foods. These foods should not be different from the local foods so as to give the semblance of interference in food habits or food practices and they should also contain all the nutrients (carbohydrate, fats, proteins, minerals, and vitamins) in a balanced form. Besides production, the food industry also has the responsibility of efficient marketing and promoting their products.

Development of Animal Sources of Protein

Most developing countries badly lack the animal source of

protein. Dairy, poultry, and livestock are the important conventional sources. Besides these, stress has to be laid on the development of resources from the oceans. Seafoods, provided they are economically and efficiently exploited, could go a long way in alleviating the present protein deficiency.

Government Action

Action on the part of the local governments is essential, not only to get the above-mentioned measures going but also in the context of subsidizing the production of nutritive foods and distribution to the needy, establishment of nutritional rehabilitation centers and public health facilities, and above all, the government funds are needed to establish agricultural universities where vigorous research in plant breeding, plant protection and pathology, development of new varieties of disease-resistant plants with higher yields and protein quality could be pursued. In the long run, it is the new research, transplanted from the laboratory to the fields, that is going to improve the quantity and quality of foods of billions of human beings.

It is evident from the outline of measures needed for augmenting the food production that to put these into practice will require a huge investment in money, materials, and trained men which most poor countries can ill-afford at their present level of resources. Accompanied by such shortages, if the population growth remains unchecked, the situation could be compounded further. In order that the lot of the living can be improved, some effective methods to slow down the arrival of new babies is extremely important. Population control at the national or international level and family planning at the individual level are essential elements in any successful fight against prevalent malnutrition. Coercive methods may be needed to convince or force the individuals who do not care to worry about figures of national population. Certain incentives, which could induce them to control the number of members of their families, are also essential.

The public health facilities in most developing countries are so meager because of their poor resources that most deaths, classified as due to gastroenteritis, measles, and several other conditions, are actually due to malnutritional states.[66] The rate of infant or child mortality is in general quite high, and under these conditions, where the risk of losing children is high, very few families will take chances of being left with one or no survivors by having the "ideal" number of two children. A campaign of family planning, therefore, must accompany improvements in public health standards so as to convince them of their most likely survival. In most developing countries, extra children are the only life insurance they have. If this attitude is corrected by instituting old age pensions or life insurance, more people could be convinced in having smaller families. As the trend goes, the average citizen is not adequately convinced about the value of a smaller family with the result that in many developing countries almost half the population consists of children. The population growth is likely to stay at a higher level, even if the children of today practice some kind of family-planning methods in their adult life, thereby making the struggle against prevalent undernutrition and malnutrition a very difficult one.

REFERENCES

1. Allen, D. M. and Dean, R. F. A.: *Trans. R. Soc. Trop. Med. Hyg., 59:* 326 (1965).
2. Altman, P. L. and Dittmer, D. S. (Eds.) : *Metabolism,* Federation of American Societies for Experimental Biology, Wisconsin Ave., Washington, D.C. (1968).
3. Altmann, A. and Murray, J. F.: *S. Afr. J. Med. Sci., 13:*91 (1948).
4. Altschul, A. M. (Ed.) : In *Processed Plant Protein Food Stuffs.* New York, Academic Press (1958).
5. Anantharaman, K., Subramania, N., Gopalan, K., and Bhetia, D. S.: In *Proceedings of Symposium on Proteins.* Central Food Technological Research Institute, Mysore, India (1961).
6. Autret, M. and Van Veen, A. G.: *Am. J. Clin. Nutr. 3:*234–243 (1955).
7. Behar, M. and Bressani, R.: *Natl. Acad. Sci. Natl. Res. Council Publ., 1282:*213 (1966).
8. Bengoa, J. M.: In *Nutrition et Alimentation Tropicales Recucil de Conferences du Cours de Formation de Nutritionistes en Afrique an Sud du Sahara organise Par le FAO.* 1 OMS et le Gouvernement Fran cais Marseille (1955).
9. Bengoa, J. M.: *J. Trop. Pediatr., 10:*63 (1964).

10. Bengoa, J. M.: In *Proceedings of the Western Hemisphere Nutrition Congress.* Chicago, (1965), p. 36.

11. Bengoa, J. M.: *J. Trop. Pediatr., 12:*169–176 (1967).

12. Bengoa, J. M.: *J. Am. Diet. Assoc., 55:*228–32 (1969).

13. Bhagavan, R. K., Doraisuvanj, J. R., Subramanian, N., *et al.: Am. J. Clin. Nutr., 11:*127–133 (1962).

14. Bressaini, R. and Elias, L. G.: *Arch. Venezolanos Nutr., 12:*245 (1962).

15. Bressaini, R., Elias, L. G., and Braham, E.: In R. F. Gould (Ed.): *World Protein Resources.* Washington, American Chemical Society (1966), pp. 75–100.

16. Bressani, R. *et al.: Arch. Latinoan Nutr., 17(3):*177 (1967).

17. Brown, L. R.: *Foreign Affairs, 46:*688 (1968).

18. Burgess, A. and Dean, R. F. A.: *Malnutrition and Food Habits.* London, Travistock (1962).

19. Chandrasekhara, M. R., Swaninathan, M., and Subrahmanyan, V.: *Bull. Cent. Food Tech. Res. Inst., 5:*25–26 (1955).

20. Cravioto, J., deLicardie, E. R., and Birch, H. G.: *Pediatrics, 38:*319 (1966).

21. Cravioto, J. and Robles, B.: *Am. J. Orthopsychiatry 35:*449 (1965).

22. Daniel, V. A., Leela, R., Doraiswany, T. R., *et al.: J. Nutr. Diet.* (India), *3:*10–14 (1966).

23. Davies, P. A.: *Proc. Nutr. Soc., 28:*66–72 (1969).

24. Daza, C. H.: Informe Anual de Labores, Secretaria de Salud Publication. Columbia, Valle del Carca (1964).

25. Dean, R. A. F.: *Natl. Acad. Sci. Natl. Res. Council Publ., 843:*77 (1961).

26. Ebbs, J. H.: In G. H. Beaton and E. W. McHenry, (Eds.): *Nutrition.* New York and London, Academic Press (1966), vol. 3.

27. Editorial: *S. Afr. Med. J.,* vol. 42, no. 29 (1968).

28. Eichenwald, H. F. and Fry, P. C.: *Science, 163:*644 (1969).

29. Food and Agriculture Organization: *Nutrition and Working Efficiency.* (1962).

30. FAO/W.H.O. Expert Committee on Nutrition, W.H.O. Tech. Rep. Serv., No. 97, Geneva (1955).

31. *Food for Us All.* U. S. Dept. of Agriculture, U. S. Government Printing Office (1969).

32. Food Stamp Program, Intern'l. Evaluation of the Pilot Food Stamp Projects, AMS—472. U. S. Dept. of Agriculture (1962).

33. Galliver, G. B.: *Proc. Nutr. Soc., 28:*97–102 (1969).

34. Gomez, F., Galvan, R., Cravioto, J., *et al.: Acta. Paediatr., 46:*286–293 (1957).

35. Howe, E. E., Jansen, G. R., and Anson, M. L.: *Am. J. Clni. Nutr., 20:* 1134–1147 (1967).

36. Howe, E. E., Jansen, G. R., and Gilfillan, E. W.: *Am. J. Clin. Nutr.*, *16:*315–320, 321–326 (1965 a, b).

37. Hunger and food stamps. *Rehabil. Health Nat. Inst. Rehabil. Health Services, 8:*2 (1970).

38. Hutchinson, J. B., Moran, T., and Pace, J.: *Br. J. Nutr., 13:*151–162 (1959).

39. Jelliffe, D. B.: *Clin. Pediatr.* (Phila.), *6:*355 (1967).

40. Jelliffe, D. B.: *J. Trop. Pediatr., 13:*177 (1967a).

41. Jelliffe, D. B.: *Infant Nutrition in the Subtropics and Tropics.* Geneva, W.H.O. (1968).

42. Joseph, K., Rao, N. M., Swaninathan, M., Indivaimma, K., and Subrahmanyan, V., *Ann. Biochem. Exp. Med.* (India), *20:*243–250 (1960).

43. Joseph, K. M., Rao, N. M., Swaninathan, M., and Subrahmanyan, V.: *Br. J. Nutr., 11:*388–391 (1957).

44. Joseph, A. A., Tasker, P. K. Joseph, K., *et al.: Ann. Biochem. Exp. Med.* (India), *23:*279–289 (1962).

45. Kapsiotis, G. D.: Food Science and Technology Branch, Nutrition Division, FAO, Rome, June, 1968.

46. Kenny, J. F., Boesman, M. E., and Michaels, R. H.: *Pediatrics, 39:*202 (1967).

47. King, M.: In *Proceedings of the Conference on the Production of Malnutrition in the Preschool Child.* Washington, National Academy of Sciences (1966).

48. Komaiko, J. R.: *Parents,* p. 30, March 1970.

49. Kotz, N.: *Let Them Eat Promises. The Politics of Hunger in America.* Englewood Cliffs, Prentice Hall (1969).

50. Lal, S. B.: *Indian J. Med. Res., 40:*471–479 (1952).

51. Latham, M. C., McGandy, R. P., McCann, M. B., and Stove, F. S.: *Scope Manual on Nutrition.* Kalamazoo, Upjohn (1970).

52. Leela, R., Daniel, V. A., Rao, S., *et al.: J. Nutr. Diet* (India), *2:*78–82 (1965).

53. Levin, B., MacKay, H. M. M., Neill, C. A., Oberholzer, V. G., and Whitehead, T. P.: *Med. Res. Counc. Spec. Rep., 296:*11 (1959).

54. Liener, I. E.: In A. M. Altschul (Ed.): *Processed Plant Proteins Foodstuffs.* New York, Academic Press (1958), pp. 79–129.

55. Lowenberg, M. E., Todhunter, E. N., Wilson, E. D., Feeney, N. C., and Savage, J. R.: *Food and Man.* New York, John Wiley & Sons (1968).

56. Mayer, J.: *J.A.M.A., 43:*85 (1969).

57. Mellander, O., Vahlquist, B., and Mellbin, T.: *Acta Pediatr.* (Stockh), *48* (Suppl. 116):31 (1969).

58. Meneghello, J., Rousselot, J., Underraga, O., Aguilo, C., and Ferreiro, M.: *Courrier, 8:*377 (1958).

59. Mertz, E. T.: *Fed. Proc., 25:*1662 (1966).
60. Mertz, E. T., Nelson, O. E., Bates, L. S., and Olivia, A., In *World Protein Resources*. Advances in Chemistry, Series 57. Washington, American Chemical Society (1966).
61. Mertz, E. T., Veron, O. A., Bates, L. S. and Nelson, O. E., *Science* 148: 1641 (1965).
62. Morley, D.: *Trans. R. Soc. Trop. Med. Hyg., 62:*200–8, (1968).
63. Murthy, H. B. N., Swaninathan, M., and Subrahmanyan, V.: *J. Sci. Industr. Res., 9B:*173–176 (1950).
64. Nelson, O. E.: *Fed. Proc., 25:*1676 (1966).
65. Nelson, O. E., Mertz, E. T., and Bates, L. S.: *Science, 150:*1469 (1965).
66. *Nutr. Rev., 27:*39–41, 133–136 (1969).
67. Osborn, G. R.: Colloques int. cent. *Natn. Rech. Scient., 169:*83 (1968).
68. Parthasavathy, H. N., Doraisway, T. R., Panemangalove, M., *et al.: Canad. J. Biochem., 42:*377–384 (1964).
69. Pecora, L. J. and Hundley, J. M.: *J. Nutr., 49:*101–112 (1951).
70. Platt, B. S., Heard, C. R. C., and Stewart, R. J. C.: In H. N. Murro and J. B. Allison (Eds.): *Mammalian Protein Metabolism*. New York and London Academic Press (1969), vol. 2.
71. Polak, H. E.: In *Rehabilitation of Children Suffering from PCM*. World Health Inter-regional Seminar on Treatment and Prevention of Protein Calorie Malnutrition in Early Childhood, Kampala (1965).
72. Puyet, H.: *Courrier, 13:*73 (1963).
73. Rao, N. M. and Swaninatan, M.: *Annu. Rev. Food Technol.* (India), *1:*73–99 (1960).
74. Rao, M. N. and Swaninathan, M.: In G. H. Bourne (Ed.): *World Review of Nutrition and Dietetics*. Basel, S. Karger (1969), vol. 11, pp. 106–141.
75. Rao, N. Rajagopalan, R., Swaminathan, M., and Parpia, H. A. B.: *Oil Chem. Soc., 42:*658–661 (1965).
76. Romeo de leon J., Jr.: An Integrated Method for the Evaluation of Nutritional Rehabilitation Services, Seccion de Nutricion Ministerio de Salud Publica., Guatemala, (1965).
77. Ross Laboratories Public Health Currents, *The Fight Against Hunger and Malnutrition in the U. S.* (1970), vol. 10, no. 2.
78. Russel, W. C., Taylor, M. W., Mehrhoff, T. O., and Hiraseh, R. R.: *J. Nutr., 32:*313–325 (1916).
79. Sauberlich, H. E., Chang, R. Y., and Salmar, W.: *J. Nutr., 51:*623–635 (1953).
80. Schneideman, I. and Bennett, F. J.: *J. Trop. Pediatr., 12:*3 (1966).
81. Scrimshaw, N. S. and Parman, G. K.: Report. U. S. Dept. State Agency Intern. Develop. Washington, (1966).

82. Scrimshaw, N. S., Behar, M., Wilson, D., *et al.: Am. J. Clin. Nutr.,* 9:196 (1961).

83. Scrimshaw, N. S., Taylor, C. E., and Gordon, G. E.: *W.H.O. Monog. Ser.,* No. 57 (1968).

84. Shurpalekar, S. R., Chandrasekhara, M. R., Lahiry, N. L., Swaminathan, M., and Indiramma, K.: *Ann. Biochem. Exp. Med., 20:* 145–156 (1960).

85. DeSilva, C. C.: *Adv. Pediatr., 13:*226 (1964).

86. DeSilva, G. C. and Baptist, N. G.: *Tropical Nutritional Disorders of Infants and Children.* Springfield, Thomas (1969).

87. Slade, P. E., Branscombe, D. J., and McGowan, J. C.: *Chemistry and Industry. 25:*194 (1945).

88. Streeter, C. P.: In *India—A Report from the Rockefeller Foundation.* (1969).

89. Subrahmanyan, V., Rama Rao, G., Kuppuswamy, S., Narayama Rao, M., and Swaminathan, M.: *Food Sci.* (Mysore), *6:*76–80 (1957).

90. Subrahmanyan, V., Bains, G. S., Bhatia, D. S., and Swaminathan, M.: *Res. Industry, 3:*178 (1958).

91. Subrahmanyan, V. Doraiswamy, T. R., Bhagavan, R. K., *et al.: Indian J. Pediatr., 26:*406–413 (1959).

92. Subrahmanyan, V., Sreenivasa, A., Bhatia, D. S., *et al.:* In *Meeting Protein Needs of Infants and Children.* Publ. 843. Washington, National Academy of Science (1961).

93. Swaninathan, M., Daniel, V. A., and Rao, S. V.: *J. Nutr. Diet.* (India), *4:*231–250 (1967).

94. Symposium: iron deficiency and absorption. *Am. J. Clin., 21:*1138 (1968).

95. Tasker, P. K., Joseph, A. A., Ananthaswamj, H. N., *et al.: Food Sci. 2:*173–175 (1962).

96. Tasker, P. K. Joseph K., Rajagopala Rao, D., *et al.: Ann. Biochem. Exp. Med.* (India), *23:*279–289 (1963).

97. Truswell, A. S. and Brock, J. F.: *S. Afr. Med. J., 33:*98–99 (1959).

98. United Nations (1968), *Report of the Economic and Social Council of the Advisory Committee on the Application of Science and Technology to Development.* U. N. Publ. E 68, XIII, 2, p. 78.

99. Vitale, J. J., Velez, H., Bustamante, J., Hellerstein, E. E., and Restrepo, A.: In R. A. McCance and E. M. Widdowson (Eds.): *Calorie Deficiencies and Protein Deficiencies.* (1968).

100. Wharton, B. A.: In R. A. McCance and E. M. Widdowson (Eds.): *Calorie Deficiencies and Protein Deficiencies.* (1968).

101. Wharton, C. L.: *Foreign Affairs, 47:*464 (1969).

102. W.H.O. Technical Report, *Nutrition Anemias.* Series No. 405 (1968).

103. Woodruff, A. W.: In R. A. McCance and E. M. Widdowson (Eds.): *Calorie Deficiencies and Protein Deficiencies.* (1968).

Chapter VIII

CLINICAL APPROACHES TO FIGHT MALNUTRITION

IT IS OBVIOUS FROM the statistics gathered by experts of FAO and WHO and the discussion of the problems in the last chapter that in countries where malnutrition is an endemic problem and fairly large sections of the population are involved, the major problem of fighting the nutritional deficiency syndromes is the prevention of malnutrition and the cure of mild forms of kwashiorkor or marasmus. However, the complete prevention of protein malnutrition which affects 70 percent of humanity requires gigantic efforts on the part of people themselves, the governments, the scientists, social workers, and the physicians. Its prevention depends largely on better education in nutrition and eliminating unspecific prejudices against foods. The important steps in the prevention of malnutrition include raising the general standard of living of the depressed populations by raising food production of traditional and nutritionally based new products, creating better employment opportunities, thereby improving the purchasing power and imparting to the masses some basic knowledge of public health and of the dietary needs of individuals at various ages, particularly those of the infants and the pregnant mothers. Medical professions can help to prevent the development of second and third degrees of protein-calorie malnutrition by recognizing its earliest signs, i.e. failure of adequate growth and subnormal stature as related to chronological age. A child provided with a well-balanced and complete diet, including adequate care by the parents, and a socially and emotionally stable environment is not likely to be a candidate for protein or protein-calorie malnutrition.[35,36]

For the development of second and third stages of deficiency syndromes, it is evident that an individual (particularly a growing child) has been ingesting low-protein foods (cereals and tubers) for prolonged periods of time, and this leads to a stage clinically described as pre-kwashiorkor. Such children would probably visit a physician due to some clinical problems such as gastroenteritis or some other infections, viral or bacterial. It is at this time that the physician can institute a rigorous diet therapy to replenish the protein reserves of the body as well as give medication for the control of infections.

In numerous places prevention of kwashiorkor or other nutritional deficiencies does not involve the lack of available food or protein but simply of education of the parents who feed the child guided by traditional superstitions rather than any knowledge of the nutritional value. For example, in Malaya, superstitions exist against giving fish to the child because, according to local belief, it causes worms. The infant food prepared by a Bantu mother contains so much water, ostensibly to facilitate feeding, that it is almost impossible to feed a baby enough calories. Such examples can be easily multiplied, and it is suggestive of the fact that mass education of the parents in dietary and sanitary methods is important. In most cases of kwashiorkor, therefore, the treatment or preventive measures are basically related to correcting the qualitative or quantitative deficiency of protein which may or may not be complicated by deficiency of available calories. The concomitant decrease in the intake of essential vitamins and minerals predisposes an individual, particularly toddlers, to bacterial infections and other forms of stress which may modify the clinical picture. In countries where malnutrition exists among the younger population, most often the reason is faulty diet which is very low in protein content of good quality. This hampers the growth of the child and keeps him underweight, shorter in stature. The child may also be using the available protein to generate energy due to lack of calories in the food.

There is evidence that in the areas where the children are malnourished and protein deficiency syndromes are endemic, the adult population is also greatly affected although not so clearly manifest because there is no growth arrest (unless the adults have suffered from PCM in infancy) as is observed in the children.[55] A clinician faced with the problem of treating mild, moderate, or severe degree of protein-calorie malnutrition has to pay the rightful attention to the infections and other clinical implications but must pay equal attention to building up the protein reserves of the body. FAO and WHO nutrition studies on calorie and protein requirements stress that any treatment of nutritional deficiency syndromes must be based on the introduction of a protein and calorie intake based on minimal requirements.[27,28]

For the purpose of initiating a successful treatment of kwashiorkor, it may be practical to follow the classification of Gomez *et al.*[35,36] into first-degree and second-degree kwashiorkor. To this could be added third-degree kwashiorkor patients who are critically ill, grossly deficient in nutrients, and have other clinical complications. The first-degree condition may be uncomplicated clinically and may be a result of simple insufficiency of food. In that case, a gradual introduction of a well-balanced diet in sufficient quantities will restore the loss of weight, improve physical appearance, and restore normal functioning of the physiological processes. In the second-degree malnutrition, the condition could be complicated clinically because of defective digestion or absorption of nutrients. In this stage the child is also susceptible to infections which could put him in real trouble because of diminished resistance compared to a healthy child. Anorexia, restlessness, and diarrhea would warrant the use of certain therapeutic procedures along with the diet therapy. The third-degree malnutrition patients are generally brought to the hospitals because of their advanced stage of malnutrition, complicated by infections and extremely unstable electrolyte balance. Despite treatment, the mortality rate in this group is still high, and more careful work is needed in this area to reduce the mortality rate. In this stage, the child is grossly underweight and shows functional, biochemical, and anatomic disturbances. The basic therapy in this condition should be to, "Provide the depleted organism with the opportunity to ingest, absorb and utilize sufficient nutrients so that it can recover its lost physiologic and biologic faculties and create the necessary reserves." [35,36] Different therapeutic measures discussed in the next section are instituted with great caution and under constant surveillance. At the same time, the diet therapy is instituted in order to accomplish weight gain and increase nitrogen and water retention. The diet therapy may be summarized in this manner: the child should be allowed foods in small amounts raised to quantities for a child of the same chronological age. The foods should be rich in proteins of high biological value in a form that is palatable, easy to ingest and digest. Because of extraordinary weakness and exhaustion not only does the food have to be in liquid form, but special nursing skill may also be required in feeding the severely malnourished child. It may be important to provide special nursing facilities in the less developed areas of the world where malnutrition is more prevalent. This procedure has the special advantage of overcoming emotional upsets or feelings of insecurity which could affect the intake of nutrients. DeSilva [60] firmly believes that kwashiorkor patients must not be allowed to gorge themselves on food, nor should the calorie or protein contents be increased unduly and hastily.

Fortunately, during the recent years a full appreciation of the symptoms of kwashiorkor has come about, and in most cases the patients are fully rehabilitated. In the early 1930s and 1940s treatments for kwashiorkor were based on an individual physician's interpretation of the condition. Some physicians tried to treat the pellagrous nature of skin lesions associated with kwashiorkor with nicotinic acid,[48] and Frontali [29] believed that he could abolish slight irregularities in the electrocardiograms by giving thiamine. Certain preparations of hog's stomach, under various names, have similarly been given and claims made for the cure of kwashiorkor. Gillman and Gillman [34] showed that 10 gm daily of a desicated preparation of hog's stomach improved the condition of a kwashiorkor patient. The diet given to the patient was unspecified. Altman [1] believed that Gillman's success with hog's stomach was probably due to the protein it contained. Gillman [33] also tried on a child 8 gm daily methionine over four days and another 11 gm over seven days in addition to a diet consisting of maize, porridge, and half-strength milk.

SIGNS AND SYMPTOMS OF KWASHIORKOR AND MARASMUS

Dermatosis and Edema

Skin changes are most indicative of the onset of kwashiorkor and may be characterized by loss of pigment and dermatosis. It gives a child's skin a pale reddish-brown color or very pale coffee color or a mottled patchwork among the colored races. Dermatosis in itself is not any indication of the condition of the patient. In numerous cases, the patients with the worst skins respond very well to treatment, and occasionally a child with better skin conditions may be worse off. No particular treatment is recommended for the skin condition, and in most instances, it heals by itself as the child responds to treatment of kwashiorkor with diet therapy. A pellagrous skin does not warrant the administration of large doses of nicotinamide or other components of vitamin B complex.[35,36]

Hair changes in kwashiorkor children are as prominent as the skin changes. Color of the hair is altered bacause of loss of pigment, and the kwashiorkor children have thin, scanty, and dull hair. The hair condition improves by itself during the course of treatment. The hair does not recover its color but is generally replaced by hair of normal color.

Edema is perhaps the most serious symptom in kwashiorkor and is of extreme importance in the prognosis. The first important indication of the initiation of cure is the loss of edema and weight gain (after having lost the excess water).[55] From a number of studies, it is evident that edema of kwashiorkor is a result of maldistribution of excess body water. The total body water is greatly increased but does not change as a percentage of body weight as edema regresses. It is the extracellular water that is increased in the edematous phase of kwashiorkor and shows a significant loss as the edema subsides. The degree of clinical edema is not related to the level of total body water concentration. As the treatment progresses, the weight of the child may not change, although there are good indications of response to therapy. It is probably because of the fact that the decrease in the quantity of extracellular water is taken up partly by the intracellular compartments and partly by the new or regenerating tissues.[41] In effect, two opposite forces are in operation during the first response to treatment. More nitrogen is retained because of building of cell solids and along with fat deposition, this tends to increase weight. The redistribution of extracellular water, however, tends to keep the weight constant and thereby the actual gain of weight by the patient is somewhat delayed. A number of workers have also pointed out that it may not be advisable to reduce edema too fast. Gomez *et al.*[35,36] explained that rapid mobilization of extracellular fluid is accompanied by electrolyte loss which may increase the risk of electrolyte imbalance. A gradual reduction of edema permits replacement of electrolytes lost in the process. In the case of adverse electrolyte status, potassium repletion becomes necessary.[55]

Occasionally the child is extremely dehydrated at the time of admission to the hospital, and this could prove fatal unless intravenous fluid therapy is given.[18] Such a child, however, would first gain weight as well as water before losing his edema.

In occasional cases, after the child responded satisfactorily to treatment and has been discharged or is ready to be discharged, the edema suddenly reappears. The reasons for this relapse are not clear, but this is a grave prognostic sign and often the cases prove fatal.

Diarrhea

The majority of children with kwashiorkor experience bouts of diarrhea at one stage or the other varying in intensity from mild to severe and for a short or prolonged time. This disorder hinders the absorption of nitrogen, and its excretion greatly increases during the time a child suffers from diarrhea with the result that the net loss of nitrogen is greatly enhanced, and as Behar [9,10] indicated, if solid foods are withdrawn from the child at that time, the physiological stress could be very much worsened. Since the exact cause has always been hard to determine, the preventive measures are not satisfactory.[16,17,54] Diarrhea is certainly a result of a number of factors acting synergistically,[55] and severe diarrhea may also develop during a treatment.[22] Any factor such as infection, enzyme lack, malabsorption, intolerance to disaccharides in the diet arising from congenital absence of disaccharides could be responsible,[11] but unless a pathogen can be isolated from repeated samples of stools and blood, infection may not be suspected and antibiotic therapy not be started.[64] Besides diarrhea of infectious origin, other contamination such as malaria or contagious diseases could also precipitate diarrhea. Emotional upsets caused by the death of a parent or some other social tragedy accompanied by lack of well-balanced food also contributes to diarrhea and to the worsening condition of an already depleted organism. Dean [23] strongly believed that in kwashiorkor patients the sugars in the food and lactose of milk contribute heavily to the severe forms of diarrhea.

In most cases, reports from various hospitals indicate that lactose intolerance does appear to be the single most important factor as a cause of diarrhea and should be verified if the pH of the stools is below 6 and they contain more than 0.5 percent of reducing substances.[12,64] It is reasonable to assume that acquired disaccharide deficiency is partly responsible for some of the cases of diarrhea in nutritional deficiency and may be due to a combination of hepatic, pancreatic, and small intestinal dysfunction. Bowie [11] listed the following as evidence for the same: (1) a carbohydrate-free diet decreases the weight of feces of a kwashiorkor child; (2) a milk diet results in large quantities of lactic acid and sugar in feces; and (3) administration of oral glucose leads to normal blood sugar curve. Bowie [13] believed that since children with diarrhea demonstrate lack of ability to hydrolyze lactose along with normal absorption of saccharides, it may be that disaccharides are not functioning normally. Wharton [69] in Uganda observed intolerance to disaccharide and glucose in kwashiorkor and reported controlling diarrhea with a diet containing fructose as a carbohydrate source. Dean [24] and Bowie *et al.*[13] in Uganda and South Africa, respectively, also reported lactose and sucrose intolerance, whereas Wharton et al [70] reported, in addition, intolerance to monosaccharides.

Removal of lactose from the diet greatly helps in controlling diarrhea. In most instances, only removal of lactose may be successful, but if the diarrhea continues despite it, the removal of sucrose from the diet should be considered. Staff [64] reported great success in lactose-sucrose-free diet. He also believed that lactose-free milk formula may prove more successful than a lactose-free soy flour diet which did not prove satisfactory for treatment of diarrhea nor was acceptable by the children. Children with diarrhea respond very favorably to a lactose-sucrose-free diet in which the main source of carbohydrtae is fructose.[56] A steady gain in weight is indicative. The stools are soft, bowel movements are at regular intervals, and lactic acid excretion drops to a minimum. After the stools are well regulated for a few days, a cereal porridge consisting of cereal flour, powder milk, and sugar is added to the diet. In the treatment of diarrhea, some educational instruction to the parents is also considered essential. It should be aimed not only at the kind of diets to be given to a diarrhea patient but at, "Avoiding the dangerous practice of using laxatives or purgatives in the treatment." [10]

In cases of severe diarrhea, which does not subside on a lactose- or lactose-sucrose-free diet, the electrolyte balance may be greatly upset, and it is of utmost importance that before any other measure is taken, the patient be relieved of the threatening acid-base imbalance at the earliest.[35,36] General recommendation is 4.7 mEq/kg/day potassium, but up to 10 mEq/kg/day potassium may be required in severe cases but should be given with extreme caution. Staff [64] successfully used a solution containing 7.9 gm KCl/100 ml = 1 mEq K/ml. During the treatment, full data should be collected on the volume of fluid intake, amount and composition of stools, urinary volume and insensible fluid losses in order to provide a diet favorable to the therapeutic regime.[35,36] Staff [64] warned against intravenous fluids without their being absolutely essential because of the risk of pulmonary edema.

Infections

In those countries where kwashiorkor is an endemic problem, the infant mortality is generally higher than in other age groups. Most often, the children who are already exhausted from the protein malnutrition succumb to an infection from which a healthy child has a chance to recover. Usually the problem is gastroenteritis, and a synergism between malnutrition and intestinal infection is well established.[58] Prinsloo *et al.*[55] postulated that one effect of an inadequate protein diet is a disturbance of the intestinal flora which plays a significant part in the clinical picture of kwashiorkor. In the majority of the fatal cases, the patients have had positive blood cultures of intestinal organisms. It is evident that these children were well below their normal weight before they contracted these infections, and because of their nutritional deficiencies, were predisposed to diarrhea, respiratory infections, and intestinal disorders.[41] According to Hansen, for every case of established kwashiorkor, there are at least 100 cases of protein deficient, malnourished children who could clinically come in the category of pre-kwashiorkor. When these children, who are physiologically quite weak, contract the infections and succumb to them, the doctors generally diagnose the terminal disease as the cause of death and fail to mention that it was the protein-calorie deficiency that precipitated it. "In England, for example, the death rate from gastroenteritis is 300 per year. In South Africa, with a non-white population that is a quarter of the size of the total population of Britain, gastroenteritis deaths amount to 11,000 in the towns alone."[41] Most of the deaths have obviously been precipitated by the prevalent protein-calorie malnutrition among the nonwhite population, especially the infants.

Wharton *et al.*[71] showed that in children admitted to the hospital, infection is universally present and gram-negative bacteria are frequently cultured from the throat while staphylococci are less common. Antibiotics, as indicated for infections, are a great help, and Behar *et al.*[9,10] suggested giving penicillin routinely for the first eight to ten days whereas Wharton felt that if the antibiotics had to be given routinely, penicillin is not the most suitable.[64] No one antibiotic can be safely given for all cases. Smythe[62] advocated the use of broad spectrum antibiotics, whereas Hansen[42] preferred the use of penicillin and sulfadiazine as a cover for bacterial infections to be given routinely even in the absence of laboratory investigation. Staff,[64] however, warned that the routine use of antibiotics without confirming the infection may lead to serious side effects. The theory of an anti-biotic "umbrella" may have a very doubtful value and leads to a false sense of security and to further diagnostic and therapeutic dilemmas. Phillips and Wharton [52] strongly emphasized that anti-biotics should be prescribed only when infection is diagnosed.

Gram-negative infections are the most troublesome. Staff [64] be-lieved that urine should be examined on admission and suggested 500 mg/day ampicillin, 15 mg/kg/day kannamycin intramuscu-larly, or 50 to 100 mg/kg/day chloramphenicol in divided doses.

Respiratory problems are also frequently present among the kwashiorkor patients. The "fruity cough" with no chest signs or chest x-ray changes may be due to pulmonary fluid rather than pulmonary infection.[71] Severe bronchopneumonia is not a common complication, and the diagnosis of tuberculosis in malnutrition is very difficult.[64] However, laryngeal swabs and gastric washings should be examined carefully. In cases of tuberculosis diagnosis, Staff [64] suggested the administration of 4 mg thiacetazone, 2 to 8 mg/kg/day isoniazid and 40 mg/kg/day streptomycin intramus-cularly.

Hookworms are occasionally observed in the stools, and 0.1 ml/kg/day tetrachlorethylene may be given for three consecu-tive days.[8] However, very little is known about the harmful effects of a small load of hookworms, and it is likely that even in severe kwashiorkor, their effect may not be of much significance. In the same way the finding of a plasmodium in the blood may not indicate a malarial condition that is likely to endanger health or to impede recovery. Antihelminths, or purgatives, should not be used indiscriminately. It is evident that it is against common sense to give a liver poison to an already-damaged liver and a purgative to an already-oversensitive gut.

Hypothermia and Hypoglycemia

Hypothermia

In critical cases of kwashiorkor, it is not uncommon to observe temperatures below 96°F sometime during the patient's stay in the hospital.[69] Brenton *et al.*[15] showed that hypothermia was quite common among children admitted to the hospital for the treatment of kwashiorkor. Subnormal body temperatures are reached particularly at night, especially when they are sleeping alone, separated from the mother, and are not fed as regularly as during the day. It may be mentioned here that in a number of underdeveloped countries, the children are used to sleeping with their mothers at home, and the mother is generally admitted to the hospital along with the child in order to keep this continuity. Wharton [69] illustrated recently that the infants which are small in size (less than 6 kg in weight, 70 cm in length or 70% of their expected weight) are most susceptible and suffer from hypothermia during the first or second nights in the hospital. The mortality rate in this group is relatively high. It has been suggested that special attention be devoted to maintain warm temperatures in the pediatric wards and also to maintain normal body temperatures in all children admitted to the hospital, particularly during the first three to four days. Whenever the conditions allow, it may be wise to let the mother sleep with the child, if it is customary for a particular child at home, since a sudden separation during the night may enhance the chances of a child getting cold. Also, care should be taken to provide extra blankets to the kwashiorkor children in the ward. Staff [64] suggested that the small-sized patients may not be washed during the first day in the hospital, be nursed away from all windows and drafts, be kept well covered, have the rectal temperatures taken every three hours and before feeding for the first four days.

Hypoglycemia

It has been shown that the children suffering from kwashiorkor have dangerously low levels of glucose in the blood. Bowie [11] believed that it may be because of (1) the inability of a poorly functioning and grossly fatty liver to absorb stored glucose, (2) the impairment of the activity of certain hepatic enzymes concerned with the glucose metabolism, or (3) failure or imbalance of the normal control. Cook [21] showed that since chronic pancreatic damage is fairly common in children suffering from kwashiorkor, it may play a significant role in the onset of hypo-

glycemia. In Uganda, Wharton [69] observed fasting blood glucose
levels of less than 40 mg/100 ml in 25 percent of the children
admitted to Mulago Hospital for treatment of kwashiorkor. A
striking feature of hypoglycemia in kwashiorkor is the lack of any
definite signs. Convulsions and sweating do not occur, and hypoglycemia is recognizable only by extreme apathy or sudden onset
of coma.[18] Kahn and Wayburne observed that hypoglycemia
often follows partial or complete failure to take food. In a severe
case of kwashiorkor, a fast as short as five hours could be hazardous.
Wharton *et al.*[70] tried glucagon for the treatment of hypoglycemia
and found it of limited value. Wharton [69] believed that "for some
hours after the administration of glucose, one of the homeostatic
mechanisms governing its level in the plasma, i.e., glycolysis is
paralyzed. Intermittent injections of glucose, therefore, carry a
great risk of severe reactive hypoglycemia for some hours after
they are given." Staff [64] believed that no treatment is indicated
unless the blood glucose level falls below 20 mg/100 ml. In that
case, according to Staff, glucose should be added to milk or 0.5
gm/kg glucose given intravenously and 50 mg hydrocortisone injected intramuscularly, followed by a continuous intravenous drip
of 10% dextrose at the rate of 100 ml/kg/day and oral prednisone
0.5 gm/kg at six-hour intervals.

PRINCIPLES OF TREATMENT OF DEFICIENCY SYNDROMES
Therapeutic Measures

Most often the patients brought to the hospital are severe
cases of kwashiorkor who would need clinical attention as much
as a proper diet. The therapeutic procedures are designed to save
the life of the patient during the early critical periods by certain clinical procedures with initiation of measures to restore the
nutritional deficiency. The former may include measures such
as routine procedures of admission, electrolyte balance, blood
transfusions, antibiotics, and vitamin therapy.

Routine Procedures

The routine procedures of admission include a thorough physical examination of the child with a view to assess the severity

of the condition, for example, the loss of weight compared to a normal child of his age and height, the extent of edema, anemia, conditions of the skin, size of spleen and temperature. According to Staff,[64] temperature is very important and may prove a vital area of attention. Laboratory tests include urine samples for sugar, protein, acetone; blood samples for parasites and estimation of hemoglobin and plasma protein and feces are examined for parasites and bacteria.[64]

Electrolyte Balance

A study of body fluids and electrolyte balance of the child is of extreme importance before any therapy is started. In numerous cases, diarrhea is a constant feature of the kwashiorkor patient causing dehydration, and if accompanied by vomiting, it could create a grave situation by upsetting the electrolyte balance. During treatment, serious attention needs to be paid, therefore, to volume of fluid intake, fluid lost in vomiting, composition of stools and fluids lost through that route, urinary volume, and the contents of the solutes and other insensible fluid losses. It is essential that the patient be relieved of the threatening acid-base imbalance as rapidly as possible.[35,36] This is attributed as the main cause of death during the first 18 to 72 hours after admission, and its correction should be one of the first therapeutic measures in treatment. In moderate cases, the appropriate electrolyte may be given orally, but in severe cases, it is imperative to resort to parenteral administration.[10] Gomez *et al.*[35,36] described that a severe case of electrolyte imbalance will show, on the part of the patient, apathy, lack of thirst, polyuria, and dehydration and edema simultaneously. Along with these clinical symptoms, the biochemical investigations indicate a relative increase in extracellular fluid volume and hypotonicity, intracellular dehydration, decrease of intracellular potassium concentration, and intracellular shifts of water and sodium.[35,36] The probability of potassium ions being deficient is quite high because of their loss through constant diarrhea and vomitting as well as by protein deficiency.[10] Similar observations have been made by Garrow[30] and Hansen,[42] and they recommended potassium supplement to the extent of at least .5 gm three times a day. Hansen [42] indicated that electrolyte solution with sodium potassium in half isotonic Darrow's solution with $2\frac{1}{2}\%$ glucose was quite effective. An effort should, however, be made to correct the electrolyte imbalance by giving a solution with precise amounts of ions as indicated by a thorough laboratory examination, and in this manner each patient should be treated as an individual. It is difficult to rely on cow's milk alone which contains good amounts of sodium and potassium but provides considerably more sodium than potassium.

Studies of the kidney function indicate a lesser amount of glomerular filtration and renal plasma flow. At the same time, there is a high clearance of osmotically free water and decreased sodium and potassium excretion.[35,36] It is suggested that in the face of the above-mentioned clinical and biochemical paradoxes, the most suitable solution may be the one which has a similar osmolarity, so that the patient's own plasma can supply the necessary ions. Hansen added that it is practical to add glucose in electrolyte solution in view of the ever-present hypoglycemia.

Magnesium deficiency also becomes apparent in numerous cases and is evidenced by muscle biopsy analysis, low urinary excretion, and prolonged positive balances of magnesium during recovery.[18] Magnesium supplements may be routinely given.

Blood Transfusions

Blood transfusions are indicated not only in cases of severe anemia but should also be used in most cases of severe kwashiorkor and marasmus because of its antishock action value. As reported from Nairobi, the liberal use of blood transfusions in severe cases of kwashiorkor has often proved a life-saving factor. Behar et al.[10] strongly believed that blood transfusions have no particular advantage over the appropriate diet therapy and should not be resorted to unless absolutely essential and unless there is an imminent danger of death due to severe anemia or some sudden shock. Arguing similarly, Behar et al.[10] also discussed the use of plasma in protein hydrolysates to combat the hypoproteinism of kwashiorkor. These transfusions could cause certain clinical complications, and if their purpose could be served by oral administration of proteins, it is best to avoid them. Gomez *et al.*[35,36] recommended the use of blood and plasma for a patient under shock or if it is difficult to keep the patient in metabolic equilibrium. According to these authors, blood and plasma are more effective in regulating and maintaining electrolyte equilibrium and in preventing the fatal relapses.

Antibiotics

Some other therapeutic procedures made necessary by the condition of the patient on admission are the use of antibiotics which should be given as indicated, depending on the infection. Behar *et al.*[10] recommended their use routinely during the first eight to ten days in order to bring the secondary infections under control.

As mentioned later in the infection section, not much is known about the harm done by the helminths or hookworms in the intestine. It is advisable that when certain therapeutic measures are being taken, these parasites should not be treated until recovery is well advanced. Most studies indicate that the presence of helminths does not hinder the treatment or recovery in any significant manner.

Some disagreement exists among physicians about the regular use of vitamin and mineral supplements. Behar *et al.*[10] believed that on a milk diet alone certain signs and symptoms, otherwise attributed to the deficiency of vitamin B complex, disappear. They did not see any benefit in giving folic acid or vitamin B_{12} because according to them macrocytic anemia responds very well to milk alone. Hansen,[42] however, did not object to the use of oral vitamins and minerals and recommended intravenous infusions if oral feeding is difficult. Fat-soluble vitamins may be administered intramuscularly. Iron may be given by either route (intramuscular or intravenous) ; if orally given, iron is not properly absorbed.

Vitamin Therapy

In kwashiorkor patients, it is often the case that they show concomitant deficiencies of essential vitamins, especially of vitamin A. The administration of vitamin A right from the beginning of treatment is recommended by most workers. In a study by Pereira *et al.*[50,51] of 175 Indian children suffering from kwashiorkor, ocular signs of vitamin A deficiency were seen in half the children, and another 28 had serum levels of vitamin A below 10 mg/100 ml. Cases of blindness have been encountered in vitamin A-deficient kwashiorkor patients. These authors have recommended the administration of large doses of water-miscible vitamin A (100,000 IU/day) for a period of seven days to these patients. With this intramuscular dose, the serum levels rose within one to two hours, and the vitamin was readily available to the depleted child. This method also facilitates hepatic storage of vitamin A as was evidenced by a few liver biopsies.

Pereira and co-workers did not suggest an oral administration of vitamin A in oil as is commonly practiced because it was poorly absorbed in children with kwashiorkor during their critical period.[51] Also, the intramuscular injections of vitamin A in oil did not raise serum levels of this vitamin in children suffering from protein malnutrition. Mahadevan *et al.*[47] have explained the reason for inadequate utilization of vitamin A in oil as being due in part to the lowering of beta-lipoprotein fraction of the serum proteins, the fraction necessary for the transport of vitamin A from the intestine. The easy availability of the water soluble vitamin A to the kwashiorkor patients suggests the decreased activity of pancreatic enzymes. The reduced beta-lipoproteins also do not hinder the absorption or transport of this form of vitamin A.

Vitamin E deficiency has also been implicated as causing megaloblastic anemia of protein-calorie malnutrition and that this vitamin plays a role in human hemopoiesis, but no conclusive proofs are yet available.

Diet Therapy

General Principles of Diet Therapy

In acute kwashiorkor, although the diet forms the main basis of treatment, controlling diarrhea, other infections, and electrolyte disturbances are of primary importance and should be brought under control. After overcoming the clinical symptoms, a diet which is adequate, well-balanced, and properly adjusted to individual requirements is the most important principle of treatment for the deficiency syndromes. The essential element of dietary therapy is the provision of high-quality protein (with all the essential amino acids in balanced amounts) in sufficient quantity and in a form that can be relatively easily digested by the patient. Approximately 2.5 gm/kg body weight should be sufficient to initiate a cure, if sufficient calories are provided and the average retention of nitrogen comes to about 40 percent.[55] There is a general agreement that whole milk or powdered milk (with varying amounts of fats) is the most convenient form of the supply of high-quality protein.

Milk is an effective source of high-quality protein, but where vegetable sources of protein are cheaper, the nitrogen retention can be brought to a satisfactory level by giving adequate quantities of vegetable protein preparations. Graham [40] observed that the children receiving more than 2.0 gm protein/kg were recovering faster from their nutritional deficiencies and indicating better weight gain compared to those getting less than this quantity. A diet devised by Dean and Swanne [25] based on calcium caseinate has been given successfully by Staff [64] and other groups in Africa and a modified table is reproduced here.

TABLE VIII

THE INGREDIENTS AND NUTRITIONAL VALUE OF THE ROUTINE
CASILAN-DRIED SKIMMED MILK-SUCROSE DIET

Ingredients of the "Dry" Mixture (gm)		Nutritional Value per 100gm of Reconstituted Diet	
Casilan	33	Protein gm	4.0
Dried skimmed milk	30	Fat gm	6.1
Sucrose	30	Carbohydrate gm	4.6
Cottonseed oil	60	Calories	90
Potassium chloride	2.7	Potassium mEq	4.7
Magnesium hydroxide	0.3	Magnesium mEq	1.3
Sodium chloride	None	Sodium mEq	0.9

1. The mixture of "dry" ingredients is prepared for use by taking 174 gm of this mixture and making it into a paste with a little cold boiled water, in scalded equipment, and

then adding, gradually, enough cold sterile water to make a total of 1,000 gm.

2. The reconstituted diet is fed at the rate of 100 gm per kilogram of body weight per day.

3. The "dry" mixture of this diet may be stored in a cool place in tins or other containers with close fitting lids, without refrigeration and without dangerous bacterial contamination for up to one month.

It is, however, a very controversial subject whether a slow recovery from a smaller quantity of protein given for longer periods is preferable to a fast recovery based on higher quantities of protein in the food. Srikantia *et al.*[63] believed that 6 gm/kg/day was probably the optimum level of protein in the diet of a child suffering from severe kwashiorkor. It may be best to generalize that the diet therapy should be initiated on smaller quantities of protein and more nutrients be added, depending on the response of the patient. Every patient should be treated individually, and different requirements may have to be recommended even in apparently similar cases. When dealing with children of vulnerable age and condition, it is of extreme importance that great precaution should be taken, even in dietary therapy, because emotional upsets caused by strange environments and strange people in a hospital may stand in the way of proper digestion. Extremely tender care is essential at the time of feeding. In some countries, the mothers are also admitted to the hospital, and I believe it must be helpful inasmuch as the child gets the loving care of the mother, and the hospital staff is relieved of some of the responsibilities. In such cases, however, the hospital staff must not lose the opportunity of sharing with the mother the dietary principles of feeding the undernourished and thereby imparting to her some useful education.

When the protein deficiency is uncomplicated, a total protein intake of 2 to 5 gm/kg/day is sufficient to promote a cure. In most instances, however, the children admitted to the hospital for treatment are those who have not only severe degrees of protein-calorie malnutrition but are also sick due to some infection. In such cases, dietetic therapy must not be rushed and in the first two or three days, because of anorexia and tendency to abdominal distensions, milk or some suitable source of protein should be prescribed in small quantities with protein content as low as 1-2 gm/kg/day. Hansen [42] gave small feeds of milk at the rate of 60 to 90 ml/kg body weight (30 ml of liquid milk contains 1 gm of protein). This may be supplemented by half isotonic Darrow's solution (lactated potassic saline) to make up the total fluid requirements of 150 ml/kg/day. Hansen stressed that with this procedure, children can tolerate full cream milk and skimmed milk, which is generally considered safer, if not necessary. Gomez et al.[35,36] suggested whole milk with 10% corn syrup ingested in quantities to provide about 35 calories/kg actual weight in kwashiorkor patients. According to them, such a low calorie and protein intake is sufficient during the first week of treatment in order to achieve a positive balance gradually. The quantity of milk can be increased in about 15 days to about 100 calories/kg body weight, to be increased more by the third week, at which time the diet consists mainly of milk, meat, vegetables, and fruit. As soon as the appetite of the patient grows, larger quantities of fruit juices, green and yellow vegetables, lean meats (partly pork or veal), and eggs can be added to the diet to make it balanced in all the nutritional requirements for a fuller recovery.

Animal Sources of Proteins and Calories

Animal sources of proteins are biologically superior and of higher quality compared to the vegetable protein. Malcolm Clark, while discussing kwashiorkor, emphasized, "I attach the greatest importance to animal protein, especially meat. The best food I have found is minced meat, mashed up with vegetables, soup and milk. Maize meal is best avoided. Meat, milk, and eggs are the most important items to be provided; after them, fruits and vegetables." During the first few days of treatment, unless clinical complications manifest themselves, a liquid form of diet is the most advisable, and the most widely accepted as well as effective is cow's milk. The latter is a convenient source of protein of very high biological value. Most recommended for the treatment of kwashiorkor and other nutritional deficiencies is the nonfat powdered milk which has a number of advantages over the fresh milk. Its use eases the problems associated with keeping fresh milk, transporting it to distant areas where local supplies are deficient, in addition to having a long shelf-life. The powdered milk contains about 34% protein, and for providing the needed 50 gm of high-quality protein for two to three-year-old kwashiorkor patients, about 150 gm of powdered milk is sufficient. Data also suggest that during inadequate protein intake from the food, proportionately more nitrogen is retained from protein in milk compared to vegetables.[59]

There has been some controversy with regard to the use of non-fat, half-skimmed milk or full-cream milk for the treatment of kwashiorkor.[10] Some prefer lower fat content of the milk on grounds that the capacity of the sick child to digest fat is seriously impaired. Gomez and his associates,[35,36] however, obtained satisfactory results with full strength whole milk, and Dean[24] went farther as to recommend 30 to 50 gm of fat to diets in order to provide additional calories for the treatment of kwashiorkor. In certain cases, where the patient cannot tolerate fat as a source of calories, bananas may be substituted. The latter are well tolerated and are an excellent source of calories.[10] DeSilva[60] stressed that when more fat is added to the diet, some of it is absorbed, and the rest is excreted in the stools, and there is no evidence that the unabsorbed fat is in any way harmful or causes losses of other nutrients.

Vegetable Sources of Proteins and Calories

In most countries where PCM is widespread, the main reason is nonavailability of high-quality animal proteins at prices that the poor can afford. In general, milk is the established choice for the treatment of kwashiorkor, but it is costly as well as scarce and substitutes must be found. The protein deficiency syndrome arises out of long-term consumption of cheaply available cereals which could satisfy the need for calories but does not provide enough protein to sustain adequate growth. This does not mean, however, that deficiency diseases like kwashiorkor cannot be treated by vegetable proteins. This does mean though that vegetable sources of protein must be judiciously chosen so that they provide balanced amounts of all the essential amino acids and then at the same time be cheap enough for the poor to afford in the underdeveloped or developing countries which have large populations of undernourished children. In vegetarian diets the protein content should be at least 20 percent of the diet. Also, the vegetable foods should be given in larger quantities because the nitrogen absorption is not so efficient with these diets as with milk or other animal foods.

A good deal of research work has been done in the last decade to show the efficacy of cheap vegetable food mixtures to see if kwashiorkor would yield to treatment with diets containing proteins exclusively of plant origin. It is evident that processed protein foods, based on blends of vegetable proteins, could be successfully used in an effective treatment as well as prevention of protein malnutrition (Fig. 18).[53] Scrimshaw[59] demonstrated that in these circumstances, when adequate proteins are provided to a child, the body is able to retain as much nitrogen from the vegetable mixtures as from an equivalent amount of protein in milk, although the nitrogen absorption as percent of intake is always less with the vegetables than with milk. Larger quantities of vegetable proteins are required, therefore, for adequate nitrogen retention, because a proportion of nitrogen consumed in vegetable mixture remains unabsorbed. According to Scrimshaw *et al.,* it is also possible at a theoretical level that a protein-deficient child is less selective in his needs for nitrogen and can use patterns of amino acids that may not be of much nutritional value to a healthy person.

Satisfactory results were obtained at Kampala by the use of diets containing banana, soya, and vitamin mixtures. A soya diet has a great advantage over milk in Asian, African, and South American countries because of its easy availability and relatively lower cost compared to a milk diet, particularly a lactose-free diet based on milk. The soya diet also reduces the complication of diarrhea that so often hinders treatment based on milk be-

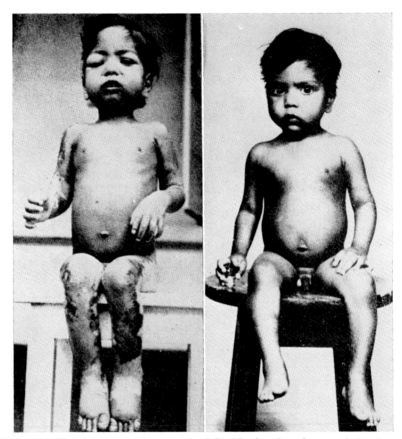

Figure 18. Kwashiorkor patient on the left side showing characteristic edema of the legs and hands, crazy pavement detmatosis, and hyperpigmented areas. On the right side is the same patient, completely cured after treatment with vegetable protein mixtures, 30 days after starting the treatment.[53]

cause of lactose intolerance. Vegetable mixtures suffer from the great disadvantage that they yield a thick porridge that is generally not well accepted, particularly in the patients showing severe degrees of anorexia. This handicap can be overcome by making a fine powder of these foods (especially those based on oilseed meals) with the help of a microatomizer.[53] This powder is easily soluble in hot water and yields a milk-like emulsion which is not only acceptable but also desired by the children suffering from protein malnutrition (PM). It may not be out of place to mention a few notable examples where plant proteins have been used for the treatment of kwashiorkor and marasmus.

Dura de Oliveira *et al.*[26] treated children with acute malnutrition in two groups, one group on a formula prepared from an aqueous extract of soybean and the other group on a milk formula, and concluded that the soy formula was as effective as the cow's milk formula in the initial treatment. In a Brazilian study, a soya formula at half strength during the first few days of treatment (1.75 gm protein/100 ml formula), gradually increasing to two-thirds strength after ten days and attaining full strength formula on the seventeenth day, was well tolerated and readily accepted, thus leading to an effective treatment. Chaudhri[19] tried a number of vegetable mixtures for the treatment of kwashiorkor and other deficiency diseases in India. The mixture used successfully has the following recipe: Bengal gram (Cicer arietinum) is roasted and ground into flour and is then cooked with molasses and fresh green vegetables and is used as a gruel. With six 3-hourly feedings (of about 6 oz at a time), a one-year-old child would get 40 to 50 gm protein and 1000 to 3000 calories. Chaudhri[19] observed that not only was the product well accepted, but the balance studies showed satisfactory absorption and retention of nitrogen with this diet. Diarrhea subsided and gain in weight and rise in serum proteins was observed. Wicks and Whittle[73] compared the effectiveness of Nutresco (a locally produced protein supplement in Rhodesia) and dried skim milk to promote the treatment of kwashiorkor and showed that the group of children on dry nonfat milk fared better than those taking Nutresco, gained more weight, and showed higher mean total serum protein levels. No difference was observed, however, in the average amount of albumin gained over a period of four weeks in the two groups. Wicks and Whittle suggested that Nutresco, if made sweeter and more palatable, is an acceptable source of protein and a good substitute for milk if the latter is not available for the treatment of undernutritional states.

It is generally agreed that although kwashiorkor children respond quite well to vegetable proteins, it is not as effective for promoting speedy treatment of PCM as milk. This is probably due to better nitrogen absorption and retention on a milk diet as Hung *et al.*[45] showed that cow's milk formula is better absorbed (89%) compared to 83% absorption with the soybean formula, but the retention as a percentage of intake is similar (28%) in both groups if the dermal losses are not calculated. When sufficient amounts of protein are made available, the body is able to retain approximately as much nitrogen from the vegetable mixtures as from an equivalent amount of protein in milk.[59] An effective use must, therefore, be made of the vegetable sources of protein in the less-developed areas of the world where there are large sections of undernourished populations and animal sources of proteins are scarce. The use of legumes, oil seeds, and oil seed meals in combination with milk for the treatment as well as prevention of kwashiorkor has been suggested by a number of workers.[3,57,65] Isolated oil seed proteins which are two to four times as rich in protein as oil seed meals and legumes may prove more suitable for treating the deficiency diseases. They can be given along with glucose or sugar and are needed in much smaller quantities (70 to 80 gm provide 50 to 60 gm of protein).[49] The isolated oil seed proteins possess a bland taste and are free from indigestible carbohydrates and odoriferous substances.[32]

Such an approach of using vegetable proteins will put to use most effectively the small reserves of animal proteins available in the developing countries. However, one particular vegetable protein source, howsoever superior in protein content in terms of percentage, may not provide protein of high biological value. For example, peanut protein isolate by itself is quite unsatisfactory but in combination with skim milk is nearly as satisfactory as skim milk.[37] The results of other studies similarly show that processed protein foods based on blends of low-fat ground nut flour, soybean flour, chick-pea flour, sesame flour and skim milk powder fortified with calcium, vitamins A and D, thiamine, and riboflavin contain protein of high nutritive value.[46,74] These authors incorporated this mixture in a rat diet at 30% level providing about 7 to 11% extra protein and found that the animals gained weight equivalent to the other group fed on equivalent amounts of powdered milk. The well-known Inca-parina produced in Central America and Multipurpose Food produced in India are the two outstanding examples of these vegetable and animal protein mixtures, which can be effectively used for the effective treatment of kwashiorkor and related deficiency diseases.

The Indian Multipurpose Food (MPF), a blend of peanut flour, Bengal gram flour, and nonfat powdered milk fortified with vitamins, has been proven to be highly effective in the treatment of kwashiorkor in children.[49,66] In small quantities (approx. 100 gm) MPF provides 40 to 50 gm of protein, and when given to the children in the form of a porridge sweetened with sugar, it causes a marked improvement in the general condition of the patient in eight to ten days. The characeristic signs of kwashiorkor, edema, dermatosis, hyperpigmentation disappear within a two- to three-week period, and the serum protein levels increase steadily.[66] The Indian MPF is made commercially in large quantities in India and is used as a supplement to the food of young children besides its use in the hospitals for the undernourished patients.

Behar[10] summarized some excellent suggestions which should be taken into consideration in planning vegetable protein mixtures for the prevention or treatment of protein-deficiency states:

(1) The amino acid content of the individual ingredients and the final product, (2) the possible presence of toxic or interfering factors, (3) the need for obtaining exact specifications for each of the components, (4) the necessity of avoiding processes that damage the quality of the protein, (5) the desirability of using products of local origin, (6) the fact that the final product must be inexpensive and easily prepared. (7) the requirement that it may be easily prepared in the home as an infant food by mothers of low-income families, and (8) the demand that it must not run counter to existing dietary habits and prejudices.

Follow-up Care

It is not uncommon to find a child released from a hospital having completely recovered and in good physical health, returning to the same hospital in worse shape than ever. It is important, therefore, that the progress made by these children with respect to their health and well-being be followed up and clinical tests be made at intervals of every few months.

Since the negligence, ignorance, or economic backwardness of the parents were responsible for the onset of kwashiorkor in the child in the first place, it seems fairly important that measures be taken not only to treat the child, but equal stress be laid on ridding the parents of the ignorance which led to this dismal state of affairs. As far as negligence or ignorance is concerned, it is best removed by making parents participate in the treatment program. Some hospitals admit the mother along with the child in the pediatric ward, and this practice may be quite sound. Given adequate instruction, the mother could be a full-time nurse as well as a source of emotional stability to the child. In the presence of the mother, the child is not scared of the unfamiliar surroundings of the hospital and hence may avoid the emotional upsets which may otherwise manifest themselves and make the treatment difficult. It may be wise to let the mother participate in preparation of milk formulas or the food for the child and simultaneously be given instructions how to use the food available to her at home. This may also be another opportunity to give her some useful education in basic necessities of good nutrition.

After the child is sent home, careful follow-up and visits by a public health nurse at regular intervals are essential to minimize the chances of relapse. Most countries have child welfare clinics, and if they are not present, the local government should pay adequate attention to build them because at the local level they serve a very useful purpose. These clinics should provide milk and other nutritious foods to the local children at subsidized prices. Hansen [42] writes that in South Africa, a demand from the people for the compulsory notification of kwashiorkor to the public health authorities has proven quite successful. Once a notification from a parent is received, the health visitor calls on the family and makes sure that either the child is admitted to the hospital for proper treatment in the case of severe form of malnutrition or attends the child welfare clinic if the complication is mild or moderate. According to Hansen, it is only those children who are not brought to the welfare clinics that suffer severely from kwashiorkor.

UNEXPECTED SEQUELAE

General

Sudden and unexplained deaths occur in patients of kwashiorkor and in many cases of children who are apparently well on their way to recovery. A number of theories exist without adequate explanation for any one of them, and the cause of many deaths from PCM remains obscure. Since very low fasting blood sugars have been reported in children with severe kwashiorkor,[5] some of the deaths may be due to the sudden fall in the concentration of blood sugar.[61] It is important that more research be done in the area of treating severe hypoglycemia and preventing death caused or precipitated by the institution of therapy.[18] Hepatic dysfunction, hypertrophy of pancreatic islets, and the effects of hyperinsulinism or potassium flux of the already potassium-depleted myocardium may also be important [30] and may be considered in the light of unexplained fetal deaths in diabetic mothers.

Endocrine imbalance [5] and defect in glycogenolysis [69] are mainly held responsible for the unexplained deaths in kwashiorkor, but special attention should be paid to general drowsiness and cardiac arrest in these patients. Such symptoms must be considered critical in view of the conflicting data available on these subjects.

Drowsiness and Coma

Drowsiness and coma have been observed in the kwashiorkor patients, particularly during the first few days of admission, by a number of physicians. In 1935, Gopalan and Ramalingaswami [38] described that some of their kwashiorkor patients became very drowsy, passed into coma and died. Trowell *et al.*[67,68] described the stages of drowsiness as, "Apathy replaced by stupor which deepens into a coma," and it is in those patients who pass into coma that death occurs. Wharton [69] described that most patients are, in general, drowsy and sleep for longer hours during their early period in the hospital. No obvious cause of this symptom is available beyond conjecture. Liver failure may be one of the reasons. Wharton described that one of the children who died had a liver "flap" which may have been caused by inability to handle the load of protein given in the early stages of treatment. In that sense, drowsiness and coma may be forms of hepatic encephalopathy.[69] In most cases, the drowsiness can be overcome with adequate care in nursing and may not need any particular therapeutic procedure.[7] Wharton also observed that the patients who were inclined to be comparatively more drowsy than the others also showed an elevated hydroxyproline index.[72] Seven out of the 22 patients with higher hydroxyproline index examined by him became drowsy, and these patients had somewhat increased chances of death.[44]

Since the etiology of drowsiness is not very clear, the best that can be done for the patients is extreme caution in nursing, gradual introduction of rich foods, and constant surveillance for any accompanying symptoms.

Cardiac Failure

In recent years there have been a number of extremely useful advances that have resulted in almost 100% treatment and recovery of a child suffering from moderate degrees of kwashiorkor or marasmus. There are still, however, 10 to 20 percent of cases of severe kwashiorkor which prove fatal, in spite of the best hospital care, that may be attributed to severe infections[42] and lack of response to medication or die due to extreme weakness. In some fatal cases, the sudden death, in spite of apparent response to treatment, eludes explanation and has been believed to be due to cardiovascular depression.

Cardiac failure during the first or second week of admission to the hospital is not uncommon among the kwashiorkor patients. Surprisingly there are a number of reports that some of the children, who later prove to be the candidates for cardiac arrest, are apparently doing very well in responding to routine treatment. It is probable that these children already have a nutritional defect in the heart muscle on a diet with or without high sodium intake,[64] as is indicated by certain histological [4] and histopathological changes in human [39] and in the cardiac muscles of experimentally induced protein-calorie malnutrition.[20] There appears to be some correlation, although at present it is of a doubtful nature, between the incidence of cardiac failure and levels of hemoglobin. In a sample of eight children with hemoglobin values less than 6 gm/100 ml, all of them had cardiac failures.[69] The work of Balmer [6] on serum enzymes and lactic dehydrogenase showed that the children with very low hemoglobin values had a prominent extra band, which disappeared with treatment.

Drastic reduction in salt intake, as practiced by Wharton *et al.*,[64,69,70] considerably reduced the incidence of cardiac failure but did not completely overcome it, and other factors will have to be looked into to understand the etiology of cardiac failure in kwashiorkor. It is, however, a wise policy to try the low sodium diet (1 mEq/kg) from the first day after admission of the patient to the hospital. Experience has shown that on low sodium diet, the chances of cardiac arrest are somewhat less, even if the hemoglobin value drops down to the dangerous level of 6 gm/100 ml. Till the time some better explanation is found for the cardiac failure, it is reasonable to look into the problems of anemia and salt retention by the body because with these factors in control, the child may be able to stand the additional stresses to its damaged myocardium. In the case of heart failure, Staff [64] prescribed 0.04 mg of digoxin per kilogram orally, increased to 0.015 mg/kg after six to 12 hours, and thereafter increased to 0.02 mg/kg/day. Also,

> Oxygen should be prescribed at once, and one of the thiazide diuretics in approximately half the adult dose, and extra potassium administered by mouth, up to 10 m Eq per kg per day. Given intravenously or intramuscularly, 10 mg of frusemide has been of great value in acute pulmonary edema, and occasionally spironolactone 12.5 b.d. has been added to the regime.[64]

RECOVERY

Clinical Changes

The treatment of kwashiorkor is often remarkably successful in the sense that as soon as the patients start responding to treatment, half the battle is won, and quite rapidly the effects of a successful treatment become evident by the improved general demeanor of the child. Ashworth [2] pointed out that, "During recovery, growth rates were fifteen times as fast as those of normal children of similar ages, and five times as fast as those of normal children of similar height or weight." But as soon as the expected weight for a height was reached, the appetite for food, a high intake of which was responsible for rapid growth, also declined by at least or comparable to that of normal healthy children; in other words, the body develops a higher efficiency in consuming foods during the early stages of recovery and slows down once the emergency of making up losses is over. Ashworth [2] concluded, therefore, that the growth rate changes are due to a reduction in food intake, and since growth-controlling mechanism is quite sensitive, the efficiency of food utilization is greatly increased during the catch-up growth, and body fat starts accumulating once the ideal weight has been reached. It is believed that body growth has a target to reach and tries to do so unless deflected from its natural growth trajectory because of malnutrition. As soon as the imbalance of food availability is corrected, the child runs fast to try to catch up to its original curve and, once having reached it, slows down to adjust its path to the old trajectory again. The recent studies of Graham [40] on measurements of total body water, extracellular water, excretion of creatinine and hydroxyproline, in nine malnourished infants of five to 30 months of age show that the nature of growth during recovery greatly differs in a number of ways from the normal growth and that some tissues suffer less and recover more promptly than others. In the malnourished children the deficits in body weight, created at the expense of body fat and cellular mass (muscle and viscera), are larger than those of height. Similarly during recovery, the gains in cellular masses were correspondingly higher. In their studies, Graham et al.[40] observed the normal production of growth hormone in the malnourished children, whereas the insulin production was greatly impaired. They speculated that the gains in cellular masses during rehabilitation may depend on insulin rather than the growth hormone.

After the patients start responding to the treatment, the sequence of changes that may be evident from that time till complete recovery is established may be termed "Nutritional Recovery Syndrome" as suggested by Gomez *et al.*[35,36] The treatment is considered successful if it fulfills the following criteria:

1. *Improvement in appetite and interest in food.* At least by the end of the first week of treatment, a child's appetite should be improved sufficiently as to accept solid food in addition to a liquid diet.

2. *Disappearance of edema.* Many research workers have commented on the rapidity with which the edema disappears as an indication of the response of the patient to the treatment and recovery. It appears, however, that its disappearance may not be of much consequence if it relapses. In the latter case it would be considered a very dangerous symptom.

3. *Healing of skin.* If the patient responds to treatment, no matter what method is employed, the pellagrous skin will peel off within ten to 20 days leaving new skin with more or less normal characteristics. It is evident from a number of studies that healing of skin takes place gradually, and it may take a number of weeks before the skin is completely normal.

4. *Hair changes.* Changes in hair may be first signs to appear and the last to disappear. The hairs that lost pigmentation are not the ones which will recover, but new hair with normal amount of pigmentation grows at the roots of the old or in the temporal patches which had become hairless under severe conditions.

5. *Changes in body weight.* The change in body weight is the most sensitive as well as objective index of the progress made by the child. Staff[64] described that a typical child, responding to treatment, begins to lose weight within three days and continues to do so during the first week. This may be attributed to loss of edema. In marasmic children with no obvious edema, this loss

of weight is less significant. After about a week's time the body weight should start increasing steadily. A large number of children responding well to treatment show a weight gain from 500 to 1000 gm a day, which may seem incredible to those not familiar with kwashiorkor.[35,36]

6. *Clear signs of well-being.* This term has been used by Gomez *et al.*[35,36] who believe that a good smile on a patient is a sign of good prognosis. At the same time, normal social behavior and neuromuscular rehabilitation appears in a child.

Biochemical Changes

The concentration of hemoglobin is probably the single most important diagnostic feature. In severe cases, it falls to as much as 1 gm/100 ml. With successful recovery, it should rise to about 10 gm/100 ml in about eight days.[64] According to Garrow *et al.*,[31] "increased serum bilirubin concentration and a decreased serum sodium concentration indicated bad prognosis, and these two factors contributed almost the whole of multiple correlation coefficient of 0.63 with respect to mortality and 0.59 with respect to the speed of recovery."

A steady increase in the total protein levels so as to reach the normal level is expected in about two weeks. Also, the protein level in the plasma should rise by 1 to 2 gm per week due to regeneration of the albumin.[64] Corresponding biochemical changes take place in all the tissues of the body. It may be summarized that recovery from nutritional deficiency accompanies increases in the amounts of serum albumin, cholesterols, nonspecific esterases, cholinesterases, pancreatic enzymes in duodenal contents, restoration of acinar cells of pancreas, and removal of fat from the liver cells.

Nature of Recovery

It is indeed a controversial subject whether or not the kwashiorkor children even catch up to their full growth potential. Garrow and Pike[32] after a study of numerous children two to eight years old believed that they were equal in height and weight for the average in the population. This kind of statement must, however, be considered in context of the control population with which the comparison has been made which itself may not have been adequately nourished. After all, the severe cases of kwashiorkor admitted to the hospitals come from a population that is in general undernourished and in which one in a hundred develops a serious and clinical case of kwashiorkor. It is probable, therefore, that both the groups, i.e. the one treated in a hospital for kwashiorkor and those "normal" children with whom the comparison is made, have not reached full growth potential. Physiologically speaking, the treatment is successful and the recovery complete as judged by the criteria that the total serum protein level has returned to normal and his serum albumin has risen to about 4 gm/100 ml and all the anatomical, functional, and biochemical lesions have disappeared completely following a reverse order from that in which they originally appeared.[35,36]

REFERENCES

1. Altmann, A.: *Clin. Proc., 7:*32 (1948).
2. Asworth, A.: *Br. J. Nutr., 23:*835–845, (1969).
3. Autret, M. and Van Veen, A. G.: *Am. J. Clin. Nutr., 3:*234 (1955).
4. Bablet, J. and Normet, L.: *Bull. L'Acad. Med., 117:*242 (1937).
5. Baig, H. A. and Edozien, J. C.: *Lancet, 2:*662 (1965).
6. Balmer, S.: Personal Communication, quoted by Wharton (1968).
7. Balmer, S. E., Howells, G. R., and Wharton, B. A.: *Dev. Med.,* (1968) (Quoted from Staff, 1968).
8. Balmer, S. E., Howells, G. R., and Wharton, B. A.: *J. Trop. Pediatr.* (1968) (Quoted from Staff, 1968).
9. Behar, M., Viteri, F., Bressani, R., *et al.: Ann. N. Y. Acad. Sci., 69:*954–968 (1958).
10. Behar, M., Viteri, F., and Scrimshaw, N. S.: *Am. J. Clin. Nutr., 5:*506–515 (1957).
11. Bowie, M. D.: *S. Afr. Med. J., 38:*328 (1964).
12. Bowie, M. D., Brinkman, G. L., and Hansen, J. D. L.: *Lancet, 2:*550 (1963).
13. Bowie, M. D., Brinkman, G. L., and Hansen, J. D.: *J. Pediatr., 66:*1083 (1965).
14. Bowie, M. D., Hansen, J. D. L., and Barbezat, G. O.: *Am. J. Clin. Nutr., 20:*89 (1967).
15. Brenton, D. P., Brown, R. E., and Wharton, B. A.: *Lancet, 1:*40 (1967).

16. Brock, J. F. (Ed.) : *Recent Advances in Human Nutrition*. Boston, Little Brown (1961).

17. Brock, J. F., Hansen, J. D. L., Howe, E. E., *et al.: Lancet, 2:*355 (1955).

18. Campbell, P. G., Rosen, E. U., Fanaroff, A., and Sapire, D. W.: *S. Afr. Med. J., 46:*605–608 (1969).

19. Chaudhuri, R. N.: *Trans. R. Soc. Trop. Med. Hyg., 57:*448–457 (1963).

20. Chauhan, S., Nayak, N. C., and Ramalingaswami, V.: *J. Pathol. Bact., 90:*301 (1965).

21. Cook, G. C.: *Metabolism, 17:*1073–83 (1968).

22. Dean, R. F. A.: *Br. Med. J., 2:*791 (1952).

23. Dean, R. F. A.: *Mod. Probl. Pediatr., 2:*133 (1957).

24. Dean, R. F. A.: In D. Gairdner (Ed.) : *Recent Advances in Paeddiatrics,* 3rd ed. London, Churchill (1965), p. 234.

25. Dean, R. F. A. and Swanne, J.: *J. Trop. Pediatr., 8:*97 (1963).

26. Dutra de Oliveira, J. E., de Oliveiro, Netto, N., and Duarte, G. G.: *J. Pediatr., 69:*670 (1966).

27. *FAO Nutr. Studies,* No. 15 (1957).

28. FAO/W.H.O. *W.H.O. Tech. Rep. Ser.* No. 301 (1965).

29. Frontali, G.: *Boll. Ed Atti Acad. Med. Roma,* 8:61 (1953).

30. Garrow, J. S.: *Lancet, 2:*455 (1965).

31. Garrow, J. S. and Pike, M. C.: *Br. J. Nutr., 21:*155 (1967).

32. Garrow, J. S. and Pike, M. C.: *Lancet, 1:*1 (1967).

33. Gillman, T.: *S. Afr. J. Med. Sci., 41:*288 (1945).

34. Gillman, T. and Gillman, Jr.: *Nature* (Lond), *155:*634 (1945).

35. Gomez, F., Ramos–Galvan, R., and Cravioto, J.: *Pediatrics, 10:*513 (1952).

36. Gomez, F., Ramos–Galvan, R., Cravioto, J., and Frenk, S.: *Ann. N.Y. Acad. Sci., 69:*969–988 (1958).

37. Gopalan, C.: *W.H.O., 26:*203–211 (1962).

38. Gopalan, C. and Ramalingaswami, V.: *Ind. J. Med. Res., 43:*751 (1955).

39. Gopalan, C., Venkatachalam, P. S., Someswara Rao, K., and Menon, P. S., *Indian J. Med. Sci., 6:*277 (1952).

40. Graham, G. G., Cordano, A., Blizzard, M., and Cheek, D. B.: *Pediatr. Res., 3:*579–589 (1969).

41. Hansen, J. D. L.: In J. F. Brock (Ed.) : *Recent Advances in Human Nutrition.* Boston, Little, Brown (1961), pp. 267–281.

42. Hansen, J. D. L.: In R. A. McCance and E. M. Widdowson (Eds.) : *Caloric Deficiencies and Protein Deficiencies.* London, Churchill (1968).

43. Holt, L. E.: *Am. J. Clin. Nutr., 11:*543 (1962).

44. Howells, G. R., Wharton, B. A., and McCance, R. A.: *Lancet, 1:*1082 (1967).

45. Huang, P. C., Tung, T. C., Lue, H. C., Lee, C. Y., and Wei, H.: *J. Trop. Pediatr., 13:*27 (1967).

46. Joseph, K., Narayanarao, M., Swaminathan, M., *et al.: Br. J. Nutr., 16:* 49–57 (1962).

47. Mahadevan, S., Malathi, P., and Ganguly, J.: *World Rev. Nutr. Diet., 7:*209 (1965).

48. McCollum, E. V.: In H. B. Glass (Ed.): *A History of Nutrition.* Boston. Houghton Mifflin (1957).

49. Parpia, H. A. B., Narayana Rao, M., Rajagopalan, R., and Swaninathan, M.: *J. Nutr. Diet., 1:*114 (1964).

50. Pereira, S. M. and Begum, A.: *Am. J. Clin. Nutr., 22:*858–862 (1969).

51. Pereira, S. M., Begum, A., Isaac, T., and Dumm, M.: *Am. J. Clin. Nutr., 2:*297–304 (1967).

52. Phillips, I. and Wharton, B. A.: *Br. Med. J., 1:*407 (1968).

53. Prasanna, H. A., Amla, I., Indira, K., and Narayana Rao, M.: *Am. J. Clin. Nutr., 12:*1355–1365 (1968).

54. Pretorius, P. J. and Smith, Z. M.: *J. Trop. Pediatr., 4:*50 (1958).

55. Prinsloo, J. G., Pretorius, P. J., Wehmeyer, A. S., *et al.: Am. J. Clin. Nutr., 20:*270–278 (1967).

56. Rutishauser, I. H. E. and Wharton, B. A.: *Arch. Dis. Child., 43:*463 (1968).

57. Scrimshaw, N. S.: *J. Am. Diet. Assoc., 35:*441 (1959).

58. Scrimshaw, N. S.: In N. M. Munro and J. B. Allison (Eds.): *Mammalian Protein Metabolism.* New York and London, Academic Press (1964), vol. 2, p. 569.

59. Scrimshaw, N. S., Behar, M., Wilson, D., *et al.: Am. J. Clin. Nutr., 9:* 196–205 (1961).

60. deSilva, C. C.: *Adv. Pediatr., 13:*213–264 (1964).

61. Slone, D., Tailz, L. S., and Gilchrist, G. S.: *Br. Med. J., 1:*32 (1961).

62. Smythe, P. M.: *Lancet, 2:*724 (1958).

63. Srikantia, S. G., Venkatachalam, P. S., Reddy, V., and Gopalan, C.: *Indian J. Med. Res., 52:*1104 (1964).

64. Staff, T.H.E.: *East Afr. Med. J., 45:*399 (1968).

65. Subrahmanyan, V., Bhagavan, R. K., and Swaminathan, M.: *Indian J. Pediatr., 25:*216 (1958).

66. Subramanyan, V., Sreenivasan, A., Bhatia, D. S., *et al.:* In *Meeting Protein Needs of Infant Children,* Publ. 843. Washington, National Academy Science (1961).

67. Trowell, H. C.: *Ann. N.Y. Acad. Sci., 57:*722–733 (1954).

68. Trowell, H. C., Davies, J. N. P., and Dean, R. F. A.: *Kwashiorkor.* London, Edward Arnold (1954).

69. Wharton, B. A.: In R. A. McCance and E. M. Widdowson (Eds.): *Calorie Deficiencies and Protein Deficiencies.* London, Churchill (1968).

70. Wharton, B. A., Howells, G. R., and McCance, R. A.: *Lancet, 2:*384 (1967).

71. Wharton, B. A., Jelliffe, D. B., and Stanfield, J. P.: *J. Pediatr., 72:*721–726 (1968).
72. Whitehead, R. G.: *Lancet, 2:*567 (1965).
73. Wicks, A. C. B. and Whittle, H. C.: *Cent. Afr. J. Med., 14:*144–147 (1968).
74. Wittman, W., Prinsloo, J. G., and Kruger, H.: *S. Afr. Med. J., 4:*959–960 (1968).

Chapter IX

NUTRITION EDUCATION

T HE PREVALENT PROTEIN-CALORIE malnutrition or other nutritional deficiency disorders are a result of insufficient availability of balanced food to more than half the human population of the world. As discussed in some of the earlier chapters, the total food output of the overcrowded underdeveloped or developing world is woefully inadequate, and everyday a losing battle is being fought between the available food and the ever-increasing number of mouths that lay claim to that food. It is an indisputable fact that a comfortable supply of food is not available, but deeper analysis of the whole situation also reveals that insufficient quantities of food could not be blamed for all the undernutrition and malnutrition in the world. Ignorance, illiteracy, and prevailing attitudes and superstitions about foods play an equally important role in perpetuating the state of malnutrition among those who suffer from it. Talking about only shortage in food supplies is a palliation and not a solution of the problem. In numerous instances, comfortable quantities of food are available but are not either properly utilized by the population or given to the most vulnerable sections of the society (the children in their periods of maximum growth) due to some prejudice.

> Food patterns and food choices often may be based less on rational interpretation of 'known facts' than on taboos, myths and misconceptions. Just because a person is poor does not mean that food is accorded top priority among purchase opportunities, any more than it means that the food choices made will necessarily be the best ones.[22]

Similarly, just because a person is rich and can afford to purchase any type of food in any quantity does not mean that he is going to buy the food that is essential for good health and vitality. As Williams [32] described

> Think for a moment of the Chinese millionaire whose child is dying

of beriberi, of the Indian rajah, dripping with diamonds and emeralds, whose wife is dying of nutritional anemia, of the Masai with their thousands of cattle and their children dying of protein malnutrition. Surely the problem is not really one of food at present but of teaching people how to use the available food and how to avoid the diseases which leads to a bad state of general nutrition.

In this context it becomes obvious that in any drive towards solving the problem of malnutrition, a comprehensive program of nutrition and health education should take priority over the other preventive measures or at least be given equal attention with regard to allocation of funds and personnel. A good food may be available, but the problem of using it is one of education, and one cannot deny that nutrition education is one of the hardest subjects to teach, particularly to the adults whose faulty food habits are often impossible to interfere with. The teaching of nutrition education in schools is an ideal approach to impart education in this vital area, but this appears to be a long-term investment. For the present, effective educational programs for the adult population need to be devised and implemented, because it is the attitude and ignorance of the adults that has resulted in the present sad state of affairs. It is the adult population that needs to be made aware of the human nutritional requirements and increased needs of children during the period of growth and that the children be given absolute priority on food consumption.[12] It is the unhygienic and unsanitary habits of the adult population that makes the semistarved ill-fed child a special target of infections. In the beginning, a nutrition education program may be faced with a lot of resistance. Unless we embark on a solid program of action, we will reach nowhere by merely talking or else we may tend to become pessimistic, as some of the nutritionists do, in view of the rigid attitudes of the people.

An effective education program must reach the people who need it the most. Generally they are the urban slum dwellers and the poor sections of the rural areas. Most often these people are not even aware that they are sick because they don't know what it is to be well. If an education program successfully eliminates some harmful dietary habits and teaches them to feel healthy within the same food budget by accepting to eat some cheap but useful sources of new foods, they will soon learn what it is to be well. Once this change has been brought about, more than half the battle is won, and probably these people will ask for more knowledge and will learn to respect the opinion of experts as they come to them or communicate by radio and newspapers.

It may be worthwhile to summarize here the conditions necessary for an acceptable education program in nutrition as outlined by Jelliffe,[16] in his excellent monograph on the *Infant Nutrition in the Subtropics and Tropics.*

The proposed program of education must appeal to the logic of the people to convince them to adopt it widely. Every culture has its own assumptions, attitudes, and beliefs about foods and the concept of nutrition, which have been passed on from generation to generation. Such attitudes may include beliefs, such as a particular food is hot or cold, heavy or light, or a particular food will make him a thief in later life or destroy his sexual ability. Fish and eggs may be quoted as examples of such foods and are not eaten in certain places in Southeast Asia because they are believed to cause worms. A proposed action based on scientific knowledge may not, therefore, appeal to the logic of the people with preset ideas. It is here that an educational program should avoid a conflict with the beliefs of the population in question and act in accord with the local standards of behavior; within these limitations, it should try to introduce new concepts of nutrition in order to improve the dietary intake of the community. For example, in an education program, it is highly undesirable to criticize their existing and established dietary systems, such as rice, bananas, potatoes, tortillas. Instead a sincere effort should be made at educating them about the nutritional requirements of the body and the desirability of adding beans, poultry, dairy, or meat products in their diets. It may be a good strategy to direct the nutrition education program first to the intelligent section of the society or community, which later could serve as an example for others to follow. It may be somewhat easier to convince the intelligent and prestigious section of the community about the increased needs of the growing children, especially of body-building foods. For effective demonstration, it may be necessary to establish a simple day nursery where children can not only be fed for adequate growth and development but also can be attracted to health-promoting foods, such as fruits, vegetables, beans, by growing them in the school backyard. An obvious gain in weight and stature of the children under the educator's care, compared to the control population outside the school, is most likely to attract attention and thereby establish a clear connection between a particular action and the desired result. Jelliffe [16] emphasized that only the education which is geared to improve the local conditions and is based on local needs and avoids the local cultural beliefs is most likely to be successful. For example, the symptom of intestinal infection in a young child may be diagnosed as "evil eye" by the local people. The educator does not have to start an argument about the diagnosis but should try to convince them to give the child boiled water for drinking. An effective demonstration will convince them that the "evil eye" is a result of drinking polluted water. Jelliffe [16] also outlined the recommendation of WHO expert committee on health education about what nutrition education must attempt to do.

    a. They should assure that the information will actually reach the individual.

    b. They should attract and hold the interest of the people.

    c. They should assure that the content and purpose of the new ideas are understood.

    d. They should be seen by the people as a means to an important goal.

    e. They should assure active participation of the people. Wherever possible it is wise to try out the chosen method on a small representative group before embarking on a large-scale education effort.

WHO expert committee on nutrition in 1962 [32] also stressed nutrition education in health services.

The objectives of nutrition education can be achieved only when a multidisciplinary approach is used. [22] At the grass-root level, thousands upon thousands of nutrition workers will have to be trained to do the field work in an affected area. They should be supported at higher levels by the local leaders, public health specialists, and nutritionists. These in turn must have the support of political leaders at the national level, the health ministry, and the scientists belonging to various disciplines. The latter should include physicians, especially trained in nutrition, teachers and research workers in nutrition, biochemistry, physiology, psychology, anthropology, agronomy, economics, and members of all basic sciences who could help in a better understanding of the role of nutrition to human growth and development and could contribute to an effective implementation of nutrition programs. A deeper involvement of local leaders and locally recruited nutrition workers is especially important for the success of any kind of nutrition education, because the policy makers at the top could do the mistake of recommending certain items of food or certain techniques of preparation, which may be impractical because of the existing economic and agricultural limitations and cultural practices.[24] The local leadership can help to modify them to suit the local conditions and make it substantial and meaningful. Moreover, these are the people who are well versed not only with the local problems, attitudes, apprehensions or misapprehensions but also the resources as well. They are also aware of certain local methods to correct a wrong situation. In countries where adequately trained personnel are not available, the highest priority has to be given to train sufficient numbers of teachers, nurses, social workers, agricultural, extension workers, home economists, and all other professionals who would carry on an effective program of nutrition education.[24]

MAIN CRITERIA OF NUTRITION EDUCATION

Education of the Mother

The most important person who needs education, if any improvement in the prevalent malnutrition has to be made, is the mother whose ignorance, illiteracy, or prejudices have often contributed to faulty feeding habits, resulting in undernutrition and malnutrition among children. The education of the mother should take the form of an elementary course given to her in practical steps, such as the following:

1. Awareness on her part about her own increased requirements of nutrients during pregnancy and lactation. It should be explained to her why she would need 20% to 25% extra protein

for the growing fetus before birth and for adequate nursing after the birth of the baby. According to the local conditions and the economic status of the mother in question, she should be advised of the protein-rich foods and other foods rich in vitamins or minerals, especially iron.[30] Beans, peanuts, green leafy vegetables, and yellow vegetables are some of the examples of foods whose nutrition value needs to be told in the simplest possible language. It may be practical to classify foods rich in protein as "body-building foods," those rich in carbohydrates as "energy-giving foods," and those rich in vitamins and minerals, such as fruits and vegetables, as "protective foods." Within these categories the mothers could be explained in a simple language the idea of a balanced diet. LeGros Clark[7] described an experiment of an organized course of instruction to the mothers in some part of India. The women were completely convinced, when explained in a simple but thorough manner, the nutritive value of low-priced foods, such as legumes and peanuts, and their beneficial effects on the dietary standards of the family when used in supplementary manner along with their traditional diets. These women gladly accepted skim milk, eggs, and green vegetables as part of their diet. After this stage not much effort was required to induce them to start a small kitchen garden or keep poultry in the backyard.

2. Next point of emphasis should be on breast feeding and an awareness of the increasing nutritional needs of the growing infants as the months pass by. It is unfortunate that mothers in certain underdeveloped countries are giving up their traditions and are resorting to bottle feeding the infants. In these countries, pure sterile milk fit for baby's consumption is hard to obtain, with the result that the child suffers from all kinds of infections unnecessarily although sterile and nutritious milk was available all the time in the mother's nipples. Bottle feeding is also an expensive proposition, and in some places it takes a laborer's daily wage to buy enough milk for a baby. In these places where mothers start breast feeding immediately after birth, the babies are healthy and well during the first six months on breast milk alone. Nutrition education should emphasize the importance of breast milk

for the baby and that no matter what the commercials say about the bottle feeding, there is no substitute as beneficial to the child as the breast milk (sterile, warm, and a source of emotional stability to the child because it facilitates desirable physical closeness to the mother). Also during the period of the first six to eight months, the mothers ought to be educated on the need for supplementary feeding. She should be taught simple methods of cooking and preparation of baby foods from the cheap and locally available vegetables and beans. An awareness that milk alone is insufficient to meet the requirements of growth of the child as well as the unsuitability of coarse adult food may convince her to make soft, easily digestible extra food for the child in the first year of life. These foods can be introduced from the fourth month. Many foods eaten by adults can be given to the infants when they are mashed, ground, and prepared in the form of a paste and not containing many spices. A child at the age of nine months can be given almost all the articles of adult diet. The mothers, however, need to be impressed upon that whereas the adults may eat a heavy starchy or carbohydrate diet without visible ill effects, the children must not be weaned on heavy carbohydrate diets. They need the "body-building foods" because of their growth. In those areas where milk and poultry and meat are expensive, the mothers should be taught the preparation of a variety of vegetable foods which are cheaper and at the same time rich in proteins. Jelliffe [16] stressed that "the most single aim of nutrition education is to persuade mothers in the tropics to make the best possible use of foods already available locally for feeding children in the early years of life."

3. The education of the mothers should also endeavor to explain, in their right perspective, some of the local social and cultural prejudices about certain foods. As explained in Chapter VI, nutritious diets, such as fish, beans, and eggs, are not given to children in numerous places because they are believed to be detrimental to their health. In certain cases irrational taboos may require specific counteraction.[25]

4. Mothers' education should also include a simple description of the common diseases of the childhood, including infections and

what causes them. Preventive measures, such as preparing foods in clean utensils away from the flies (which are carriers of diseases), boiling water before giving it to infants, maintaining hygienic surroundings, disposal of excretion, must be stressed upon. Mothers can also be taught to recognize the early signs of protein or protein-calorie malnutrition in terms of certain physical signs, such as inability to gain weight or height, and should be able to take the child to a doctor or public health agency in the earlfer stages of an infective diarrhea or common intestinal worms or malaria or any other infectious disease. She must understand that a purgative to a child suffering from diarrhea, which may be given under the belief that it would get rid of the worms responsible for it, could be dangerous and could worsen rather than help the child.

The elementary education of the mothers will go a long way to improve upon the prevalent malnutrition within the same resources, because more than anything else, the ignorance and illiteracy of the mothers lead to faulty handling and feeding of the babies who suffer the consequences of malnutrition at a very critical stage of their growth. Williams [33] described the mother as the "main gate keeper" whose personal values of food determine the health standard of the family, and if she is given balanced information on the locally available weaning foods, is encouraged in prolonged breast feeding, and is taught the elementary principles of hygiene, the purpose of nutition education can be well served. Sebrell and King [25] have given an excellent description of the role of mother craft centers in order to combat malnutrition. These centers, as the places of educating the mothers, can change the whole life style of the community in terms of their dietary habits in a short period of one to two years. Staffed by dietitians, nutritionists, and public health nurses, the centers can impart sound knowledge in the areas discussed above to most of the mothers of the communities they serve. Sebrell and King [25] described the operation of 14 mother craft centers in Haiti at an annual cost of only $1,000 to $2,000 with each center effectively serving a community of 3,000 to 4,000 people.

Participation of the People

In any program of education designed to improve the health and dietary standards of a population, full cooperation and participation of the people is essential. Good dietary habits and a vigorous health cannot be given to the people. They have to work to get it. Once the people learn to participate in the educational programs designed to improve their health, they suddenly realize how unwell or unhealthy they are and how urgent it is for them to improve their health. With most of the people, particularly in the developing countries, suffering is so much a part of their existence that they are simply unaware what it is to be healthy.[16] Since they don't understand how diseases are caused, they put the blame of their occurence not on the unhygienic way of their life and grossly unbalanced diet but to factors such as "will of God" or "evil eye" or simply to bad luck. Any program of nutrition education will be incomplete and unsuccessful if it does not envisage a wide participation of the people and does not seek to enlighten them on their beliefs with respect to standards of health. All methods of persuasion need to be used to bring about changes in attitudes and values and convince the people that their economic and personal lives will not change unless they feel the need to do it or have the desire to change for the better. Dictation to the people to change could prove very dangerous, and as Margaret Mead [18] once said,

> Every time we fail to tell the people the reasons for our actions, we are reducing the status of the people and their state of responsibility. Too often in the past, we have not accorded to the people whom we are attempting to change, full dignity and full rights to change in every respect.

It is the people themselves who have to recognize the existence of nutritional deficiencies and the associated diseases and that their attitudes on nutrition are mainly responsible for it. Once attitudes are changed and the people feel the need for this or that article of food, they will always be willing to struggle to get those things economically. Awareness of need should take precedence over the creation of purchasing power, or else they will not know how to manage their budget in order to give the best possible foods to their family. Sudden improvements in the purchasing power without prior educational programs about their nutritional requirements and needs in terms of hygienic and sanitary dwellings often lead to spending money on things like alcohols, gambling, and litigation. The real need in most poor countries is proper education and dispelling ignorance and false prejudices and teaching them how to make the best of the available budget. Once the desire to change has been firmly rooted, the available extra money will always be utilized to fulfill the newly created desires to feel healthy and see the children healthy and well.

Any course of instruction or education must not be abandoned after it is completed. A follow-up study on a continuing basis is as essential as starting the program. If an education program is not followed up, it is ill conceived and does not take into consideration the powerful impact of the old beliefs and prejudices which it intends to uproot. A nutrition education course is only a beginning or a kind of orientation; its beneficial effects can be obtained only by close follow-up for a prolonged period of time, until something from inside triggers them on to continuous action in the desired direction.

Overcoming Cultural Prejudices and Superstitions

The economy of a community greatly influences the availability to its members of the foods that are nutritious and health promoting, but at numerous occasions, these beneficial foods are not eaten because of certain social and cultural taboos, prejudices, and superstitions. When these prejudices are applied on the foods to be offered to the younger member of the family, it results in malnutrition, growth retardation, and permanent damage to his personality. Social prejudices are sensitive issues and have been discussed in detail in Chapter VI. But it is true that it is because of such prejudices that one can see marasmic children in wealthy families who could economically afford any amount of food. Children in these families are not given meats, beans, and eggs in the belief that they are harmful. When meat is cooked for the family, it is not given to the child because it is considered unsuitable for him. Behar *et al.*[1] described that "instead of giving the weaned infant special foods, a selection is made among those received by the rest of the family, which tends to eliminate foods richest in protein."

It is under these circumstances that nutrition education to the community assumes a role equal to the economic development plans. To put it in the right manner, the success of the economic development plans may depend on the nutrition education of the community. The ignorance about nutritive value of foods and social prejudices about them will not only perpetuate malnutrition but will affect the economic fabric of the community. The productivity of an underfed and weak agricultural or industrial worker will be far less than a healthy man eating a well-balanced diet. When social prejudices prohibit eating "body-building foods" by the weaning and preschool children, the effects could be very disastrous in terms of future of the community. A well-organized campaign against some of the harmful practices should be the top priority of a balanced education program because unless the hold of the unnecessary prejudices on the minds of the people is broken, a course in nutrition education is bound to fall on deaf ears. Such a campaign may try to acquire a place of prestige for a protein-rich food, which is presently occupied by a carbohydrate staple; for example, banana is revered in many parts of Africa.

Food faddism is another form of prejudice or superstition which has often resulted in poor health and conditions of malnutrition among people of the economically wealthy classes of technologically advanced countries. An appropriate program of nutrition education is essential for the victims of these fads. In the United States many of the special foods advertised to lose weight or create a slim figure are deficient in certain nutrients essential for good health. The person patronizing such foods may lose weight as desired but may also lose body vitality and become a victim of some form of malnutrition.

Sometimes ignorance, faddism, quackery, or combinations of all three lead individuals to consume, or give to their children, excessive quantities of some nutrients. For example, toxic reactions result from excessively large doses of Vitamin D[9,23,29]; and children develop carotinemia from consuming too many carrots or too much African palm oil.[8] Pathological alterations also result from excessive intakes of Vitamin A.[5,15] In essence, harmful food faddism and quackery flourish because of ignorance of the principles of nutrition and sound dietary practices.[24]

FORMAL EDUCATION IN NUTRITION

Schools

School age is the most appropriate age for teaching new ideas in nutrition and developing in the youngsters the concept of a well-balanced diet. School children are always the most receptive audience, and if this education is not a mere dull book routine and is accompanied by practical demonstration and field trips, it will prove very useful. Instruction in nutrition in the school is not merely a course like algebra, geometry, or arithmetic but should be conducted in a manner that the children get their parents involved in the program. It should be aimed at teaching the parents through the children, and a number of trials in different countries of the world have shown that this approach brings rich dividends. It was observed in Israel that families with school children receiving education in nutrition ate better (i.e. ate well-balanced food) compared to those families with no children of the school age. In many other developing countries, the nutrition education of communities through schools is becoming more and more important. McWilliams [17] has given a good account of the aims of nutrition education to the elementary school children. The following approach in teaching this subject may be tried.

1. *Formal instruction* on the function of proteins, carbohydrates, fats, and different vitamins and minerals should be carried out, with an emphasis on what the deficiency of each could lead to. During this instruction, a firm idea should be developed as to which of all the common foods familiar to children are body-building foods (rich in proteins), energy-giving foods (rich in carbohydrates or fats), and protective foods (rich in vitamins and minerals), and that it is essential to eat daily some food of each category in order to insure proper body growth and development. It may also be important to point out the

importance of quality of proteins in terms of their utilization by the body and why the essential amino acids in balanced proportions have to be provided in the foods. This will help to emphasize the importance of dairy, poultry, and meats as a part of the diet. In the developing countries of the world where animal proteins are scarce and very expensive, this instruction may include the appropriate intake of cereal and legume proteins so as to balance the intake of essential amino acids. The details of these have been given in Chapter VII.

2. *Practical instruction* should include feeding experiments on the laboratory animals, such as guinea pigs, white rats, or rabbits. To the control group should be given a well-balanced diet having foods in the body-building, energy-yielding and protective category, whereas to the experimental group one category of foods should be omitted. The absence of body-building foods, for example, will create protein deficiency and result in loss of weight, stunted growth, and reduced activity level. The deficiency of protein in the diet also inhibits the appetite with the result that the total food intake is also reduced. Experiments could also be designed to demonstrate specific deficiencies, such as vitamin C or some other vitamin or mineral. The demonstration of such deficiencies in the animals could carry quite a personal message to the child and make him careful about his diet.[17] Along with this theoretical and practical instruction, students can be made a part of planning menus for the school lunch based on the nutritive value of each item to be included. They may be encouraged to keep a complete record for a month of what they ate with every meal and analyze later the quality and quantity of food eaten over that period. This could then be correlated to their nutrition requirements according to their individual weight and age. School meals have an especially great practical educational value.

3. The children, especially in the lower grades, must also be encouraged to maintain a vegetable and fruit garden in the backyard of the school with the assistance of the teacher. Trips may be planned to local bakeries, grocery stores, dairy, poultry, and meat farms. In this manner, the students will develop a greater

appreciation of the variety of foods in each category necessary to maintain health and will also give them the incentive to add their variety to their daily food intake.

4. Audio visual aids can also be used to develop a better appreciation of the problems of good nutrition. Public libraries may have films available of the prevalent malnutrition in various parts of the world. The faces of children suffering from nutritional deficiencies, such as kwashiorkor or marasmus, will bring to light the nutritional problem of the world. The films can also demonstrate how in some countries people become blind for lack of vitamin A in their diets or become scorbutic for lack of vitamin C.

The above-mentioned approach could make instruction in nutrition a very lively and fascinating subject. Due importance should be given to this study because it is probable that a child may not make use of the trigonometry learned at school in his adult life, but he sure will use the nutrition knowledge to his benefit all his life. The teachers responsible for this type of instruction in the schools must receive during their training advanced courses in nutrition, school meal planning, and horticulture so as to be effective teachers. A well-trained school teacher could also teach adult classes in the evenings so as to make better use of his training and also earn some money, thereby making the job of a nutrition teacher somewhat more attractive.

Colleges

Advanced courses in nutrition at the college and university level are essential not only for the select few who would like to specialize in this field but also for students belonging to other disciplines as well. Fortunately in home economics most of the schools of higher education give an adequate number of nutrition courses. A survey of Cederquist [6] showed that out of the 12 Michigan schools of higher education in home economics, all of them offered one to seven courses in nutrition, and 11 of the 12 schools offered nutrition courses without any prerequisites. Mueller [19] at the Nutrition Symposium of the Federation of American Societies for Experimental Biology made a strong plea for the inclusion of adequate instruction in nutrition in the medical schools and medical sciences and suggested that nutrition education be made essential for the purpose of adequate well-rounded training of physicians. Mueller [19] outlined the recommendation of the American Medical Association's council in food and nutrition which may be summarized as follows: A medical school should prepare an integrated teaching program of nutrition through an interdisciplinary curriculum committee, which should avoid duplication as well as coordinate the efforts of different departments. Hospital internships or residency programs should be determined by the quality of facilities available, and the various granting agencies should provide funds to develop additional training programs in nutrition. A continuing postgraduate education in nutrition should be available for the benefit of practicing physicians as well as postgraduate students who could explain the scope of research in this area. The medical as well as dental schools need to improve the education standards in the area of nutrition.

Nutrition Career

In order to attract brilliant students into the field of nutrition, a career in this specialty not only needs adequate recognition but needs promotion in terms of professional and monetary rewards. The prevalence of widespread malnutrition all over the world and the need to cope with the gigantic task of fighting it bring to light the importance and needs of professional nutritionists. Such programs as Food for Peace, Supplementation Programs under AID, Head Start have already brought to light the need for recognition of nutrition specialists and properly trained physicians, who have a sound background in basic sciences.[19] The problem of widespread malnutrition also indicates the necessity of having a sizeable number of well-trained nutrition workers and dietitians in all countries of the world who could carry out at the grass-root level the nutrition policies decided by the professionally trained nutritionists. The dietitians are intermediaries between the scientists and others who participate in nutrition education.[13] The nutrition workers and dietitians need not go through a postgraduate training in this field but may be able to function satisfactorily with a limited number of courses in nutrition with emphasis on practical aspects of nutrition besides adequate instruction in home economics, agronomy, and marketing. Such an individual will be an asset as a social community nutrition worker in a community which is faced with the problem of malnutrition among its members: he also has the task of simultaneously setting their economy straight with respect to production and marketing of the different items of food essential to improve their nutritional status. The nursing training schools and the teacher training colleges should impart theoretical as well as practical nutrition orientation to the trainees and create well-trained nutrition nurses or nutritionists who could effectively teach and promote the concepts of good nutrition in the hospitals and the educational system of the community. In India, over 60,000 persons have been given special instructions under the applied nutrition program,[28] and these workers are greatly instrumental in carrying out the nutritional policies of the government.

INFORMAL EDUCATION IN NUTRITION

Mass Media

The mass media can play a very important role in the nutrition education of communities.[16] Television is a very effective medium in imparting education by giving visual displays and demonstrations, but this medium has not been used widely, where it is needed the most. In most underdeveloped countries, where the problem of malnutrition is most acute, the television facilities are either absent or are present in a very limited way, confined to a few centers. Also, the television receiving sets in those places are so expensive that they can be afforded by a wealthy few. However, other means of mass media, such as informative articles in newspapers and magazines, could be as useful. Films, posters, and other visual aids, such as advertisements using attractive colors, or oral propaganda can also go a long way to make people aware of the need for dietary education. The mass media should be used to explain certain diseases as well as principles of hygiene along with a few simple facts about nutrition. Film documentaries about the role of various nutrients and demonstrations of menus based on cheap locally produced foods can also be shown. Compulsory showing of documentary movies in all theatres as is generally done in India could prove a good vehicle of instruction, if some excellent films are produced and regularly exhibited in the theatres. Faulty food habits among countries suffering from malnutrition are more of a result of ignorance rather than nonavailability of needed foods, and an informal but effective campaign through the mass media on the basic principles of nutrition can go a long way to eradicate some of the nutritional problems.

Hospital Staff Nurse and Public Health Agencies

The hospitals and public health agencies get ample opportunities to learning firsthand the food habits and socioeconomic condition of the parents, whose children are brought to them for treatment of protein malnutrition or other nutritional deficiencies. Through appropriately trained personnel, such as a staff nurse or a nutrition worker, a good deal of practical education in nutrition can be given to the parents in an informal manner. During the time their child is being treated, the mothers can be made part of the cooking schedules in the hospitals or can be given detailed instructions about what to feed the child and ask them to cook it at home and bring it for the child under hospital care. Keeping mothers away from the child while the latter is being treated will not only lose the opportunity to educate the parents in the much needed nutrition education but will also amount to half the treatment, because on discharge from the hospital, the child will go back to his previous dietary intake and may relapse his condition and come back to the hospital. Jelliffe [16] has a lifetime of experience in many developing countries, and he complains that in many cases the doctors and nurses are impersonal to the point of frightening the patients, which may stem from their idea of class and status prevalence, especially in Latin America.[11] Such a hospital staff is simply oblivious of the necessity of educating the parents. Such an apathy or lack of appreciation on the part of the medical staff may be removed only by a well-organized educational program in nutrition during their medical and nursing training. The hospital nurse and public health nurse should make it a part of her duties to instruct the parents in whatever she feeds to the child under her care, and as an extension of the same, she may be asked to make regular home visits after the child is discharged from the hospital. Nutrition education can be much more effective if carried out in the accustomed home circumstances, using actual examples from the kitchen and locally available foods.[4]

Whereas the hospital nurse or public health nurse may concentrate on the mother, the public health nutrition worker can concentrate on the male population. The topics of instruction to the adult male popualtion must be wider than the instruction in food value of certain common foods, and the desirability or amounts of their consumption. The nutrition education to the adult male population of a community through a public health nutrition specialist may include the following items.

1. Human nutritional requirements and how they can be satisfied by the variety of foods available in a particular community.

2. Methods of food preservation, which may help to make them available through the year without losing their nutritive value.

3. The importance of raising crops of beans, nuts, and fruits along with those of cereals and an attempt at educating them on the value of eating cereals and beans together.

4. The nutritional importance of raising dairy and poultry products and what it means to eat proteins of high biological value. The public health specialist can supervise a rural demonstration in how to raise and vaccinate chickens or how to produce better rabbits or bigger eggs.

5. Basic facts about food adulteration as well as the presence of certain toxic agents in the foods.

6. Finally the most important part of nutrition education should include the principles of sanitation and public health practices. The effectiveness of this pattern of education will de-

pend entirely on the proficiency of the public health worker and the informal manner in which this education is imparted.

Women Clubs, Churches, and Other Civic Groups

Clubs for women, where they gather for social and cultural activities, could become centers for educating them in nutrition as well as modern methods of child rearing. Churches and certain other civic groups, such as civic and professional associations, adult education centers, health and nutrition centers, consumer and producer cooperatives, youth clubs, national and international social welfare organizations,[26] can achieve the same objective, i.e. "enable people to promote and protect their own health and well being, and that of their children and community in which they dwell." [16] Since the biggest aim of nutrition education is a change in the dietary pattern that contributes to malnutrition, these social organizations can do a lot to create a desire to learn and change because of their intimate relationship with the social life of the community. The social organizations can make sure that the information reaches the members of the community along with its contents and purpose. This may prove better and more effective than formal teaching institutions, such as schools or government-organized adult classes. For example, the widespread use of banana as a food of prestige in Africa has the sanction of the Church and other cultural or social organizations, and if the latter preach to the people the poor food value of this food, and suggest a nutritious locally produced substitute, they are likely to be more successful than any government agency.

Food Industry

Although not a recognized forum for education, the food industry can render a great service to the community and can impart effective nutrition education in the course of promoting their products. In the developing countries, the food industry has a special responsibility not to market and advertise those products which do not contribute to the health and well-being of the community. In the case of protein-rich or vitamin- or mineral-rich foods, the commercials sponsored by the food industry could lay special emphasis on the ingredients of a particular product and present it to the public in an informative manner. The label on the product should contain the minimum daily requirements of protective and body-building nutrients. Special recipes on these labels suiting the local conditions could also bring about an awareness of the nutritional needs. For example, soybean flour is readily available in India. It could be usefully used along with rice and wheat cereals, and together they will provide proteins of high biological value. But the product has not become very popular for lack of imaginative advertisement on the part of the food industry. It is for the manufacturer to make attractive packages with explanation of nutrients as well as simple ways to use the products in a manner that does not interfere with their cultural pattern of cooking and eating. Food industry by its efforts could render a great service, besides promoting their products.

EDUCATION IN FAMILY PLANNING

The biggest problem in nutrition at the present time is not that millions in the developing countries do not have enough to eat, and half the population of the world goes to bed hungry, but the exploding human population on this planet. The problem of supplying food to the existing population as well as to the newcomers is truly staggering. At the present rate the human population threatens to double every 25 years. The yearly increase in population amounts to more than 60 million, which may be equal to the combined populations of Poland and Spain. A country like India, with two fifths of the land area of United States and about three times its population, is expected to cross the billion mark in population by the turn of the century. Can she adequately feed that many people? Already more than 300 million children suffer from protein-calorie malnutrition with about 100 million on the Indian subcontinent alone. The race between the number of people and the food supply is becoming more and more difficult every day. The situation is not very bleak when we take the world population as a whole. During the recent years the world population has increased at about 1½ percent annually, whereas the net food production has grown at the rate of 2 percent.[21] But it is the lopsided production of the food that upsets the balance. Most of the advances in food have been achieved in technologically developed countries of the West, whereas Asia, Africa, and Latin America, which contain the bulk of human population, have shown a slow rate of increase in food production.[10,21] Unless this imbalance is corrected and the situation changes significantly, it will be extremely difficult or rather impossible to avert food shortages or famine conditions in the over-populated areas of the world.[2] With about a billion population in India 25 years from now, if a draught or crop failure take place as happened in 1966–67, all the external aid in the form of food ship-ments or the surplus of the entire developed world will no longer be sufficient to avert famine or widespread malnutrition.

It is unwise, therefore, to discuss the food supply or the nutri-tional standards of the people without simultaneously tackling the problem of population stabilization. "It is essential that a major program on population control proceed concurrently with any nutritional program. To do otherwise would in the long run almost certainly result in an increase in total human suffering." [14] It is also imperative that the program to stabilize human popu-lation be started right now and an education campaign in the art and necessity of family planning be started on an emergency basis. It must be remembered that even the most successful family planning education and implementation of its objectives is at best a long-term solution. Optimistic estimates on the success of family planning programs will only reduce the needs of extra food by only 20 percent over the next 20 years. The impact of food requirements will be significantly felt only after the year 1985 if a vigorous campaign in family planning is started right now. But what if we don't take concrete and effective steps now for a long-term control of population! In that case the popula-tion will double over the next 25 years along with double the amount of food needs, and the problems arising from a geo-metrical increase of population growth will be beyond com-prehension. It is imperative that without any further delay, the greatest possible effort be expanded to curtail the increase in the number of people, while working simultaneously to satisfy the needs of the present population and of those babies who arrive in spite of the family planning programs. Spengler [27] calculated on the basis of 1965 figures that, "Whereas the world supposedly will need only something like 60% more calories in 1985 than in 1965, India will need 100% more, Pakistan will need at least 150% more, China will require some 50% more, and Brazil at least 75% more."

Such grim figures should be enough of an incentive to make the maximum possible efforts to curtail the growth of human populations. A number of options are available. The major ones being (a) totalitarian methods, and (b) Socrates methods. The former will use authority of the government to force the people not to have more than one or two children and subjecting them to harsh treatments for failure to obey, such as penalties in the form of extra taxes, reduced food rations. In this system the government may legislate for the compulsory sterilization of all adult population after they have the set number of children. The Socrates methods would advocate persuading the people while respecting their dignity and their right to procreate according to the fulfillment of their social, cultural, and emotional needs. Whereas the former methods may be more efficient and bring about the desired results in a short span of time, I would rather advocate the adoption of persuasion methods in spite of the great urgency to plug the population explosion as soon as possible. It is here that we need a comprehensive program of education in family planning. An enlightened population fully aware of the needs of the program and its impact on the economy of the country and personal well-being of the individuals is preferable to a population which practices family planning and controls the number of children under duress. Burton [3] explained how the Socrates methods work.

> Socratic educational methods assume that the people already possess information, feelings, interests and beliefs which profoundly influence the learning process. Socratic methods are concerned less with direct teaching than with creating situations where people learn by experience—that is, take part in some activity, either intellectual,

manual, or administrative, with preferably some expert guidance at hand to pose problems, answers, questions and set initial standards.

A campaign of education in family planning may approach the problem in the following manner:

1. Schools. In order to enlighten the parents of tomorrow it is practical to educate the children of today. At the junior and senior high school level, a comprehensive course in reproductive physiology of the human should be accompanied by detailed instruction in the economy of the community and the nationality to which they belong. The aim of this education should be to emphasize that the human numbers, agricultural and industrial production, state and national economy, employment opportunities, and the individual prosperity are closely linked. An unplanned increase in human numbers could adversely affect everything. If this instruction at school is properly organized, its effects will be felt in the homes of these children as well.

2. Public health and civic groups can make a similar effort to enlighten the adult population. Public health nurses, nutrition workers, staff of the maternal child health centers, churches, women clubs, or the representatives of the local government are ideal agencies to undertake the task of educating the people in the art and necessity of family planning. The child health programs must review all possible channels of education of the mothers. Adequate attention needs to be given to integrate family planning into maternal and child health services.[20] Prenatal care of the mothers and regular checkups should include lessons on how to space the children and the methods of family planning. Child spacing is also an important factor in maintaining the nutritional status of the mother. Visiting the families at home and discussing with the couples the problems involved will be very helpful. The home visits for the purpose of nutrition education can be combined with instruction on family planning.

3. As in case of promoting a product, advertisements on mass media could be effective in bringing an awareness for smaller and happier families. Newspapers, movies, television, posters, and even the organization of family planning fairs could prove helpful. Posters on the walls in convenient places as well as in residential areas, radio broadcasts, and documentary films have

played an important role in India to make the people conscious of the need, and there are useful indications that people are getting the message.

4. Finally, a distributing system for the family-planning aids (pills, condoms, jellies, foams, intrauterine devices) and medical facilities for voluntary sterilizations must be organized on a sound basis. Mobile medical units, which could bring these services to the homes of the people living close to big cities or in remote areas, should be organized to provide help and education on a continuing basis.

Every cent spent to promote family planning is one of the best and sound investments that any country can make these days. It is an investment in the future of our species as well as in the prosperity and well-being of our future generations.

REFERENCES

1. Behar, M., Viteri, F., Bressani, R., et al.: *Ann. N.Y. Acad. Sci., 69*:954–968 (1958).
2. Bennett, I. L.: In G. H. Bourne (Ed.): *World Review of Nutrition and Dietetics*. Basel, S. Karger (1969), vol. 2, p. 1.
3. Burton, J.: *Health Educ., 12*:131 (1954).
4. Byrne, M.: *J. Trop. Pediatr., 8*:22 (1962).
5. Caffey, J.: *Ann. J. Roentgenol. Radium Therapy Nucl. Med., 67*:818 (1952).
6. Cederquist, D. C.: *Fed. Proc., 26*:170 (1967).
7. Clark, F. LeGros: In G. H. Bourne (Ed.): *World Review of Nutrition and Dietetics*. Basel, S. Karger (1968), vol. 9.
9. Cohen, L.: *Ann. Intern. Med., 48*:219 (1958).
9. Debre, R.: *Am. J. Dis. Child. 75*:787 (1948).
10. FAO *Third World Food Survey*. Rome (1963).
11. Foster, G. M.: *Hum. Org., 11* (No. 3):5 (1952).
12. Gomez, F., Galvan, R., Cravioto, J., et al.: *Acta Paediatr., 46*:286 (1957).
13. Harper, A. E.: *Am. J. Clin. Nutr., 22*:87 (1969).
14. Howe, E. E., Jansen, G. R., and Anson, M. L.: *Am. J. Clin. Nutr., 20*:1134 (1967).
15. Jeghers, H. and Marraro, H.: *Am. J. Clin. Nutr., 6*:335 (1958).
16. Jelliffe, D. B.: In *Infant Nutrition in the Subtropics and Tropics*. Geneva, W.H.O. (1968).
17. McWilliams, M.: *Nutrition for the Growing Years*. New York and London, John Wiley & Sons (1967).

18. Mead, M.: In A. Burgess and R. F. A. Dean: *Malnutrition & Food Habits*. London, Travistock (1962).
19. Mueller, J. F.: *Fed. Proc., 26:*167 (1967).
20. Petros–Barvazian, A.: In P. Gyorgy and O. L. Kline (Eds.): *Malnutrition is a Problem of Ecology*. Basel, S. Karger (1970).
21. Rao, M. N. and Swaminathan, M.: In G. H. Bourne (Ed.): *World Review of Nutrition & Dietetics*. Basel, S. Karger (1969), vol. 2.
22. Read, M. S.: In P. Gyorgy and O. L. Kline (Eds.): *Malnutrition is a Problem of Ecology*. Basel, S. Karger (1970).
23. Reed, C. I.: *J.A.M.A., 102:*1745 (1934).
24. Scrimshaw, N. S. and Behar, M.: In G. H. Beaton and E. W. McHenry (Eds.): *Nutrition Vol. II, Nutrient Requirement and Food Selection*. New York, Academic Press (1964).
25. Sebrell, W. H. and King, K. W: In P. Gyorgy and O. L. Kline (Eds.): *Malnutrition is a Problem of Ecology*. Basel, S. Karger (1970).
26. deSilva, C. C.: *Adv. Pediatr., 13:*226 (1964).
27. Spengler, J. J.: In G. H. Bourne (Ed.): *World Review of Nutrition and Dietetics*. Basel and New York, S. Karger (1968), vol. 9.
28. Tepley, L. J.: In P. Gyorgy and O. L. Kline (Eds.): *Malnutrition is a Problem of Ecology*. Basel, S. Karger (1970).
29. Tumulty, P. A. and Howard, J. E.: *J.A.M.A., 119:*233 (1942).
30. W.H.O. Program in Nutrition. *W.H.O. Chron., 19:*429 (1965).
31. *W.H.O. Tech. Rep. Ser.,* 245 (1962).
32. Williams, C.: In R. A. McCance and E. M. Widdowson (Eds.): *Calorie Deficiencies and Protein Deficiencies*. Boston, Little, Brown (1968).
33. Williams, S. R.: *Nutrition and Diet Therapy*. St. Louis, Mosley (1969).

INDEX

371